AF799757

present to the reader the whole chain, including the technical support, ergonomics, working technique, and workflow of the treatment steps. All while giving scientific arguments and personal opinions on different theoretical knowledge or working techniques. We have tried to keep the language simple, non-sophisticated, so that the work is easy to read and understand. The iconography is represented by diagrams and photographs from personal case studies.

The tremendous support offered by my family, friends, and colleagues made this work possible. I greatly valued and took into consideration our collaborators' pertinent suggestions when on different topics discussed in this book: Dr. Stefan Jitaru (magnification), Assoc. Prof. Sanda Cîmpean, Dr. Radu Bulat and Dr. Sergiu Spătaru, Dr. Razvan Pop (endodontics)—Chaps. 1, 2 and 3, Assoc. Prof. Ada Delean—Chaps. 1, 2, 3, 4, 5 and 6; Dr. Mircea Mureşan (periodontology)—Sect. 3.2; Dr. Pieter-Jan Swerts, Dr. Andrei Voicu, Dr. Ionuţ Aiordachioaei (restorative and prosthetic dentistry) Chaps. 5, 6, 7, 8 and 9. Special thanks to our colleague Dr. Tudor Secasan for correcting the English text.

Cluj Napoca, Romania Marius Bud

Contents

Part I

Preparing the Dental Office and the Patient for Restorative Treatments

Equipment, Ergonomics and Magnification Workflow

1

The basic principles of restorative dentistry have not changed significantly in the last 30 years. Aesthetic, biological, and mechanical criteria are now strictly respected by dentists in the spirit of refinement based on scientific arguments, the evolution of materials, and the general worldwide trend toward aesthetics and biomimicry. This trend has been helped by the rapid development of materials and equipment and bringing many elements of technological progress while generating contradictory evidence. The abundance of instruments and materials in recent years has led to a competition for aesthetic, faster, more predictable, and minimally invasive treatments as close as possible to the natural situation and with an increasing success rate. All these requirements, which imply precision and finesse, are challenging for the operator to meet without using magnification accompanied by good lighting. This chapter will be focusing on the dental operating microscope, the dental loupes, minimally invasive instruments for tooth preparation, dental matrices, instruments and materials for finishing and polishing, lamps for light-curing materials, and photo/video documentation of cases.

1.1 Tools and Equipment

1.1.1 Dental Operating Microscope (DOM): Overview and Brief History

Since the early 2000s, the principles of minimally invasive dentistry have been increasingly and widely promoted in dentistry [1]. David Clark, founder of the Academy of Dental Microscopy and one of the pioneers of dental microscopy, stated: "the greatest indicator of long-term tooth retention is the volume of healthy natural tooth tissue that remains after we finish treating a tooth."

Supplementary Information The online version contains supplementary material available at https://doi.org/10.1007/978-3-031-55899-3_1. The videos can be accessed individually by clicking the DOI link in the accompanying figure caption or by scanning this link with the SN More Media App.

© The Author(s), under exclusive license to Springer Nature Switzerland AG 2024

M. Bud, *Direct Restorations*, https://doi.org/10.1007/978-3-031-55899-3_1

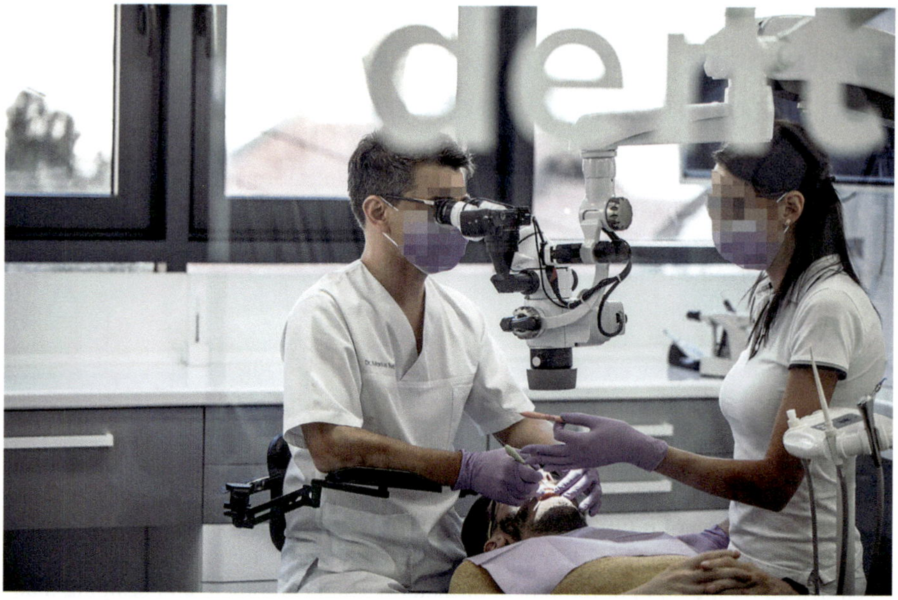

Fig. 1.1 The clinical use of a dental operating microscope

The use of magnification helps to achieve this. In recent years, the dental operating microscope has become increasingly common in dental offices, being used both for endodontic and restorative, prosthetic, or surgical treatments (Fig. 1.1).

The components of a dental operating microscope (DOM) are the stand and arms, the optical body, the light source, and various accessories.

1.1.1.1 Stand and Arms

The dental operating microscope can be placed above the patient by attaching it to a stand using articulating arms. The stand and arms represent the optical body's balance and stabilizing devices. There are several different ways of mounting: on the floor, on the wall, on the ceiling, or on the dental chair.

The floor stand is the most popular mounting method because it is equipped with wheels that allow easy movement and the positioning of the DOM for ergonomic adjustment in the dental office. The floor stand's weight is considerable, in the order of tens of kilograms, and it has a pillar to which the rest of the construction is hinged to. In this way, it can ensure the stability of the DOM. Disadvantages include the taking up space on the floor and the fact that it can propagate vibrations from the floor to the optical head, causing discomfort to the dentist. The floor stand is usually placed on the dentist's nondominant hand side (most often the left side), as far away as possible from the patient's head, in order to free up space for the dental assistant's chair and to facilitate access from other parts in the room.

Attaching the microscope to a side wall frees up floor space but makes it difficult for the dental assistant to reach the working position. As a rule, the wall opposite to the dominant hand is preferred, as far away as possible from the patient's head, for ergonomic benefits.

Attaching DOM to the ceiling is one of the best solutions in terms of freeing up space in the office, but like wall fixing, it has the drawback of it being permanently fixed and not allowing any changes in position.

Articulating arms keep the optical head in the optimum vertical and horizontal working position. The horizontal position is maintained by several short arms that move in the horizontal plane and whose movements are controlled or blocked by mechanical or electromagnetic brakes. The mechanical brakes are based on the pressure principle exerted by a handle of a softer material, usually brass, over a rigid metal pinion. The pressure is applied by tightening a screw until the arm stays in place when no force is exerted, but it can be pulled easily when the operator desires. It is neither desirable nor practical for the brakes to be fully tightened during work or between patients, as this will lead to wear of the brass handle. However, the breaks can be locked entirely for transport. The electromagnetic brakes can be found on modern, more expensive models, which allow complete joint locking and are operated with a push of a button. This ensures a higher level of stability during work.

A pantograph arm handles vertical movement with a mechanical or gas spring. The weight of the optical head varies depending on the accessories mounted on it. The gas spring obtains tension with a spring to maintain its variable weight. It must be adjusted so that the optical head remains balanced in the desired position to easily allow movement to another position.

1.1.1.2 Optical Head

The optical head is the most important part of the whole microscope from the dentist's point of view. The optical head is a mechanical-optical construction that allows observation of an area of the operating field at the desired magnification. The optical head consists of all the elements attached to the DOM arm: eyepieces, objective lens, and magnification changer (Fig. 1.2).

The eyepieces consist of two tubular structures whose position can be adjusted to match the interpupillary distance. Each eyepiece is equipped with a pair of lenses with a standard parameter, coded with the letter ×: 10×, 12.5×, and 16×. The eyepiece lenses allow dioptric adjustment and adjust the light projection according to the length of the viewer's eye. Eyepieces usually have detachable or telescopic rubber extensions called cups. The cups intend to standardize the position of the eye relative to the eyepiece lens to a comfortable distance.

The letter × stands for the eyepiece magnification power, which is different from the magnification power of the microscope, and choosing it has practical importance: the higher it is, the greater the depth of the image, but the smaller the size of the field of view. The 12.5× magnification factor is considered an average parameter that provides sufficient depth and a wide field of view. Some professionals prefer 10×.

Hinged are the two eyepieces to the optical head body, and they are either fixed or have the possibility to change the angle. If fixed in their position, it is usually at

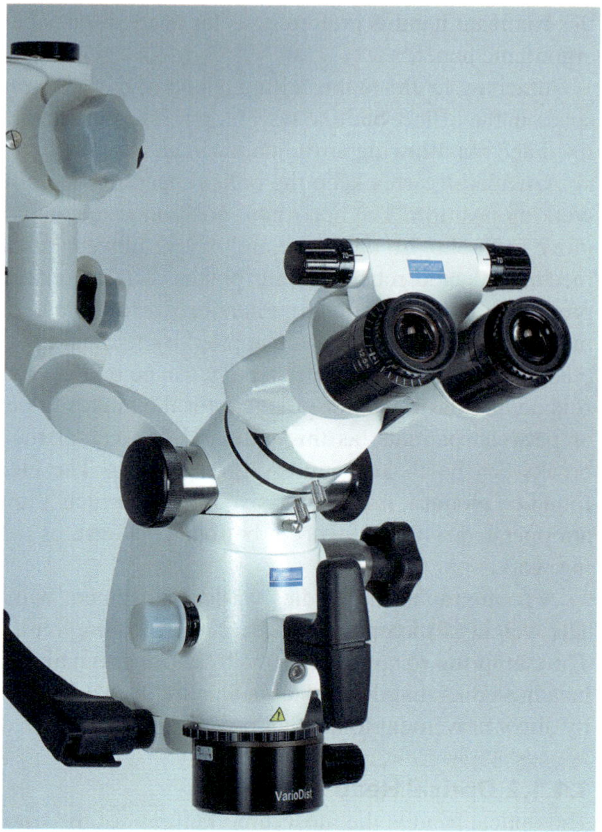

Fig. 1.2 Optical head of a dental operating microscope

an angle of 45°. Variable position eyepieces can usually be set from 0° to 180°, having the advantage of increased ergonomics.

The lens allows the light to enter the microscope and it is coded with the factor "f." This represents the distance to the object to be examined, which can be fixed or variable.

The fixed lens can be f 170, f 250, f 320, and more, which means we can place the object to be examined at the distances measured in millimeters to get a sharp and focused image. The lens will be chosen according to the practitioner's need for space, the specific practice (endodontics, restorative dentistry, periodontology, and others), and the dentist's height. These lenses allow for fine adjustments, similar to the micro vision of laboratory microscopes, by operating a rotary knob.

Variable magnification lenses usually bear registered trade names, e.g., *VarioFocus*, *VarioDist*, etc., and can cover a broader range of distances, such as 200 to 400 mm. Variable objective lenses, although expensive, provide clear ergonomic benefits and ease of operation.

The magnification step changer represents the segment in the optical head that allows the total magnification power to be changed. Two types of design allow this: a Galilean step changer or a continuous step changer.

The Galilean changer involves a pair of lenses inside the optical head, fixed in a cylinder, operated from the outside by a rotary knob, with magnification factors indicated on the side. The pair of lenses increases or decreases the image according to its position, coded by a magnification factor notation: 0.4, 0.6, 1.6, and 2.4. The digit 1 marks the absence of a pair of lenses in the beam path (optical path). Therefore, we can have configurations with a fixed number of magnification steps, such as "three-step," where we have a pair of lenses and an accessible path—so we will have the magnification factor 0.4 and 1.6, which are the pair of lenses and the digit "1" that is marked twice, indicating the free optical path. There are also "five-step" configurations, i.e., two pairs of lenses (0.4 with 2.4, 0.6 with 1.6) and an accessible path (marked with the number 1), or six-step, where there are three pairs of lenses.

The continuous switch is activated by pressing a pedal or using a rotary knob, moving a lens vertically. This increases or decreases the overall magnification. This is a less commonly chosen construction setting for dental microscopes.

1.1.1.3 Light Source

Obtaining the magnification involves focusing the light reflected from the object under examination, which requires appropriate illumination. Ambient light is not sufficient, no matter how bright it is. A significant advantage of the microscope over loupes is how light is transmitted. Microscopes allow the beam of light emitted into the field of view to be projected through the objective lens, through which it returns on a parallel path. This method of illumination is called coaxial illumination and allows no shadow viewing.

Several light sources are commonly used: halogen, xenon, and LED. The first two are sources that emit intense heat and must be placed away from the optical head—the light is conducted using optical fiber. LEDs have become increasingly powerful and capable of emitting light without generating high temperatures, and they have been increasingly integrated directly into the optical head. LED sources also have the advantage of a long operating time, with light emitted constantly throughout the procedure, and have the possibility of choosing warm, cool, or neutral tones.

Because the light projected by the DOM is very bright, the ambient light in the office must also be bright to balance the difference. Otherwise, the dental assistant's gaze, which is focused directly on the brightly lit operating field during the assist, will suffer.

Light sources are usually provided with green or orange filters. The former increase the contrast of blood vessels and are helpful in surgical procedures, while the latter prevent premature polymerization of composite resins during work. Some filters prevent polymerization without radically changing the color of the microscope light.

1.1.1.4 Accessories

DOMs are modular devices, and there is always the possibility to add other accessories. Manufacturers can continuously improve the offer and, thus, the dental practices. There are many types of accessories, but the most important ones are those that allow the installation of a camera or bring ergonomic improvement.

Photo-video capture systems are essential accessories that can be added to a basic optical head. They consist of an optical splitter or *beam splitter* (Fig. 1.3) and a *camera-video adapter*.

The optical splitter is a device that removes a part of the light from one of the two optical paths (each corresponding to one of the eyes) and redirects it to the optical camera sensor. The ratio between light going to the eyepiece and light going to the camera differs from manufacturer to manufacturer, e.g., 50:50 or 80:20. The eye should receive as much light as possible, so the 80:20 ratio is preferred. *Global Company* owns the patent on a *Virtual Beamsplitter*™ that sends less than 5% of the light to the camera, while the rest going to the eyepiece.

The camera adapters are specific to a particular brand, so they must be chosen from the start. Sony's Alpha cameras have become very popular among dentists using the DOM because they are lightweight and reliable. DSLR cameras are becoming less used because they are heavy, and their sensor breaks down faster if used for live transmission or long video shooting. Moreover, some cameras can switch off after several minutes to prevent the video sensor from overheating.

DOM manufacturers offer the possibility of embedding a video sensor in the optical head, which is more cost-effective but is usually technically inferior and without the possibility of further improvement.

Installing a camera on the DOM allows real-time transmission of the treatment on a monitor, which helps the dental assistant. Photo-video captures are also a good way of communicating with the medical team or explaining the details of diagnosis or treatment to the patient.

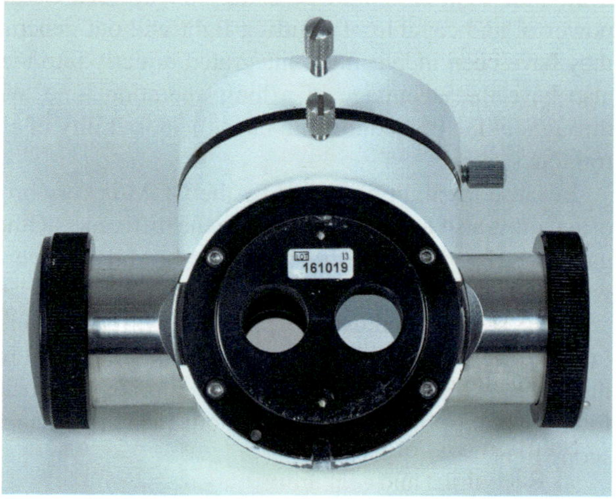

Fig. 1.3 The beam splitter, an accessory that allows the attachment of some accessories (camera/video adapter, spy eyepiece)

Ergonomic accessories improve the working position, and they can help either position the dentist further away from the patient with the help of the standard *extension arm* or angulate the optical head to the left or right without the operator's repositioning.

The benefits of a DOM use in dentistry are many and unanimously accepted [2]: increased visibility, increased treatment quality, decreased occlusal fitting of direct restorations, ergonomic working position, dentist's safety and motivation, better communication with patient and assistant, and avoidance of iatrogenesis [3, 4].

The main critical points in the working steps for direct and indirect restorations that get the benefits of magnification are the following:

(I) Examination:
- Assessment of occlusal anatomy.
- Identification of small demineralized enamel areas and incipient caries.
- Identification of enamel cracks, which are impossible to detect without magnification.
- Assessment of remaining enamel wall thickness and strength.
- Checking the marginal sealing of old composite fillings or other materials.
- Identification of small, incidental pulp chamber openings.

(II) Cavity preparation:
- Identification and minimally invasive removal of the remaining materials from old fillings.
- Identification and removal of enamel cracks most commonly located on the gingival edge.
- Minimally invasive dentin removal and minimally invasive cavity preparation.
- Assessment of thickness and strength of remaining enamel walls after cavity preparation.
- Identification of small, incidental pulp chamber openings.
- A gentle approach to pulp chamber perforations without mechanical pulp injury.
- Circular enamel sealing checking of preparations for *inlay/onlay*.
- The evaluation of preparations for direct composite veneers.

(III) Direct restoration:
- Controlled application of MTA at the opening point of the pulp chamber for direct pulp capping.
- Checking the sealing of sectional or circular matrices.
- Checking the matrix fitting and the custom ring from the dental embrasures with the *custom ring* technique.
- Controlled application of the liner for pulp protection.
- Surface inspection after etching.
- Uniform application and surface inspection when the adhesive system was applied.
- Removal of excess adhesive/extruded material outside the matrices in the proximal and oral areas.

- Identification and removal of voids and impurities from the filling materials.
- Controlled application of composite materials and prevention of excess materials.
- The possibility of fine modeling of occlusal morphology.
- The possibility of fine layering and controlled application of the characterizations in direct anterior restorations.
- Achieving good-quality restoration finishing due to surface texture magnification evaluation.

Additional benefits:

- Installing a beam splitter for a second eyepiece (spy eyepiece) or attaching a DSLR photo-video camera. The camera is mounted below the eyepieces and allows bilateral accessory mounting (Fig. 1.4). This camera can connect to an external monitor and allows the assistant or dentist to view the operating field in order to assist the treatment or to observe the procedure.
- Attaching a photo/video camera that allows taking photos/videos needed for case documentation or education of the medical team and students.

Several factors limit the widespread use of the microscope, the most important being the very high cost, but there are also space limitations or dentist's low motivation. Whatever the impediments are, microscopy is gaining momentum, a rewarding development both for patients and dentists.

Surgical, dental loupes can be an excellent magnification alternative for restorative treatments. Postural correction using loupes is not as effective as when using a microscope. Learning to use loupes has a shorter learning period, and it is appreciated to provide better adaptability for beginners [5].

Proper posture has challenged dentists since their undergraduate years [6]. The microscope helps the dentist achieve a correct working posture relatively quickly.

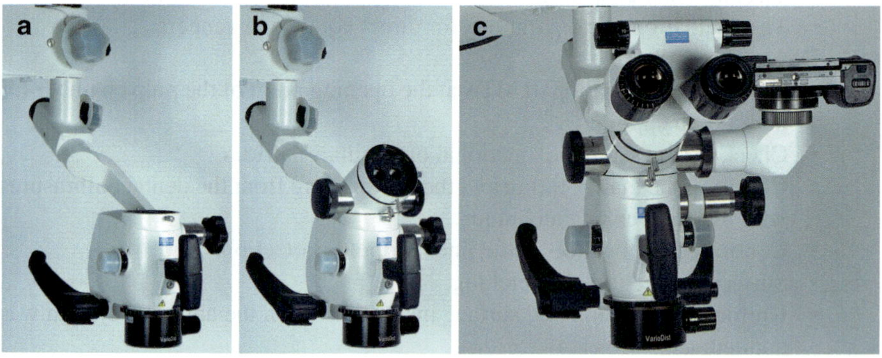

Fig. 1.4 Microscope body without eyepieces (**a**); optical body with attached beam splitter (**b**); optical body with beam splitter, video camera, and eyepieces (**c**)

Since the optical head will always remain fixed on the stand, the dentist must maintain a correct working posture throughout the treatment.

Ergonomic recommendations for working with DOM [7]:

- Position the DOM above the patient's face.
- Place the working area right in the center of the spotlight.
- Tilt the binoculars at approximately 135° to the microscope body.
- Adjust the minimum focal distance.
- Choose the lowest magnification step to start with.
- For body position adjustment, keep the back straight (sagittal head position, cervical spine has to be in continuation of the thoracic spine; lateral head position, bipupillary line has to be perfectly horizontal).

Once the operator has set up his working position and established the correct posture, the next step is to adjust the microscope to get a clear image of the operator's field. This image should remain clear regardless of the chosen magnification level. This adjustment setting is called parfocality.

Parfocality is the ability of a lens to remain in focus when the factor of magnification changes. It is imperative in microscopy because, during treatment, the operator will frequently need to change the magnification level.

To achieve parfocality, choose a clinically relevant area (reference area) on the operating field (e.g., a dental surface) or mark on a sheet of paper the letter "X" on the headrest of the horizontally positioned dental chair and then follow the following steps:

(I) On the *lowest* magnification level:
  - Turn on the DOM and light source from the ON/OFF button.
  - Adjust the diopters to zero for each eyepiece.
  - Position the light beam centrally on the reference area.
  - Bring the eyepieces to eye level and pinpoint the reference area.
  - Raise/lower the dental unit to obtain an approximately clear image.

(II) On the *highest* magnification level:
  - Raise/lower the dental unit until there is a clear image.

(III) On the *lowest* magnification level:
  - Obtain a clear image by adjusting the diopter for each eye separately while covering the other eye with a hand.
  - Check the *interpupillary* distance to obtain a single image when looking with both eyes simultaneously through both eyepieces.
  - Change the magnification level and examine whether the image *remains* clear on all magnification levels or just on some of them.

1.1.1.5 Dental Loupes

The loupes (Fig. 1.5) are more straightforward, cheaper, and more mobile optical devices, but they have the disadvantage of poor ergonomics and loss of coaxial illumination. Because the operator is constantly moving, the eyes will eventually become tired when working with magnifiers, even though they are trying to remain still.

Fig. 1.5 Dental loupes

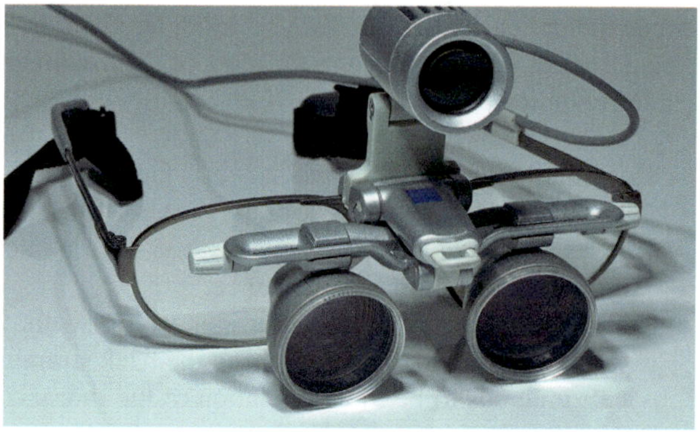

In terms of construction, there are two main categories of loupes: Galilean and prismatic. Depending on the mounting method, they can be classified as spectacle-mounted (through-the-lens/TTL), sliding (flip-up), or head-mounted.

Like microscopes, magnifiers require a light source because the ambient light is insufficient, especially at higher magnifications.

The loupes can have a predefined working distance or a custom-made working distance tailored to the dentist's needs. It is also preferred to have the two tubes custom-mounted so that the interpupillary distance is correctly respected (some loupes allow manual adjustment).

The Galilean loupes are so-called because they are constructed of a convex lens (objective lens) and a concave lens (ocular lens), a structure invented by Galileo Galilei. Having a simple construction, they are lighter and cheaper, yet they allow comfort and clarity at lower magnification levels. The field of view decreases while the magnification power increases. The Galilean loupes generally offer magnifications of 2.5× and do not go beyond 3.5×. Another advantage of the Galilean loupes is that they allow a slight deviation between the line of sight and the center of the eyepieces, making them easier for beginners to wear.

The prismatic loupes, also called the Keplerian loupes, are constructed of two positive lenses with a prism between them. This design allows high magnifications without narrowing the field of view and superior image clarity. Prismatic loupes usually magnify up to 6×, but 8× magnification is also available. Since prismatic loupes have more optical elements than other loupes, they are heavier and more expensive. Due to their heavier weight, they are sometimes preferred to be head-mounted. Another initial disadvantage is the need to align the line of sight with the center of the eyepiece lens, so they are a little more demanding to use, and more experience is needed, especially as they typically have a higher magnification power.

Orascoptic Company manufactures loupe models with changeable magnification power so the user can choose between three available magnification steps: 3×, 4×, and 5×.

The available light sources for magnifiers use LEDs. The most qualitative ones provide good illumination but are expensive, often as expensive as the magnifiers themselves. The LED light sources are installed next to the magnifier so that the light spot casts shadows. Rechargeable batteries are used to power the LEDs, which can be carried on a belt or in a pocket or attached to the magnifier less often because they are heavy.

Conclusion

The history of other medical areas has already shown us that new equipment has a variable, sometimes even a long, period of widespread acceptance, balancing three significant factors: the benefits to the treatment, the cost of acquisition, and the effort put in by the operator/dentist.

In the case of microscopes, so far, only the first factor is unquestionable. The costs and reluctance to change continue to be significant impediments to the widespread magnification usage in restorative dentistry.

The introduction of magnification and the operating field's illumination improvement are among the most dramatic changes in restorative dentistry in the past 30 years. Illumination is the key factor that adds to the lens's magnification so that the treatments can be safely performed and to high-quality standards.

Review Questions

1. What are the components of a DOM?
2. What are the main working steps to achieve direct and indirect restorations that get the benefits of magnification?
3. What accessories may be additionally mounted on a DOM?
4. What are the ergonomic recommendations for using the DOM?
5. How is parfocality achieved?
6. How many types of dental loupes are there, and what are the characteristics of each type?

1.1.2 Minimally Invasive Instruments for Tooth Preparation

The cavity preparation is most commonly done with high-speed (turbine-mounted) and low-speed (contra-angle-mounted) dental burs. In addition to this classic method, there are other methods of preparing or enhancing the internal surfaces of the cavity in order to increase the adhesion of restorative materials: ultrasonic, air abrasion, laser, and chemical dissolution of carious dentin. We will now refer to some minimally invasive methods for cavity cleaning and mechanical improvement of adhesion.

1.1.2.1 Sonic and Ultrasonic Instruments

Ultrasound (US) is commonly used in dentistry. As early as 1957, Richman reported the use of a US generator for the preparation of access cavities, as well as endodontic therapy [8]. Diamond tips (Fig. 1.6) can have different shapes. Since ultrasound tips do not function by rotation like dental burrs, they can be active only on one side, depending on their shape and type, thus protecting adjacent teeth when class II cavities are prepared [9].

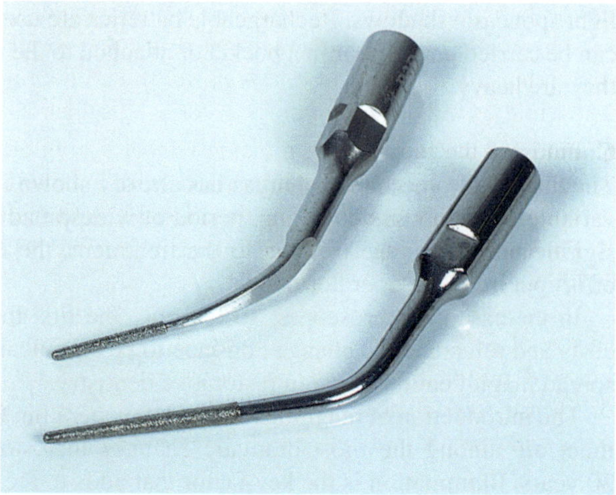

Fig. 1.6 Ultrasound diamond coated tips

Advantages of using diamond US tips compared to conventional diamond dental burrs [10]:

- Diamond US tips have better cooling compared to conventional diamond dental burrs. The cold water flows along the rod, reaching its end without interfering with its trajectory. It does not form a water and air cloud around the active tip because they have cooling holes pointing toward the tip's working direction. It does not block the view and does not distract from cutting.
- Low noise only occurs when it comes into contact with the tooth.
- Better visibility and access, thanks to different lengths and angled shapes.
- More efficient cutting.
- Long-term durability.
- The method is more conservative.
- Less fear and more readily accepted by patients, including children.
- Less need for local anesthesia.
- Effective cavity cleaning due to the phenomenon called cavitation.
- Correct use minimizes the pulp-dentinal complex's damage potential due to the active surface's low friction coefficient.

Pedro et al. reported that fewer enamel fractures occurred when preparing cavities with US than in conventional diamond burr preparation. Problems related to US tips correlate with improper use: usage at higher power than recommended, high force application, and lack of sufficient irrigation.

1.1.2.2 Air Abrasion Technology Based on Aluminum Oxide Powder

The air abrasion method was introduced in dentistry in the 1950s by Black [11], but it was neglected due to the emergence of high-speed turbine burr preparation. Recently, the method has been reintroduced as a minimally invasive alternative to turbine burr preparation because it is well accepted by patients, especially young ones, generating less noise, less sensitivity, and vibration. Air abrasion has proven to be relatively effective in removing infiltrated dentin and occlusal pigmentation [12]. Moreover, it has been reported that occlusal caries' diagnosis is better after air abrasion use [13, 14]. The working principle is simple, consisting of a jet of particles made from abrasive powder (e.g., aluminum oxide) impacting the tooth surface under the action of compressed air used with cooling to reduce the aerosols of powder in suspension. The device can be mounted at the end of a dental unit or can be a stand-alone device (Fig. 1.7).

The most widely used abrasive powder is aluminum oxide (Al_2O_3), with a particle size of ~27.5 μm. Under the effect of this jet, small amounts of dental tissue are removed, producing a cavity with an irregular contour [15]. The lack of the operator's sense of touch and low specificity in removing carious tissues are still a barrier to the widespread application of this method [16].

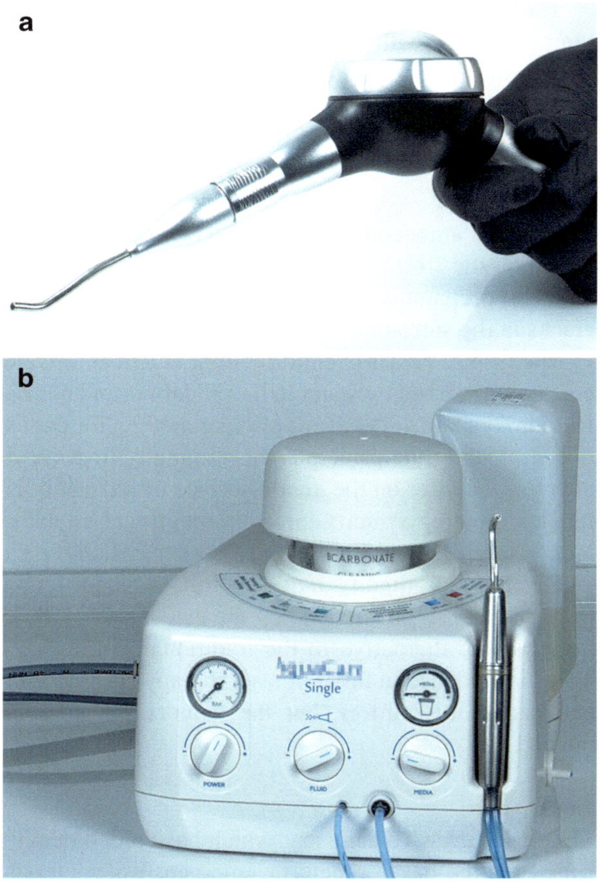

Fig. 1.7 Air abrasion tool (**a**); minimally invasive dentistry equipment used for air abrasion and polishing (**b**)

Given the minimal temperature rise during operation and the other advantages mentioned, this method is recommended for small cavity preparation when more cleaning of the internal cavity surface is needed [17].

Given these downsides, new powders such as bioactive glass powder (BAG) and glycine have appeared on the market.

BAG has a higher hardness than enamel (7 GPa compared to 3.5 GPa enamel) but lower than aluminum oxide—the particles' shape is round, making it less invasive [18]. BAG is effective for removing extrinsic pigmentation and desensitizing exposed dentin, and it is much more selective between enamel and dentin, making the preparation more conservative than aluminum oxide [19, 20].

Glycine is an amino acid. The powder is water-soluble and has less than 63 microns particle size, making it a finer powder than aluminum oxide and preparing soft tissues. Glycine is used as a powder in periodontal therapy. It removes tartar and dental plaque much more effectively than other powders, such as sodium bicarbonate or calcium carbonate. It has been demonstrated that minimal damage to gingival tissue occurred when the tip was directed perpendicular to the dental surface, compared to other powders [21–23].

The study by Giacomelli et al. [24] discussed the treatment of composite restorations by airflow with glycine powder and demonstrated that a smoother surface with more minor surface defects (1–2 microns) could be obtained compared to using sodium bicarbonate (5–10 microns). The adhesion is directly proportional to the microretentions' quality [25].

1.1.2.3 Laser

The laser is a noncontact method to prepare the tooth structure and desensitize the odontoblastic fibers from the dentin, eliminating the sensitivity typically reported with burr preparation. Laser tooth preparation does not generate vibrations or microcracks in the surrounding enamel.

The Er:YAG laser is emitting light at a peak wavelength of *2940 nm*, the laser's energy is absorbed by water in the epidermis and dermis, and it is also well absorbed in hydroxyapatite [26]. It is a popular method for caries removal and cavity preparation, following the principles of minimally invasive dentistry [27]. Moreover, the effect of the laser on the dentin surface of the cavity is one of opening the dentinal tubules, creating a microscopically rough surface with micromechanical retentions, ideal for adhesion [28].

Given the low quality of the scientific evidence found conducting a meta-analysis, Montedori et al. concluded that the evidence was insufficient to support the use of lasers as an alternative to the traditional milling method for cavity preparation. There is evidence in favor of laser therapy for pain control, the need for anesthesia, and patient discomfort, but the authors judged this to be insufficiently documented [29].

Conclusion

Minimally invasive dentistry, which has guided dental practice in recent years, has called for the development or emergence of methods that are as conservative as possible with dental tissues. However, the literature hardly accepts their equivocal effectiveness or, moreover, their supremacy over the traditional method of cavity preparation with burs. There is no foolproof method of cavity removal and cavity preparation. However, any new method has the undeniable advantages of using drills, which still have the advantage of the age of the method, easy protocols, quick and cheap implementation compared to any other minimally invasive method, extensive research in studies, and verification of long-term results.

Review Questions

1. What are the advantages of using US diamond tips compared to conventional diamond burs?
2. What is and how is cavity preparation by blasting/air abrasion achieved?
3. What are the characteristics of using a laser for cavity preparation for restoration?

1.1.3 Instruments for Direct Restorations with Composite Materials

The tools that are commonly used for handling, forming, shaping, finishing, and polishing composite materials are:

- Composite modeling kit.
- Modeling brushes.
- Wetting agents.
- Dental light-curing lamp.
- Sectional and circular matrices.
- Composites' heating oven.
- Finishing and polishing tools (see Chap. 7).

Besides these, the medical industry provides dentists with various other instruments and accessories necessary for direct restorations, all adopted by dentists according to their personal preferences and desired beliefs.

1.1.3.1 Modeling Kit

The composite layering and shaping steps require special tools in terms of shape, elasticity, and surface properties to make the handling of composite resin materials as efficient as possible and the operator's effort as little as possible and within ergonomic standards. Dentists now have at their disposal a multitude of tool kit variants that are designed specifically for composites clinical work or that are borrowed from dental technology. Most of these kits more or less mimic the classic PKT kit. We have selected one kit from this multitude of kits that will be presented below.

LM-Arte is a tool kit for layering and modeling composites developed by a company in collaboration with Style Italiano Group. The tools are made of surface-treated steel, so composite materials do not easily stick to them. Each tool has a

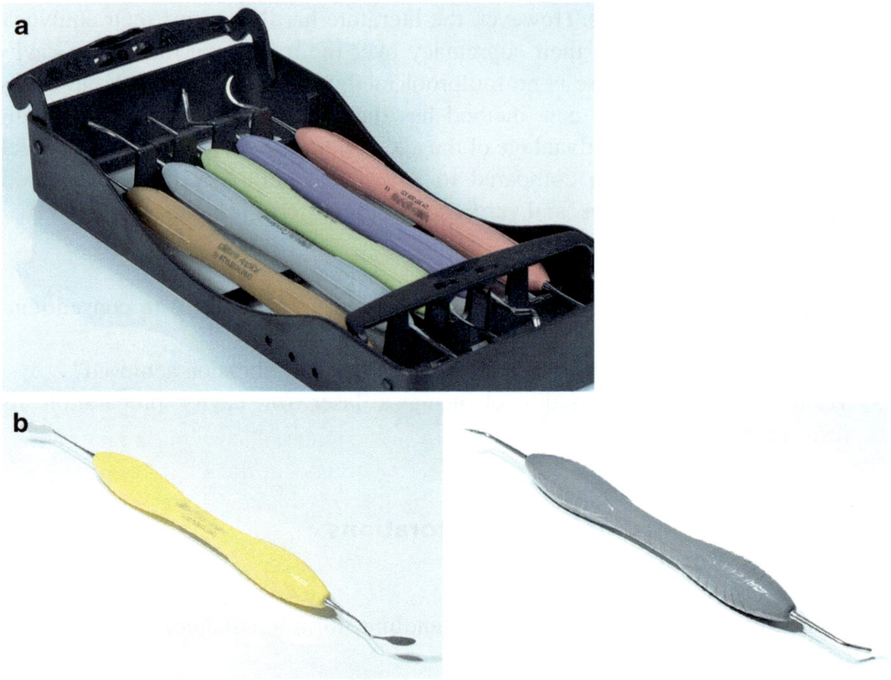

Fig. 1.8 LM-Arte modeling kit (**a**); LM-Arte Solo Posterior and Solo Anterior for composite restorations (**b**)

silicone handle of a different color and a name depending on its purpose. The LM-Arte Basic Modeling Kit Set includes the following tools (Fig. 1.8a):

- LM-Arte Applica, the dental spatula mainly used to apply portions of composite in the cavity.
- LM-Arte Condensa, an obturator mainly used for condensing the composite in the cavity.
- LM-Arte Fissura, a specific modeling tool used for sculpting the occlusal anatomy.
- LM-Arte Misura, an instrument for measuring the space kept free for a layer of composite or measuring the thickness of the applied layer
- LM-Arte Eccesso, scaler used for removing the excess of light-cured composite.

In addition to the complete kit for posterior teeth, single instruments try to emulate the role of other instruments by shape and indications, such as LM-Arte Solo Posterior and Solo Anterior (Fig. 1.8b).

Today, the equipment market has an abundance of instruments for handling composite resins and occlusal anatomy modeling. From all these instruments, we have selected a few innovative examples that have been released in recent years, their popularity varying among clinicians by country, region, and specialty:

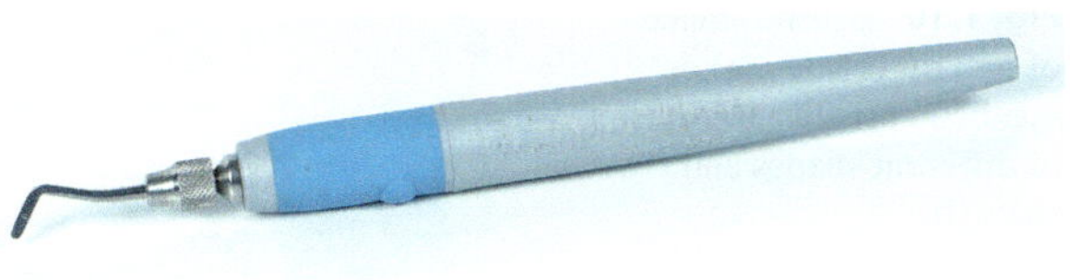

Fig. 1.9 Dental composite modeling instrument: Compothixo

- *CompoRoller (Kerr Company).* CompoRoller™ is an innovative composite shaping tool that provides complete control when layering and contouring a direct composite restoration into its final shape. The tool has seven differently shaped silicone tips that rotate around a central axis.
- *CompoThixo (Kerr Company).* The tool consists of a handle and four different tips. Due to the vibrations transmitted to the tip, the tool optimizes the composites' thixotropic properties by modifying the viscosity without changing the chemical and mechanical characteristics of the material. The vibration frequency is 100 Hz. The instrument allows superior composite adaptation to the cavity walls, reduction of air bubbles, composite layer's thickness control, and a good adaptation of the bulk composite (Fig. 1.9).
- *SonicFill Handpiece (Kavo Dental).* It plugs into a terminal of the dental unit and allows sonic activation of the composite, significantly reducing the viscosity of the material—allowing for effective filling. The piece is part of a concept that includes the bulk *SonicFill* composite *(Kerr Company)* with an increased degree of filling. As the sonic energy is applied through the handpiece, the viscosity decreases to 84%, increasing the flowability of the composite. This increases the resin's adaptation to the cavity shape, improving marginal sealing and eliminating air bubbles. When the sonic energy is turned off, the composite returns to a more viscous consistency, allowing the occlusal morphology to be achieved.

1.1.3.2 Modeling Brush

Dental technicians successfully use composite modeling brushes in laboratory work. Their integration by dentists into clinical practice is relatively recent and has been quickly encouraged by the advantages of using composite modeling brushes, even if relevant studies do not yet back these up.

Special brushes have been designed for composite materials, but the brushes used by technicians, even particular cosmetic, or fine art brushes, can also be used successfully (with limitations and reservations). These modeling brushes can be made from the following materials: natural bristles, synthetic bristles, or silicone pieces, and the active part can have different shapes (Fig. 1.10): brushes with different shapes of the active part made of natural bristles, synthetic bristles, or silicone. Straight brushes can be used for anterior teeth, but in the posterior area, the active part needs to be curved to access the molars. They can be for single-use, and they can be fixed in a reusable handle, or they can be classically nonremovable (and they need to be cold disinfected between uses).

Some of the brush designs have several shapes of the active part that can be changed by detaching the handle. One such product was developed by Styleitaliano

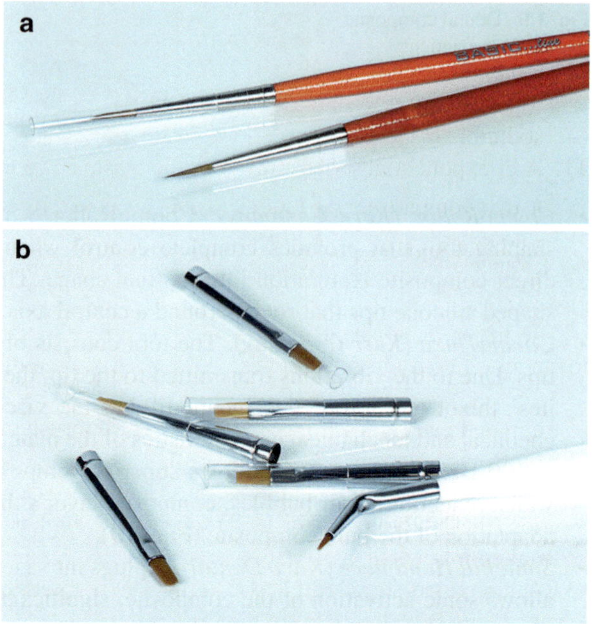

Fig. 1.10 Brushes made of natural bristles (**a**) or synthetic bristles; brushes of different shapes and sizes (**b**)

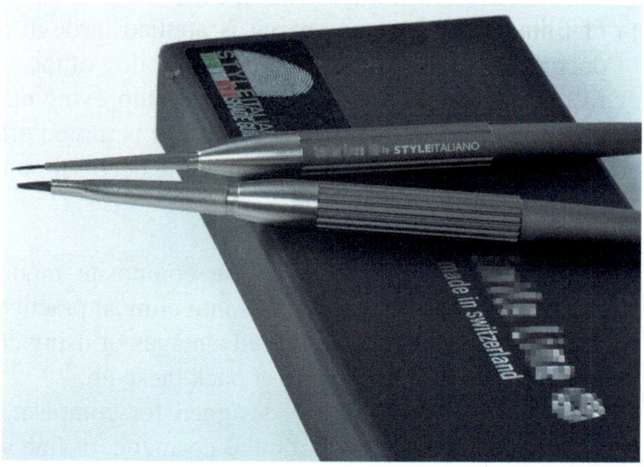

Fig. 1.11 Compo-Brush Composite Brush Kit

and Smile Line (Switzerland) under *Compo-Brush* (Fig. 1.11). They are made of black synthetic fibers, which provide extreme precision and the best contrast when applied to composite materials. The brush tip can be easily bent by the user for better access to the back areas. The Compo-Brush set contains two complete brushes and two replacement brush tips for each model.

Modeling brushes can be used dried or dipped in modeling resins.

Using modeling resins can cause maintenance problems for reusable brushes that are difficult to clean and disinfect after wetting in modeling resins. The brushing movement only takes place in one direction, from composite to tooth.

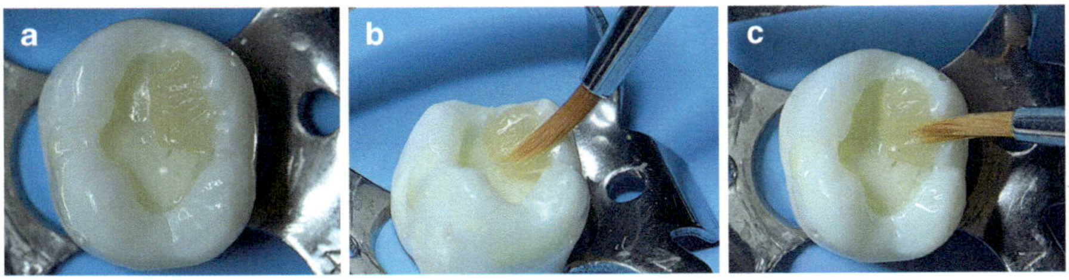

Fig. 1.12 Direct restoration: composite resin modeling (**a**), (**b**), and (**c**)

The use of a brush for composites modeling is associated with the following advantages (although not all of them are backed by published studies to this day):

- Improved marginal sealing of the composite (brush movements should always be from composite toward tooth).
- Cleaning excess composite material occlusally placed outside the cavity boundaries (the effectiveness of this procedure is higher when the brush is dry and smaller than when the brush is wet).
- Rounding and surface finishing of the unpolymerized composite obtained from metal tool modeling (Fig. 1.12a).
- Shaping smooth anatomical structures such as grooves and fissures (by applying pressure with a sharp brush, you can create grooves and fittings or accentuate certain fissures (Fig. 1.12b, c).
- Smoothing the grooves and trenches before light-curing. When using the successive cusp buildup technique or other sequential techniques to restore occlusal morphology, grooves with irregular and retentive areas may result. Brushing the grooves with the tip of a thin brush could improve their shape.

The use of microbrushes is widely adopted by clinicians for composite compaction, excess removal, or even shaping. The micro applicators are already in use on the working field, since the application stage of the adhesive. They are easy to use and create the composite's smooth and glossy appearance on the surface layer. Good modeling, however, is difficult to achieve with these; the modeling brush gives improved results. Although widespread, the usage of adhesive-impregnated micro applicators for shaping the last layer of the composite is contested by some studies because it was shown that filling the composite microfissures with adhesive has unfavorable mechanical effects due to its low filler loading.

1.1.3.3 Wetting Agents

Some composite materials stick very effortlessly to the modeling tools, and a wetting agent is required to allow for proper handling. The composite adhesive is probably the most widely used and studied wetting agent used successfully by clinicians [30]. Modeling resins are special wetting agents that have been developed to prevent composites from adhering to instruments and facilitating modeling (Figs. 1.13 and 1.14). The scientific world has investigated the application of patterning resins

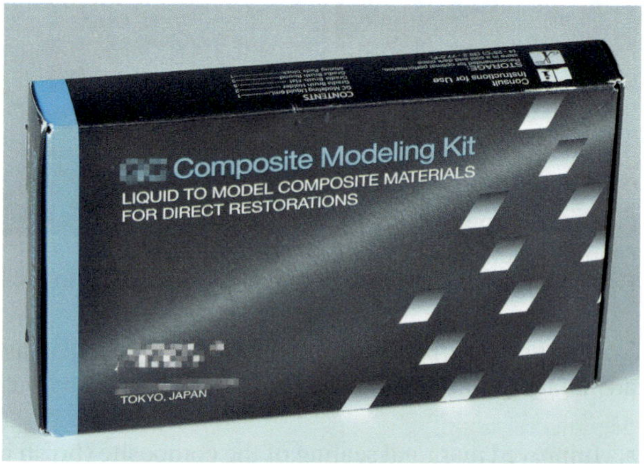

Fig. 1.13 Composite modeling kit for direct restoration

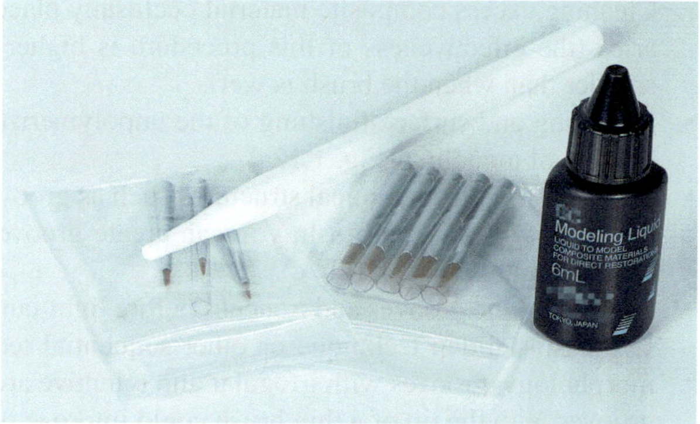

Fig. 1.14 Modeling brushes and modeling liquid

between layers of composite materials from the following perspective: introducing color changes to composites and their behavior over time. Good maintenance of aesthetic properties [31] and stability of physical properties [32] have been proven, while, on the contrary, other studies had shown a decrease in the restorations' surface strength when modeling resin was applied to the surface [33].

We conclude that modeling resins or wetting agents should only be used when necessary. The decision whether or not to use a wetting agent or a modeling resin may be specified in the package leaflet of the composite material itself, or the dentist has decided to use it or not. If a composite of softer consistency is used, which shows adhesion to instruments that is more than average, then a modeling resin may be helpful.

If, on the contrary, the composite has a firm consistency and does not adhere very well to the instruments, then the dentist can skip the modeling resin.

1.1.3.4 Composite Syringe Heater

The composite syringes can be heated to temperatures of 40–70 °C, before use, in special heaters that have slots for multiple syringes. The heater is intended to increase the composite resin's adhesive properties and fluidity.

Many dental professionals still have questions about heating composites. However, if the composite is approved for heating by the manufacturer and is backed by safety and effectiveness tests, then there is no reason not to use heated composite.

Studies have shown that composite resins preheated to 60–70 °C for a limited time will not only have adverse effect on mechanical properties (such as torsional or tensile strength) but will also not affect the polymerization depth [34]. Similar or even lower contraction forces are generated compared to composite resins heated at room temperature [35].

Conclusion

Although handling the composite resins can ultimately be accomplished with unspecialized tools, developing specially dedicated tool kits improves the shape, design, ergonomics, surface treatment, functionality, and flexibility. All these things contribute to increased quality, efficiency, and comfort care. The ideal size, the composition, and the shapes of the most efficient tools for handling and shaping composite resins will always be a matter of debate because all these characteristics imply a dose of subjectivity that depends on the experience, practical skills, and knowledge of each practitioner.

Using a composite modeling brush is becoming increasingly common among dentists due to the immediate visible results while modeling. Furthermore, the studies confirm the following advantages: an increase in marginal integrity, a decrease in excess material, and a decrease in voids in the composite body.

The wetting agents should be used when the composite resins' manufacturers recommend them or when the dentist considers, based on his own well-reasoned experience, that he/she can obtain better results by using a particular dental composite resin in combination with the wetting agents.

Review Questions

1. What tools can a composite resin modeling kit contain, and what are their characteristics?
2. What are the characteristics of composite resin modeling brushes, and how can they be used?
3. What are the wetting agents/modeling brushes, and how are they used?
4. What is an oven, and how is it used for heating composite resins?

1.1.4 Dental Matrices

Main idea: The matrix holds the place of a proximal wall until its restoration. The aim is to create a wall made of composite material that follows the proximal tooth anatomy, being in proper contact with the adjacent tooth without any excess material (in the gingival, oral, and buccal embrasures) and of appropriate height (marginal ridge level).

In the 1800's dentistry, one treatment meant cleaning the carious tissue and filling the cavity with a material (amalgam or gold) without paying much attention to anatomical and morphological structures. It was only toward the end of the nineteenth century that dentists began to pay close attention to the concept of restorations *to be as anatomically accurate as possible*, including the proximal walls and the contact point [36].

The traditional matrix consisted of a thin, straight metal strip surrounding the tooth. One of the best-known and most popular matrix systems still used by dentists today is the Tofflemire matrix retainer, introduced by Dr. Joseph Tofflemire in 1946 based on the Ivory No. 9 model. Its main advantage is that it can tighten firmly and can nicely fit a matrix on the tooth.

The matrices can be classified into circular matrices (which surround the entire tooth crown) and sectional matrices (which only target proximal areas).

To deal with various restorations, the clinician needs to have as many matrix systems as possible, in order to be able choose the best one for each case. One single matrix system cannot serve all clinical situations.

1.1.4.1 Circular Matrices

The studies published up to this date show that circular matrices lead to inferior results compared to sectional matrices when the latter are used for proximal cavity and contact point restoration [37–39], including MOD cavity restoration [40].

Although the earliest versions of circumferential matrices used a flat metal tape installed in the matrix retainer (e.g., Tofflemire, Fig. 1.15a), the pre-curved tapes appeared later on the market to better reconstruct the proximal anatomy, allowing the contact point to be lowered (e.g., Slick Bands Tofflemire—Style, Garrison Dental Solutions). A significant disadvantage of these systems is that the matrix retainer remains attached to the tooth throughout the treatment and limits the working space (e.g., Tofflemire; Omnimatrix-Ultradent). Some systems have solved this problem by replacing the holder with a screwdriver-like clamping device that is removed after the matrix is fixed to the tooth (e.g., SuperMat—Kerr Company). Other systems have even directly incorporated the miniaturized clamping device into the matrix without needing a screwdriver (Palodent 360—Dentsply Sirona).

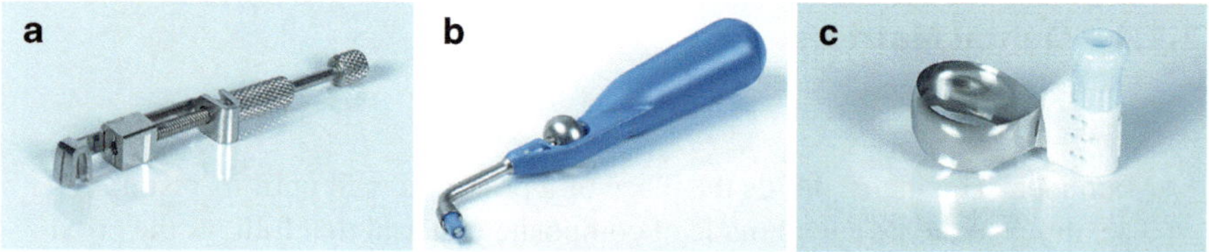

Fig. 1.15 Tofflemire matrix retainer (**a**); tensioning instrument (**b**); circumferential matrix system Palodent 360 (**c**)

The significant advantages of the circular matrices refer to:

- Ease of use.
- The versatility of the cases that can be solved.
- Relatively low price.

The disadvantages are related to:

- The presence of the matrix retainer that could limit movement during work and could be uncomfortable to the patient.
- Restoring the proximal anatomy.
- Difficulties of adaptation, especially in the cervical area.

The circular matrices can be classified according to several criteria, the main ones being the following:

1. The material: whether a matrix band is made from plastic or metal, it can influence the light-curing process and how the matrix is firmly fixed to the tooth.
2. The shape: flat-tapped or pre-curved matrices. The tape's shape is the most important so that a flat tape will not be able to restore a pre-curved anatomical proximal wall with convex morphology that can restore a correct contact area with the adjacent tooth.
3. Matrix installment modalities: with fixed matrix retainer (Tofflemire, Fig. 1.15a), with removable matrix retainer (SuperMat, Fig. 1.15b), or without matrix retainer (Palodent 360, Fig. 1.15c).

It is recommended to avoid using flat tapes without pre-curved contours that cannot restore the anatomical convexity of the teeth. They can be successfully used for temporary restorations, prosthetic bridges, and pre-endodontic reconstructions, but not for definitive proximal restorations. The pre-curved pre-fabricated metal strips installed in the universal matrix systems or other circular or sectional matrices are preferred.

Among the main disadvantages of straight metal strips, or moreover, of any flat matrix that is not pre-curved, it can be mentioned:

- Straight proximal wall without anatomical convexities.
- Occlusal displacement of the contact point.
- Difficulties in tight adaptation.

The restoration of the proximal walls with the flat matrices raises two significant problems:

1. High gingival embrasure is much extended toward the occlusal, with the risk of the papilla not filling it. The occlusal displacement of the contact point increases the distance between it and the alveolar bone level. If this distance exceeds 5 mm, according to Tarnow's law [41], the papilla will not grow up to the contact point to fill the entire embrasure (Fig. 1.16).

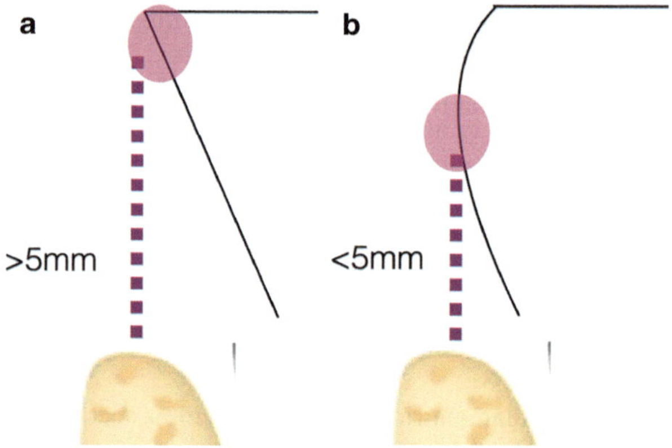

Fig. 1.16 Graphic representation of the distance between the interproximal contact point and the alveolar bone level: proximal wall restored by flat matrix (**a**) versus contoured matrix (**b**)

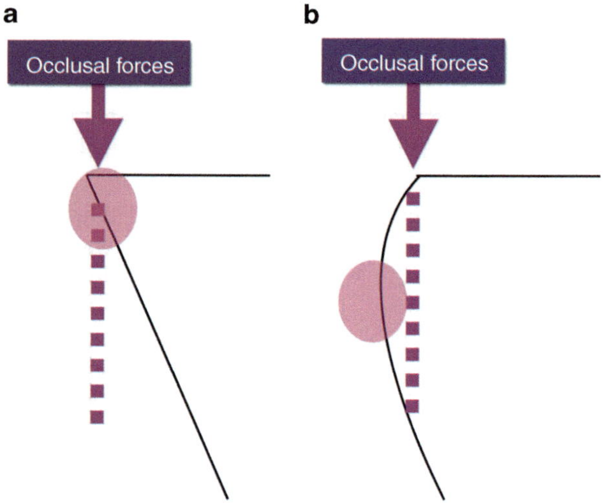

Fig. 1.17 Graphic representation of occlusal force transmission on the marginal ridge for proximal wall restoration with a flat matrix (**a**) versus contoured matrix (**b**)

2. Decreased mechanical strength of the marginal ridge that is not sufficiently supported by the material, as in the case of a pre-curved matrix restoration (Fig. 1.17). The marginal edge takes up a significant proportion of the occlusal forces [42]; therefore, it must be strong and supported by a sufficient composite mass. The obtained marginal edges will not have the necessary support because they have a significantly low mechanical fracture strength [43].

1.1.4.2 Sectional Matrices

The sectional matrices can be manufactured from a metal or celluloid (Fig. 1.18). The metal sectional matrices are 38–76 micron thin foils [44], fixed with the wedges in the gingival edge area and fixed with rings in the buccal/oral embrasures. The studies conducted for the restoration of class II cavities indicate tighter contact points when sectional matrices are used together with rings rather than circular matrices [45].

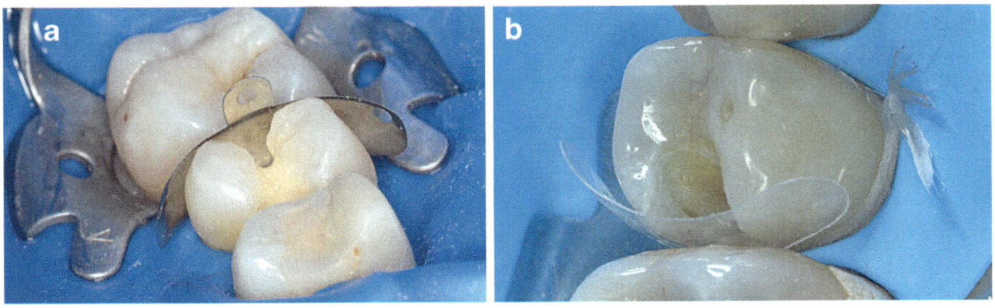

Fig. 1.18 Sectional matrix made of metal (**a**) or clear celluloid (**b**)

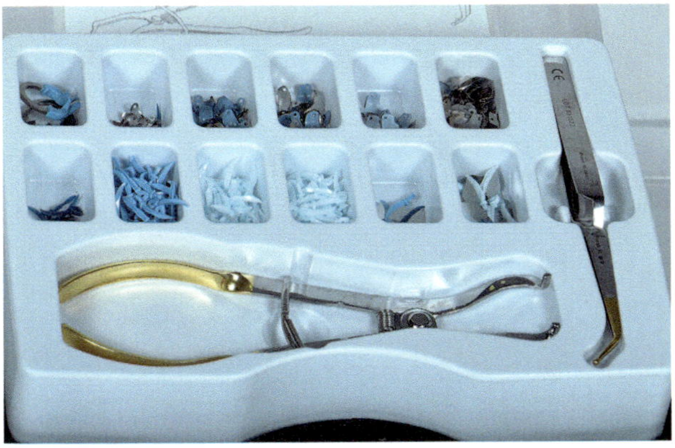

Fig. 1.19 Palodent V3 Triodent sectional matrix system

1.1.4.3 Sectional Metal Matrices

A professional matrix system offers the clinician several size options for matrices, rings, and wedges, as well as the accessories needed to handle them: matrix ring forceps and unique autolocking matrix pin tweezers (Fig. 1.19) (*V3 Triodent—Dentsply Sirona; Composi Tight 3D Fusion Garrison—Henry Schein*) (Fig. 1.20).

The Palodent V3 Triodent matrix system (Dentsply Sirona, Germany) consists of the following:

1. Matrix ring forceps (Fig. 1.21) for ring handling. The forceps has ring-holding tweezers so that the ring does not rock in the tensioned forceps. After clamping on the ring, the forceps can be locked by sliding a rod. This allows the ring to be handed to the operator, with the tweezers spread apart, under tension so it can be applied to the buccal and oral embrasures. The inner side of the forceps handles has a notch that is necessary to activate the ring by squeezing it when it is likely to expand after multiple uses and steam sterilization.
2. Self-locking pin tweezers (Fig. 1.22) for handling matrices, dental wedges, and WedgeGuards. The pin tweezer has a pin that fits into the perforations of the matrix or the dental wedges, or WedgeGuards, allowing firm fixation without

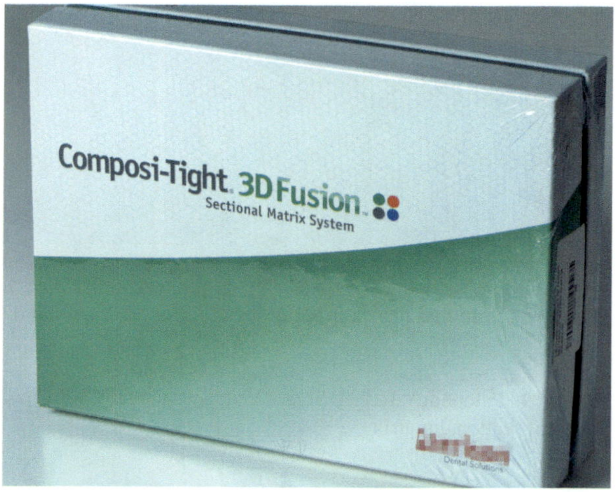

Fig. 1.20 Composi Tight 3D Fusion Garrison sectional matrix system

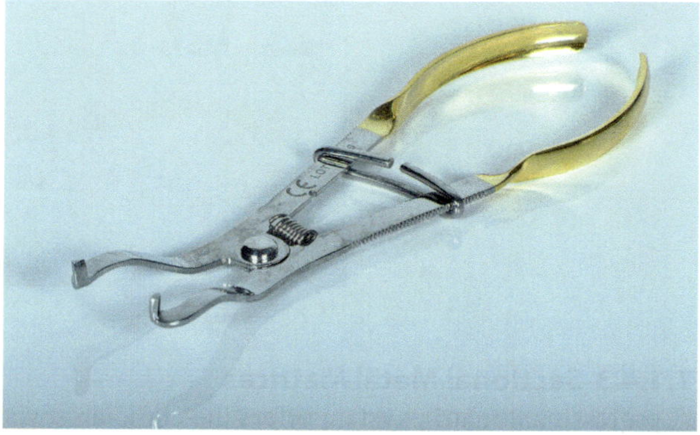

Fig. 1.21 Matrix ring pliers (Palodent)

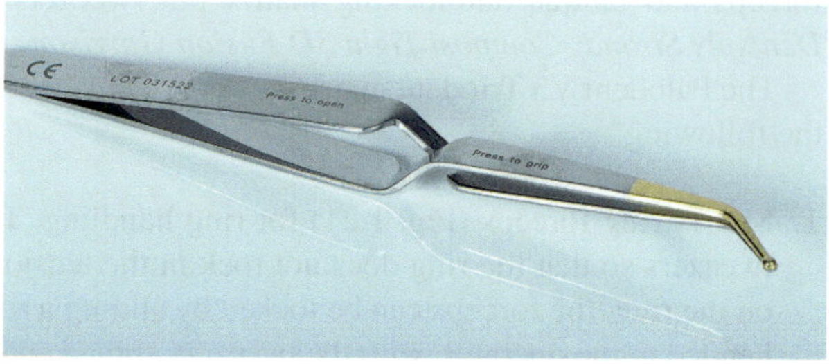

Fig. 1.22 Auto-locking tweezers for sectional matrices (Palodent)

deforming the metal surface (in the case of matrices). The principle of the self-locking pin tweezer is that it remains with its jaws closed at rest when not pressed by the operator.

3. Pre-curved sectional metal matrices. These have different sizes for accommodating various types of premolars and molars (Fig. 1.23). They are made of stainless steel, with an average thickness of around 50 microns, and may have a polished surface or a PTFE-coated surface (Fig. 1.24). PTFE (Teflon) prevents the matrix

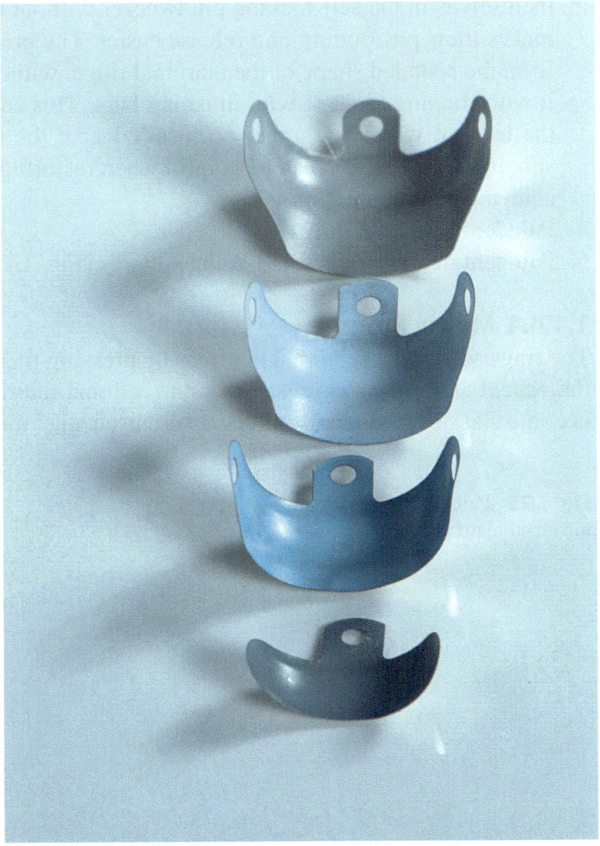

Fig. 1.23 PTFE-coated sectional matrices in various sizes

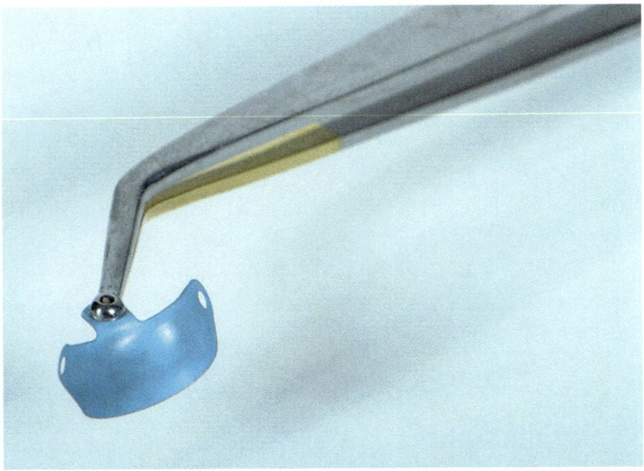

Fig. 1.24 Palodent PTFE-coated sectional matrix

from sticking to the composite and helps to better unstick the matrix after light-curing. Furthermore, the color coding of the PTFE layer helps to identify the desired size quickly. The lateral and occlusal pin tweezer holes help to secure themselves in the self-locking pin tweezer without the risk of deformation. This makes their positioning and release easier. The pre-curved occlusal edge helps form the rounded shape of the marginal ridge, without needing to shape or adapt it with shaping tools or with finishing burs. This edge is positioned precisely at the level at which the upper occlusal edge of the marginal ridge is desired. A subgingival extension can be helpful when restoring cavities extended below the cementoenamel junction.

4. Palodent ring (Fig. 1.25).
5. Palodent dental wedges and WedgeGuards (Fig. 1.26).

1.1.4.4 Matrix Rings

The rings secure the sectional matrices by pressing them tightly against the tooth in the buccal and oral openings. The first sectional matrix systems, which have now become classics (Palodent and Garrison), used steel metal rings (Fig. 1.27a, b).

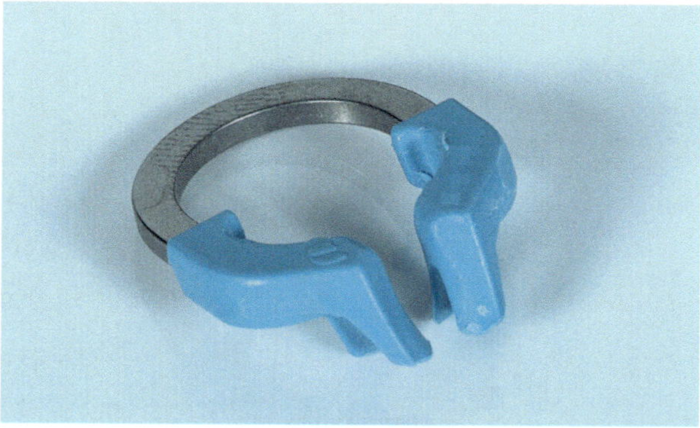

Fig. 1.25 Palodent universal matrix ring

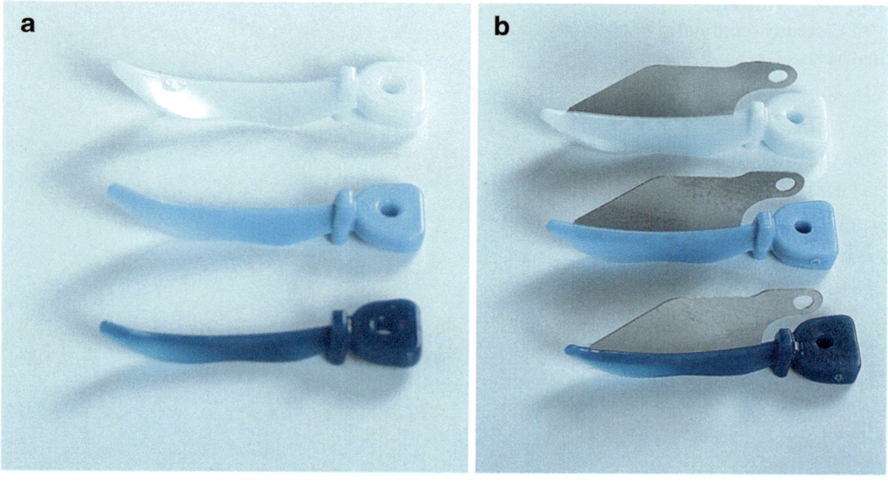

Fig. 1.26 Small, medium, and large Palodent plastic wedges (**a**); small, medium, and large WedgeGuards (**b**)

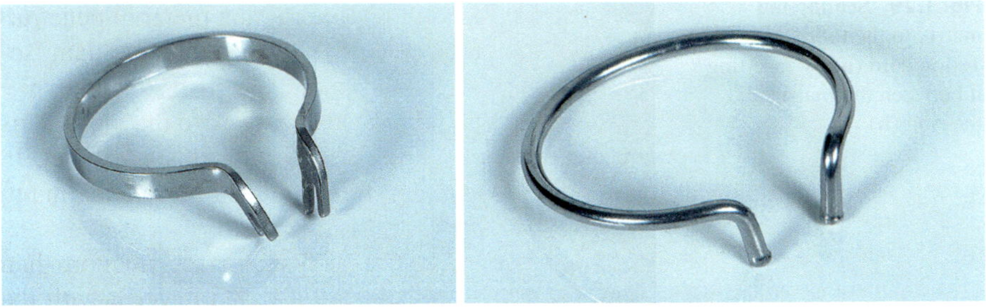

Fig. 1.27 Metal rings for sectional matrices

Fig. 1.28 Garrison matrix ring

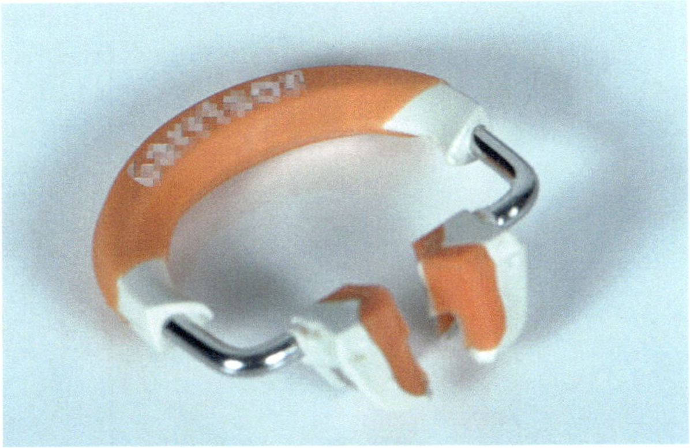

Modern matrix systems have different types of rings compared to older systems. For example, the Palodent ring is made from titanium, and the tines are plastic-reinforced glass fiber, with each tine coming into contact with two teeth. The ring provides a good tooth separation of about 60–80 microns [46], which is about the thickness of two matrices (Palodent V3), and, in addition, there is an excellent fit of the metal matrix on the tooth. Moreover, the tine shape prevents the ring from entering more extensive proximal cavities. Tines are V-shaped, so they allow removal of the dental wedge or insertion of the dental wedge to be replaced with another size when necessary.

Other models of fixation rings for sectional matrices are Garrison (Fig. 1.28), Triodent with transparent tines, TOR-VM, etc.

The shape of the ring tines is standard and may not adequately be used in all clinical situations. In some cases, it is necessary to fix them with a liquid dam for more stability or to insert a liquid dam, or PTFE, between the tines and the matrix to improve matrix adaptation (Fig. 1.29).

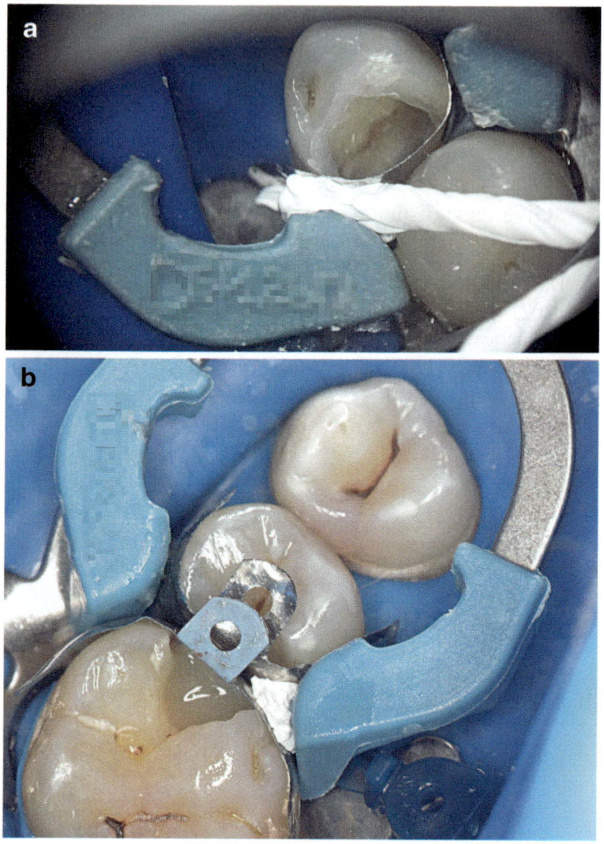

Fig. 1.29 Sealing the matrix to the tooth with a Teflon cord (**a**) by inserting it between the matrix and the ring (**b**)

Difficulties that may occur	Potential solutions
Matrix deformation during its application, due to heavy forces applied	Changing the matrix with a new, nondeformed one and spacing the teeth (with a dental wedge, matrix ring, or dedicated spacer instrument). Finalizing the cavity preparation until there is the possibility of a matrix insertion
Ring instability	Liquid dam fixing
Matrix not fitting on the tooth	Fill the space between the ring tines and the matrix with a PTFE tape or a liquid rubber dam to press the matrix onto the tooth (Fig. 1.29)
Failure to insert the dental wedge	Thinning the dental wedge with a dental burr or a surgical blade

1.1.4.5 Dental Wedges

Dental wedges can be classified by material *t* and design (Fig. 1.30):

- Wooden dental wedges.
- Plastic dental wedges.
- Plastic dental wedges that can be filled or are hollow inside (V-shaped).

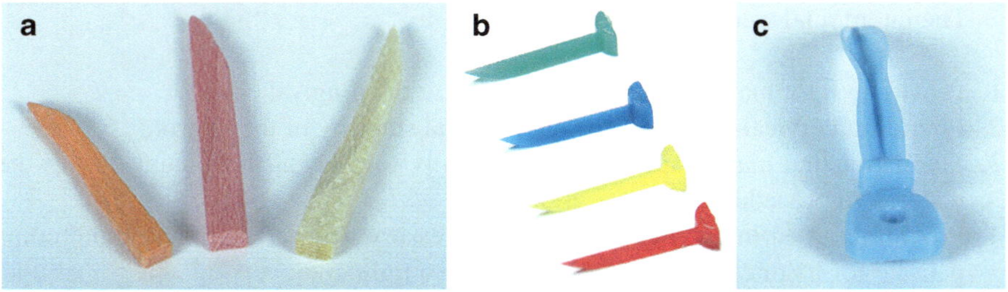

Fig. 1.30 Wooden wedges (**a**), plastic wedges (**b**), V-shaped plastic wedges (**c**)

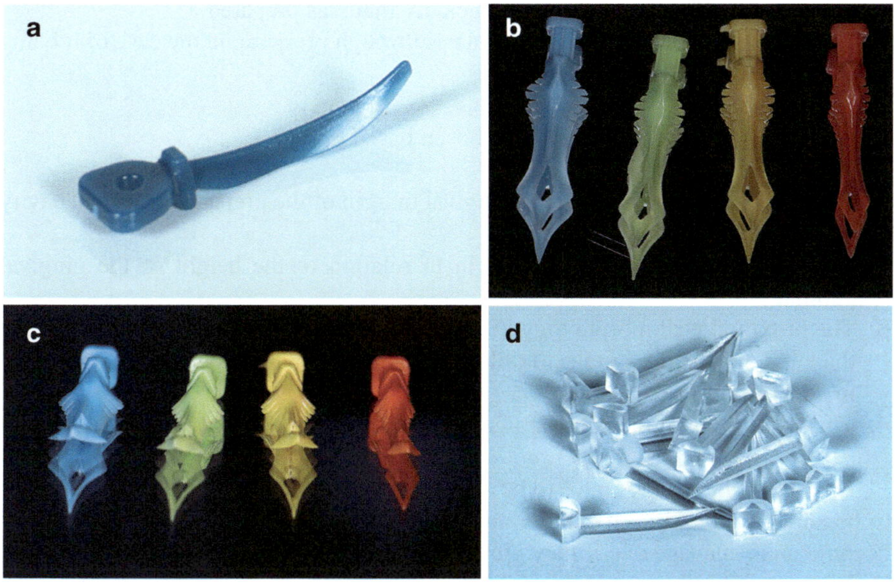

Fig. 1.31 Wedges of different shapes and sizes

The wedges designed in different shapes were in order to be used more straightforwardly and to achieve better results:

- Dental wedges that have the shape of a yataghan with the tip of the wedge slightly raised so that there is no risk of the tip protruding on the opposite side under the rubber dam sheet or piercing the dental papilla during the insertion (Fig. 1.31a).
- Anatomical-shaped dental wedges to allow the matrix to be tightly fixed on the tooth (Fig. 1.31b, c).
- Transparent plastic dental wedges such that when they are used together with transparent celluloid matrices, they can allow a better composite material light-curing by the passage of light during the process (Fig. 1.31d).
- Light-reflecting interdental wedges to improve the composite's polymerization in the gingival edge area.

The interdental wedge's roles are:

1. Providing tight matrix sealing on the tooth at the gingival edge.
2. Providing cervical-occlusal, buccal, and oral stability of the matrix.
3. Stabilizing the matrix and securing it firmly to prevent movement during the restorative procedure.
4. Providing a fast interdental separation necessary to insert the matrix and compensate for its thickness in order to achieve a tight contact point.
5. Preventing material extrusion.
6. Keeping the space for the interdental papilla free.
7. Repositioning the gingival margin and the rubber dam sheet more apically, near the gingival margin of the proximal cavity that was prepared.
8. Producing temporary papilla hemostasis through pressure, in the case of it being swollen.

The dental wedges to be used are chosen based on:

1. The size of the gap between the gingival margin of the prepared proximal cavity and the adjacent tooth.
2. The position of the gingival margin in relation to the height of the gingival papilla.
3. The proximal wall morphology in some teeth which may be concave, indicating thicker dental wedges in the middle portion or personalization by being wrapped in a PTFE tape.
4. The positioning of the contact area.

Therefore, the wedges have to be selected for specific individual cases, in order to be suitable in width, thickness, and taper. The insertion of dental wedges may become more manageable if they are moistened or lubricated. The insertion of the wedges may be more accessible from the oral side because the oral embrasure is broader, but each practitioner can decide on the most suitable option.

Interventions on dental wedges:

1. Even though most manufacturers produce standard-sized dental wedges, these do not satisfy all clinical cases. Depending on the case, the wedges can easily be customized with a scalpel blade or burs.
2. The presence of the interproximal wedge may influence the position of the contact area. If the upper margin of the wedge interferes with the curved portion of the matrix, there is a risk of deforming the matrix, resulting in a flattened proximal morphology or an abnormal concavity in future restoration of the proximal area. If there is no possibility of lowering the level of the wedge, then it must be adapted by cutting it using a burr in the interference zone [47].
3. In the case of concave proximal walls in the cervical area, a PTFE-wrapped wedge can be used. This can be achieved by wrapping a strip of PTFE tape

around the wedge's central area to become more pronounced and push the matrix into the concave area of the proximal wall (Fig. 1.32).

1.1.4.6 Mounting the Sectional Matrix Systems

In the first phase, the matrix size is chosen and the possibility of a subgingival extension is assessed (Fig. 1.33). To choose the size of a matrix, the distance between the edge of the matrix and its point of maximum convexity is measured

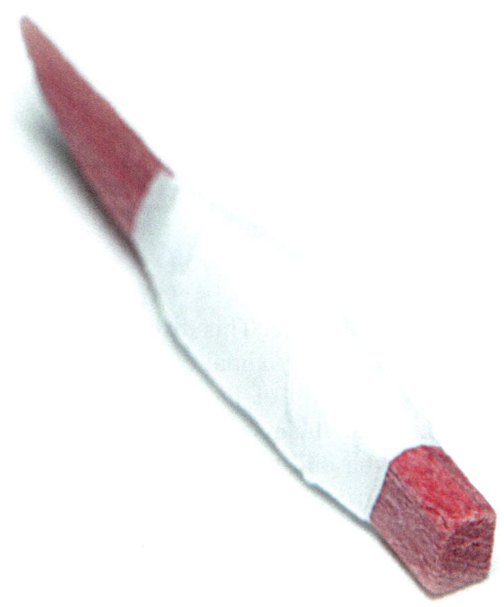

Fig. 1.32 Personalized interdental wooden wedges, wrapped with PTFE tape, to fit the sectorial matrix on concave proximal areas

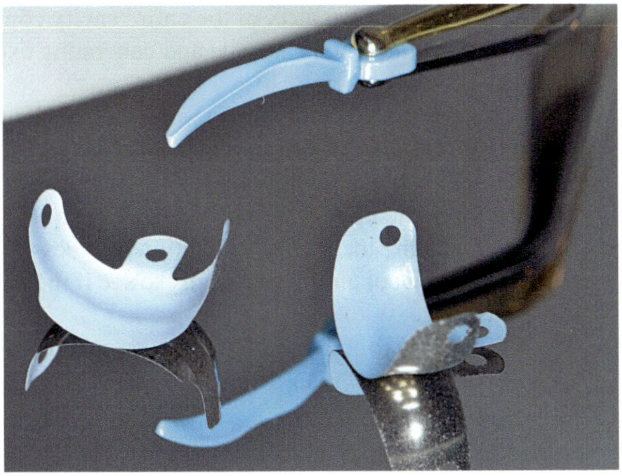

Fig. 1.33 Matrices with or without subgingival elongation

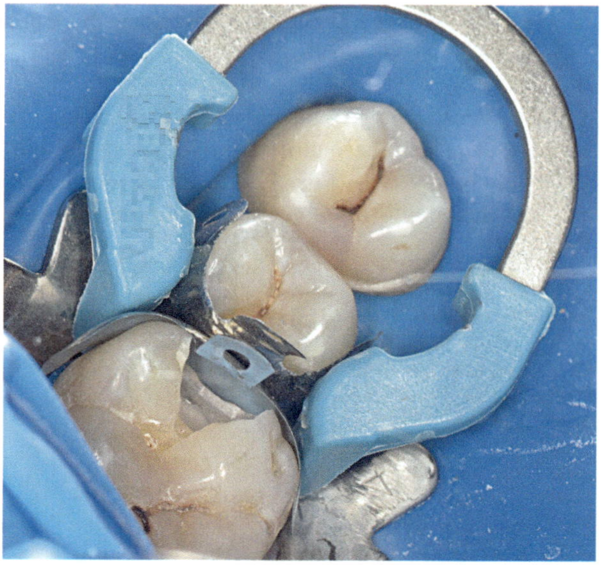

Fig. 1.34 Palodent matrix centered oro-bucally, positioned at the level of the future marginal ridge

with the periodontal probe. This distance must coincide with the distance between the point of maximum proximal convexity of the adjacent tooth and the bottom of the sulcus where the tip of the periodontal probe is placed. The elements to be checked when fitting the matrices are (Fig. 1.34) the following:

1. Centering in the oral-buccal direction [48]. When inserting the interproximal wedge, the matrix can quickly move from the correct position.
2. Matrix's occlusal edge should be placed at the tooth's marginal edge level, for those matrices with a curved shape toward the marginal edge (e.g., Palodent). For matrices with a straight occlusal edge, they should be placed above the tooth's marginal edge by 0.5 mm (e.g., TOR-VM). Placing the matrix in a position that is too high-occlusal placement—or too low-cervical placement—dislocates the contact point in an incorrect position.
3. Adapting/sealing the matrix of the entire cavity contour so that it does not allow the composite material to extrude and generating excess material in the interdental area.
4. Positioning the matrix in contact with the adjacent tooth by pressing it with a rounded, preferably plastic, pointed instrument (e.g., obturator). Sharp instruments might scratch the thin matrices, which might poorly shape the composite causing food retention.

Ways of checking the matrix adaptation tightness:

- Blow a strong jet of air into the cavity to see if the matrix is moving or it has been dislocated.
- Trace the internal contour of the cavity in the contact area with an explorer with a sharp tip or a "Fisura" instrument to detect areas where the sealing is not tight (Fig. 1.35).

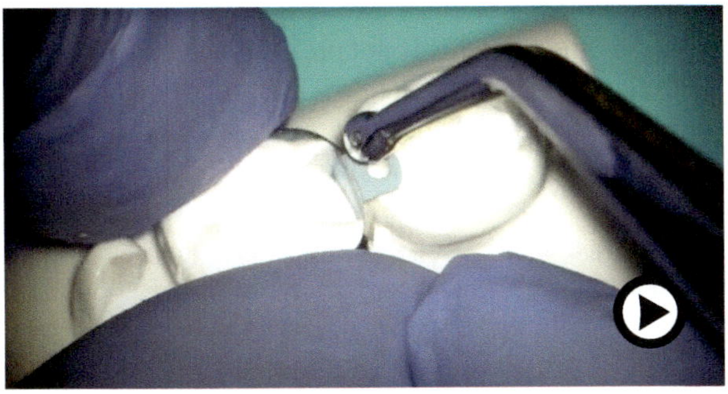

Fig. 1.35 Mounting the sectional matrix system—Palodent plus (▶ https://doi.org/10.1007/000-bqg)

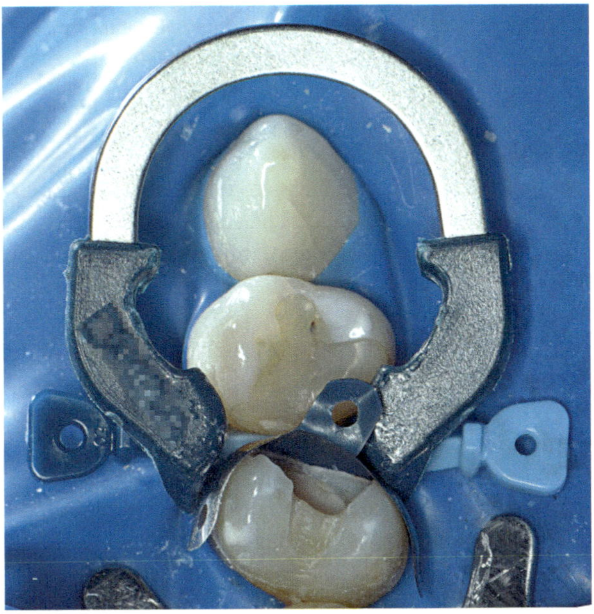

Fig. 1.36 Fitting a sectorial matrix using two wedges that are inserted from the buccal and oral side

1.1.4.7 Mounting Two Wedges Simultaneously

The wedges can be inserted either from the buccal or the oral side [45]. They are usually inserted from the side where the embrasure is wider. There is also the possibility of mounting the two wedges simultaneously from opposite directions (buccal and oral) (Fig. 1.36) to ensure a better adaptation of the matrix at the gingival margin to the buccal and oral embrasures. In these situations, whether the two wedges have sufficient proximal space in the gingival margin area is examined. The same thing can be successfully used in cases of teeth with cervical concave morphology.

If hollow V-shaped plastic wedges are used on the inside, two wedges can be stacked on top of each other, but this is not preferable because the top-placed wedge may interfere with the matrix in the area of the future contact point, resulting in a damaged proximal surface (as a shape).

Difficulties that may occur	Potential solutions
The wedge does not seal the matrix well to the tooth	A larger wedge can be used, or a PTFE tape can be wrapped around the wedge
The wedge deforms the matrix because it is too high in the occlusal direction	Wedge reduction with a scalpel blade or a burr
The top of the wedge protrudes on the opposite side under the rubber dam	Reinsert the wedge while the rubber dam is stretched and molded onto the palate (apically positioned)
Due to the rubber dam's elasticity, the wedge is pushed out of the interdental space	When the wedge is inserted from the buccal side, the rubber dam can be stretched (pulled) to the proximal area so that the rubber dam withdraws as the wedge penetrates

Conclusion
The use of an appropriate matrix system is essential for restorations that aim to restore interdental contacts. The shape, the size, the material, the correct fit, and the proper adaptation can strongly influence the clinical outcome.

Review Questions
1. What are circular matrices, their advantages and disadvantages, and how are they classified?
2. What are the two main problems with using flat/straight/uncontoured matrices?
3. What does the Palodent matrix system include?
4. What are the main characteristics of matrix rings?
5. What are the main functions of interdental wedges?

1.1.5 Instruments and Materials for Finishing

The finishing is performed differently on the posterior teeth compared to the anterior ones. Anterior teeth require a more elaborate working protocol to achieve pleasing aesthetics.

The working protocol for finishing anterior teeth involves several steps, each requiring specific tools. The working protocol is detailed in Chap. 7.

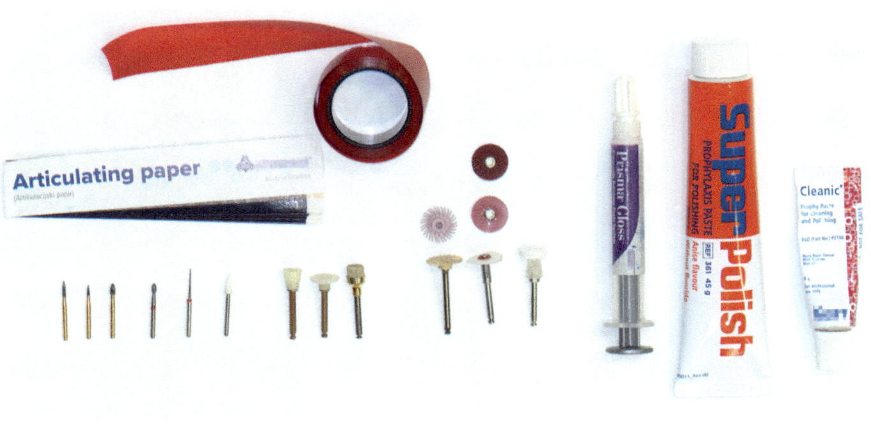

Fig. 1.37 Basic instruments and materials for occlusal adjustments, finishing and polishing in a direct restoration

Fig. 1.38 Small grained diamond dental burs set

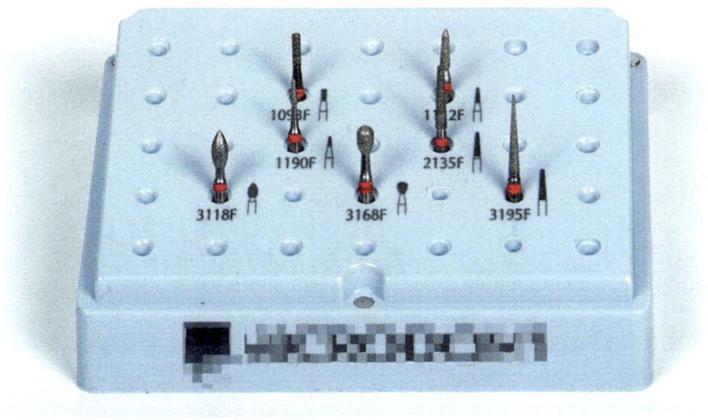

The necessary occlusal adaptation, finishing, and polishing tools can be (Fig. 1.37):

- Occlusal paper.
- Small-grained, yellow or red, oval- or flame-tapered diamond burs (Fig. 1.38).
- Multi-bladed burs (Fig. 1.39).
- Arkansas burs/stones, abrasive discs, and silicone spirals or rubber spirals (Fig. 1.40).
- Rubbers (Fig. 1.41).
- Rotary brushes for composites (Fig. 1.42).
- Polishing cotton buff wheels.
- Polishing pastes.

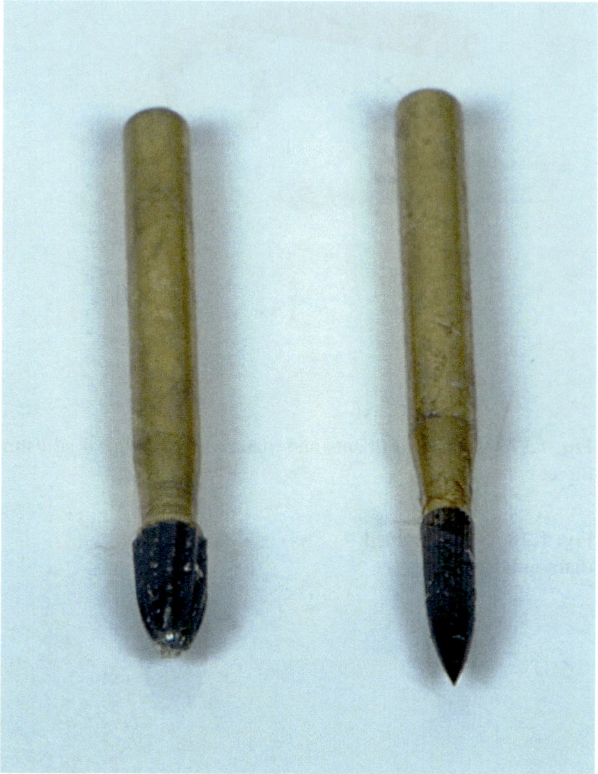

Fig. 1.39 Multi-bladed burs

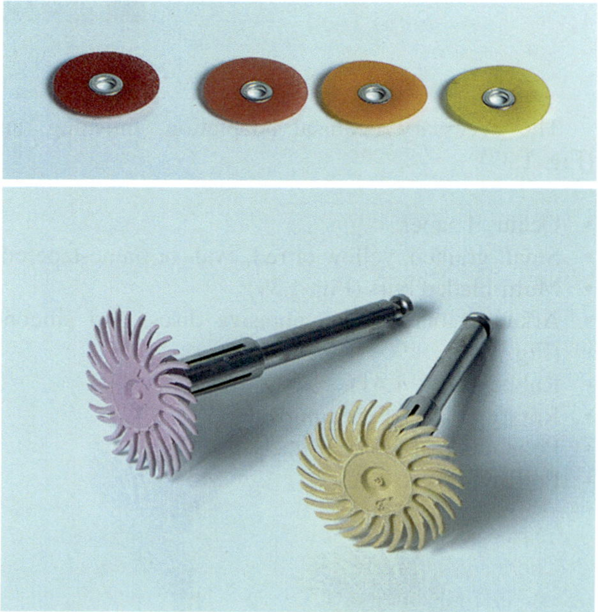

Fig. 1.40 Abrasive discs; silicone or rubber spiral wheels

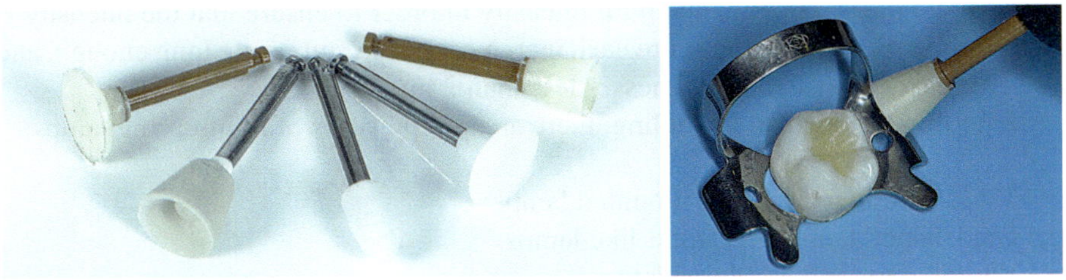

Fig. 1.41 Polishing rubber

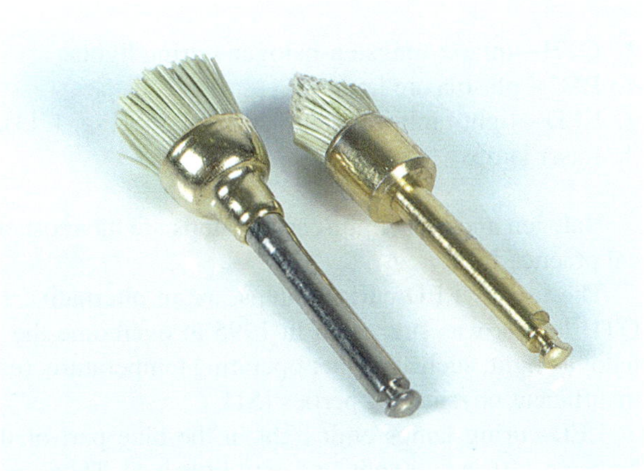

Fig. 1.42 Aluminum oxide-impregnated brushes for composite resin polishing

1.1.6 Lamps for Light-Curing Materials

1.1.6.1 Technical Characteristics

The light-curing materials allow the dentist to initiate the light-curing process voluntarily; this represents a significant advantage compared to the self-curing materials with a shorter working time, whose duration cannot be influenced by the operator.

Proper material polymerization plays an essential role in the long-term success of direct composite restorations. In the case of self-curing materials, the polymerization process is triggered by mixing the material components, and the operator can no longer influence it. In the case of light-curing materials, the polymerization technique is strongly influenced by the device used (lamp) and the operator, so the possibility of introducing errors increases.

The first generations of light-curing lamps used quartz-tungsten-halogen (QTH) bulbs as a light source, which overheated and needed a built-in fan to be cooled (their power was 400–600 mW/cm^2). Their lifetime was limited to some hours determined by the bulb's characteristics. The light emitted by this bulb gradually decreases with use, so constant measurement of the lamp output is mandatory.

There are relatively straightforward guidelines for clinicians based on three variables: the light intensity, the exposure duration, and the incremental lamination of the composite material. Thus, the dentists have been advised to constantly monitor, by periodic measurements, the light intensity in order to ensure that the intensity is above 600 mW/cm^2, to light-cure each increment of the composite long enough, and to layer the composite in thicknesses less than 2 mm [49].

In terms of design and handling, there are several types of light-curing lamps:

- Table-mounted and chair-mounted lamps.
- Gun-shaped lamps and wand-like lamps.
- Wired lamps and cordless lamps.

There are four main types of light sources that have been developed for light-curing dental materials:

1. QTH—quartz-tungsten-halogen-curing lights.
2. PAC—plasma arc lamps.
3. LED—light-emitting diode-curing light (Fig. 1.43).
4. Laser lamps.

Halogen and LED light-curing lamps are the most commonly used in daily clinical practice [50].

The use of LED-curing lamps, as an alternative to photopolymerization with QTH lamps, was suggested in 1995 to overcome the problem of quartz-tungsten-halogen light, such as higher operating temperature, reduced efficacy over time, and insufficient physical properties [51].

LED-curing lamps emit light in the blue part of the visible spectrum, usually between 440 and 490 nm, and emit little heat. They can be powered by rechargeable batteries, which require low power, and are quieter than QTH units because they do not need a cooling fan. Early versions of LED units emitted lower light intensity, while the newer versions incorporate multiple LEDs with various wavelength ranges to broaden the spectrum of light emitted and increase the overall intensity to adequately light-cure all dental materials.

The polymerization time reduction is limited by the need to keep the Vickers hardness values of the light-cured composite as high as possible [52]. A low-energy density with an increased exposure time may be more recommended than a high-power intensity at a depth of 3 mm [53].

The newer light-curing lamps have higher intensities, above 1000 mW/cm^2 up to 2000 mW/cm^2, which allow either shorter curing times or thicker composite layering. Using these higher-intensity lights may produce higher shrinkage

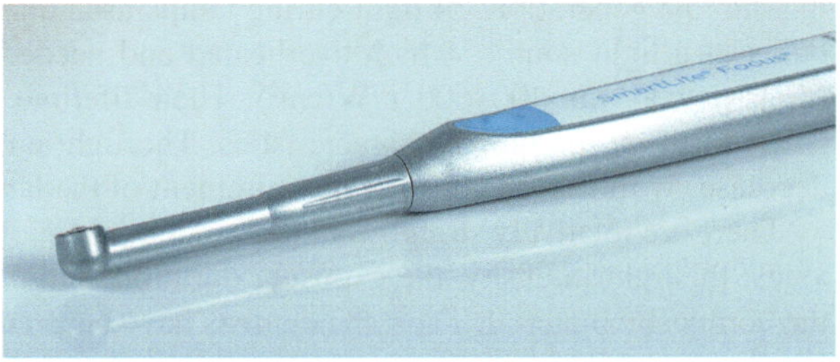

Fig. 1.43 Light-curing lamp for composite resin

stress inside the restoration, but it can also increase the temperature in the pulp chamber [54].

It is always important to consider the type of light-curing lamp and the polymerization method used to influence the light-curing kinetics, the light-curing shrinkage, and the associated stresses, composite surface micro-hardness, the depth of polymerization, the degree of monomer conversion, the color change, and the microleakage of the light-curing composite restorations.

Light-curing quality is influenced by:

- The properties of the composite material that is being light-cured.
- The technical characteristics of the curing lamp: power (minimum 600 W/cm^2), diameter of the light guide, number, type, and distribution of LEDs.
- The distance between the composite material and the tip of the light guide which the light is emitted from the light-curing lamp.
- The positioning of the light beam (angle, access to the desired surface).
- The type of light emission pattern (e.g., continuous, pulsed, and in increasing steps).
- The existence of possible obstacles that prevent the light from reaching the desired surface and depth (metal matrices, wedges, matrix rings, etc.)

Most light-curing problems occur in the deep cavity and gingival margin areas and are associated with pulp disease and marginal secondary caries. Possible explanations for incomplete composite polymerization at the gingival margin could be the following:

- The long distance between the light guide tip and the material. The removal of the light guide tip at about 3–6 mm away from the surface to be light-cured can decrease the power of a lamp up to 50% [55] and can cause the light-curing incompletion of the composite.
- Presence of metal matrices and wedges that may prevent the light beam from reaching into the entire composite mass.
- Difficult access of the lamp tip to the posterior area. Access is facilitated by the straight direction of the lamp with the side opening of the light guide (Fig. 1.44).
- Operator's inattentiveness in positioning and directing the light beam emitted at the tip of the light guide.
- Light-curing lamp technical problems (e.g., insufficient power, too small diameter of the light guide).
- Improper application of the working protocol: decrease recommended light-curing time and saliva contamination before or during light-curing.

The stress caused by the light-curing contraction may exceed the adhesion strength between the composite and the tooth structures, leading to adhesion defects [56], more precisely to gaps between the composite and the tooth [57]. These adhesion defects can generate two categories of problems:

1. Bacterial microleakage [58].

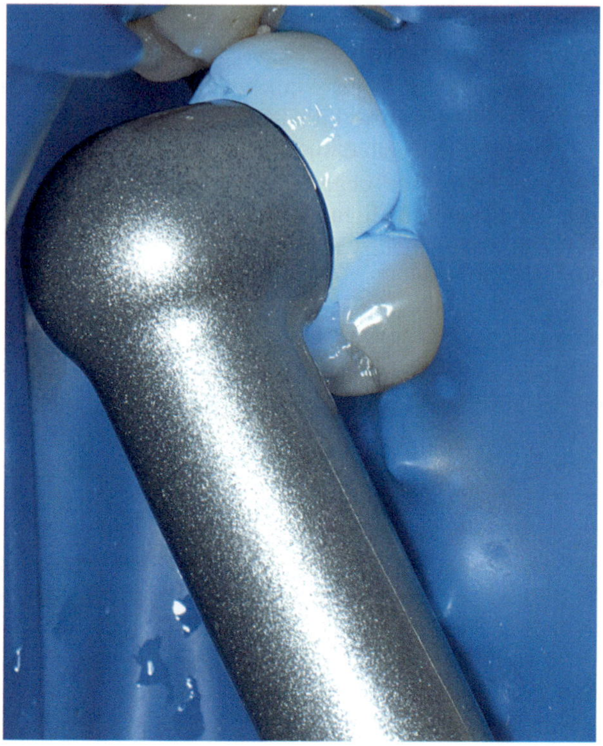

Fig. 1.44 The light-curing lamp has a lateral light emission for easy access to posterior teeth

2. Damage to mechanical strength through micro-cracks or cracks in enamel and cusp bending [59].

The bacterial microleakage may be one of the causes of postoperative sensitivity. This may disappear in the first few weeks [60], or it may persist for a longer time leading to pulp inflammation and restoration failure [61].

Insufficiently light-cured composite monomers can lead to more permeable void areas (in the material) that allow bacterial infiltration and, subsequently, generate pulp inflammation.

1.1.6.2 Temperature Developed at the Pulp Level

Many current clinical procedures can cause an increase in pulp temperature, with the subsequent development of symptoms such as hyperemia, dentinal hypersensitivity, and characteristic spontaneous pain of acute pulpitis due to pulp heating and sequential trauma [62, 63]. The amount of heat that is transferred to the dental pulp during a composite light-curing procedure is dependent [64, 65] on:

- The type of light-curing lamp (halogen/LED).
- The lamp power density (mW/cm^2).
- The light-curing scheme (continuous, pulsed, increasing).

- The distance between the pulp and light guide tip.
- The composite nuance.
- The thickness of the composite layer applied to the base of the cavity.
- The thickness of the remaining dentine on the cavity base.

Studies indicate an increase in temperature at the pulp chamber level of 1.5 °C up to 23.2 °C, probably depending on the specific experimental settings of the study [66], but other studies have found values of up to 3.2° [67]. In addition to the heat produced by the lamp at the pulp level, heat from the exothermic reaction of composite materials during light-curing is added.

However, the energy density generated by the lamp plays the most critical role in increasing the intra-pulpal temperature, as opposed to the heat generated by the exothermic reaction of the composite. This is because the composite resin layers added to a restoration act as insulators rather than heat generators.

In 1965, Zach and Cohen demonstrated in an animal model that a temperature increase of 5.5 °C in the healthy pulp induced necrosis in about 15% of teeth. When the intra-pulpal temperature was maintained with 11.1 °C higher for 10 s, approximately 60% to 70% of the teeth developed irreversible pulpitis [68]. Pohto and Scheinin showed that the critical temperature for irreversible dental pulp damage starts between 42 and 42.5 °C [69], so the increases are similar. Although the actual value of the critical temperature rise that causes the pulp damage is still controversial, the heat produced by different types of lamps is debatable. It can be assumed that the increase in pulp temperature during light-curing of the composites above the threshold of 5.5 °C should be kept away to avoid any risk of pulp inflammation.

Methods of lowering the temperature transmitted to the pulp during light-curing of materials:

- Shortening light-curing sessions.
- Blowing the cavity with a gentle air jet during light-curing.

The optimum light-curing process of each material is achieved when the manufacturers' guidelines for composite material are followed precisely and also when the light-curing lamp usage instructions, regarding the use in conditions of isolation and the correct application of the adhesive system, are taken into account.

The light-curing errors can lead to compromised restorative treatment. Thus, choosing a good-quality lamp and its use according to correct working protocols contributes to restoration success.

Conclusion

The light-curing lamp represents a critical piece of equipment because improper curing can compromise the results of a treatment performed with the best composite materials and working techniques. It is the responsibility of each practitioner to ensure that the safety instructions of the used lamp are respected: the power generated, the time of action, the heat developed and transmitted to the tooth, etc.

Review Questions

1. What factors can influence the quality of the lamp polymerization?
2. On what does the amount of heat transferred to the dental pulp during a composite polymerization procedure depend?

1.1.7 Video and Photographic Documentation of Cases

More and more dentists include photographs in their working protocols regardless of the specialty they practice. Taking photographs is essential for communicating with patients but also with other colleagues. It allows the documentation of the performed cases or can be used for other purposes (social media or marketing, teaching, educational purposes). The professionalism of photographs taken must correspond with the purpose for which they were taken, and it can reach the level of art depending on the talent and passion of each doctor. The minimum level of recording and archiving is very easy to achieve, and efficient communication with the patient can be achieved by any practitioner.

Dental photography allows patients to visualize their smile and the status of each tooth from the same perspective as the doctor. This helps the patient better understand the rationale for the recommended restorative treatment [70]. The imperfections not readily visible to the patient in a mirror will be noticeable in photographs. The patient may be more motivated to replace the old, inadequate fillings that he or she can observe more clearly in photographs or treat asymptomatic carious lesions.

The following summary includes minimal information about the necessary equipment, accessories, and a simple protocol for taking photos. This chapter does not aim to exhaustively cover the subject of dental photography, which currently contains an abundance of high-quality literature for dental photography enthusiasts.

Before taking photographs, obtaining written consent for photography and ensuring that all measures are taken to protect the patient's confidentiality is essential. These are, moreover, also mandatory legal measures according to the national (Law no. 202/1998, republished as amended, Law no. 190/2018) and European (Regulation 2016/679/EU, Directive 2016/680/EU, Directive 2002/58/EC) legislation in force. The consent for taking photographs can be easily added as part of the patient documents that are filled in at the first visit when the patient comes to the dental practice.

1.1.7.1 Smartphone Photography

For intraoral and extraoral photography, unique cameras are recommended, as not all dental practices own a DSLR camera. Many dentists use their mobile phones to take dental photos. Mobile phones now use advanced technology, with high-resolution, high-megapixel cameras. It could be said that nothing beats the convenience of a smartphone camera. Chances are a phone is already handy, so it is easy to find and take a quick photo in the office anytime. Moreover, there already exist easy-to-use

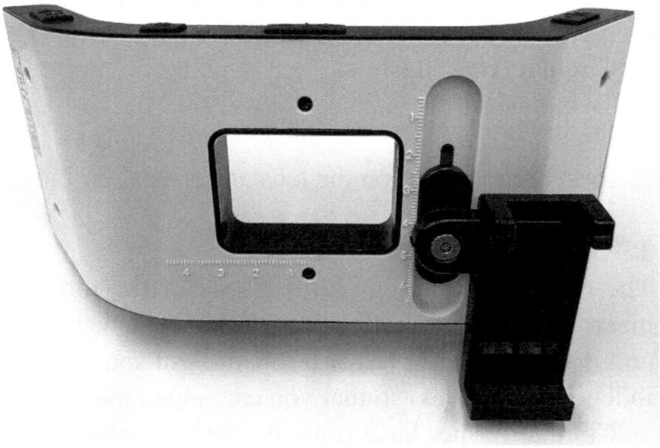

Fig. 1.45 Mobile phone flash for dental photography

accessories that help doctors install special lenses and flashes on their phones to get good-quality dental photos (*SmileLite MDP, Styleitaliano*) [71] (Fig. 1.45).

Features of dental photography with smartphones:

- Small aperture due to small size and diaphragm, regularly achieving a wide field of view.
- Good ISO setting, higher light sensitivity with less noise.
- Good resolution when it comes to displaying details.
- Wide monitor for previewing and viewing images.
- White balance, magnification, focus, ISO, metering, and shutter speed are requirements for taking pictures that the latest generation phones meet.

1.1.7.2 Photo Equipment Required

Choosing the most suitable equipment for extraoral and intraoral photography requires some knowledge about digital photography, and this thing can lead to confusion for doctors because there is a wide variety of cameras available on the market. The camera and lens hardware play an essential role in obtaining good-quality photographs, but knowing color and light in photography is crucial. Investing in a DSLR camera will result in significantly better image quality than a smartphone; however, many variables are at play.

The DSLR camera is the best option for taking predictable dental photographs [72]. The DSLR camera should be equipped with a macro lens (85–105 mm) and an on-camera external flash for high-quality intraoral macro photography.

1.1.7.3 Camera Lens

The most commonly used macro lenses for dental photography are those between 60 and 105 mm (60, 70, 85, 90, 100, and 105 mm).

1.1.7.4 Flash

Two types of flashes can be used for dental photography:

- Circular (ring) flash.
- Twin flash.

Both are mounted on the lens and have their indications.

1.1.7.5 Circular Flash (Ring)

The circular flash (Fig. 1.46) is one of the most common lighting solutions for macro dental photography because it offers the best price/performance combination and is easy to use. It has two sets of light sources (the light ring is divided into two independent halves) so that you can adjust the power of each half individually.

Circular flashes have some limitations, which can be explained as follows:

- They produce a circular capture light. Although this is a good aspect, in the case of glossy surfaces, especially at the front teeth, shiny areas could appear, which mask surface details.
- They are not recommended for color transfer.
- They require a lens adapter ring.

This flash provides good illumination and is relatively inexpensive and easy to purchase; it is an ideal solution for dental photography, even for beginners.

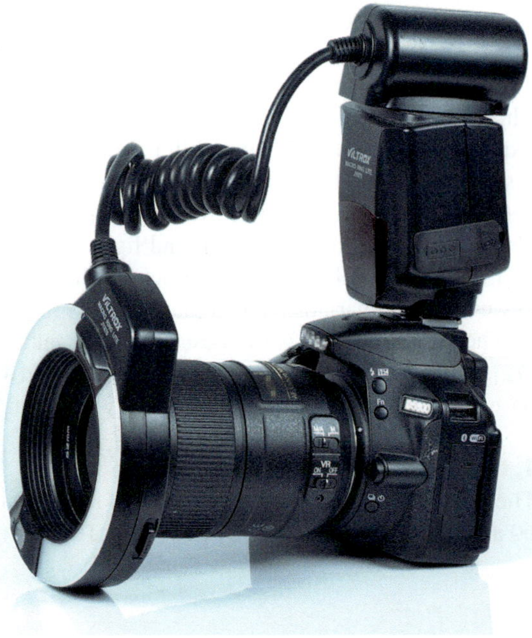

Fig. 1.46 Circular flash attached to a DSLR camera

1.1.7.6 Dual Flash, Twin Flash

Controlling the light and shade is the easiest way to show tooth texture; this is recommended especially for front teeth or portrait photos. Using a dual flash provides an easy way to position the direction of the two flashes' light and set their power individually. The best results are achieved when it is used with appropriate diffusers to achieve good light quality.

The double flash is one of the flash types designed for macro photography. The main difference between a ring flash and a double flash is the flexibility in positioning the flash heads. The ring flash has flash tubes permanently embedded in a ring, which is attached to the lens. The dual flashes are constructed differently: they have two flash heads mounted on a separate ring or each arm (Fig. 1.47).

The most significant disadvantage of a dual-flash solution is the price and that it requires perhaps more skills.

1.1.7.7 Minimum Required Accessories

The lip retractor contributes significantly to the final result of intraoral photography. These essential accessories are used to retract the lips, labial, and buccal mucosa to expose the dental arches and help light penetrate the oral cavity. They can be made of plastic or metal, unilateral, bilateral, or circular (Fig. 1.48). The bilateral double-headed retractors have two variants: a slight curvature or a large curvature. This shape allows the adaptability to a variety of mouth sizes. The transparent plastic retractors are less visible in the photo; their complete removal from the image is sometimes impossible when taking a photo.

The intraoral mirrors are essential when taking occlusal and buccal photos because the photographic angle does not usually permit capturing these photos from a direct view. Intraoral mirrors are available, and a standard set should include buccal and occlusal mirrors. Mirrors can be made of glass or metal, with or without a

Fig. 1.47 Twin flash

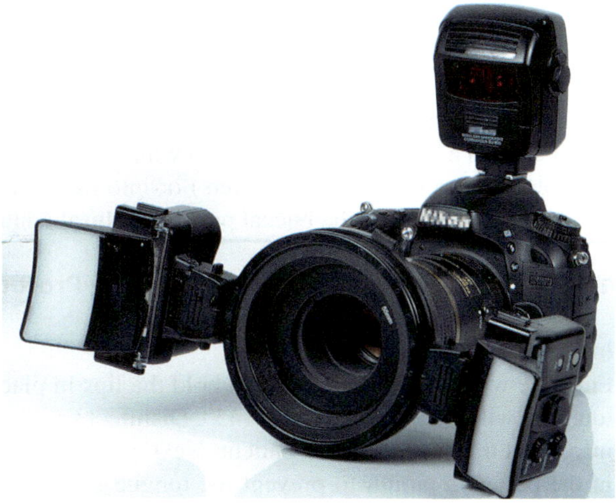

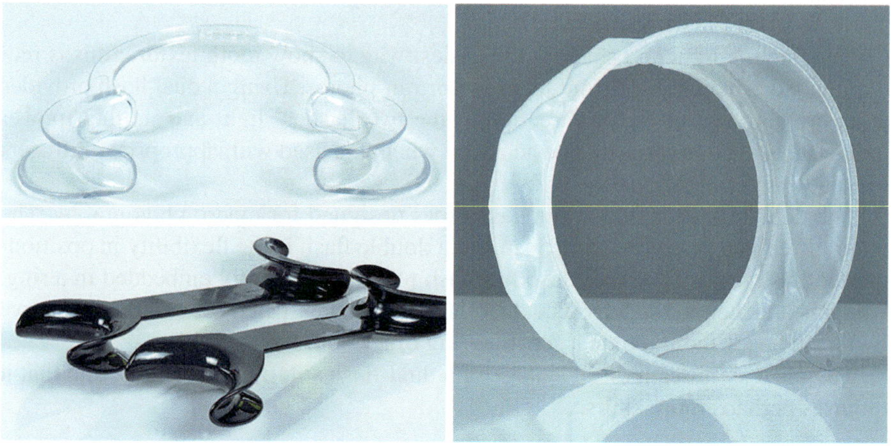

Fig. 1.48 Different types of lip retractors for intraoral photography

Fig. 1.49 Intraoral photography mirrors

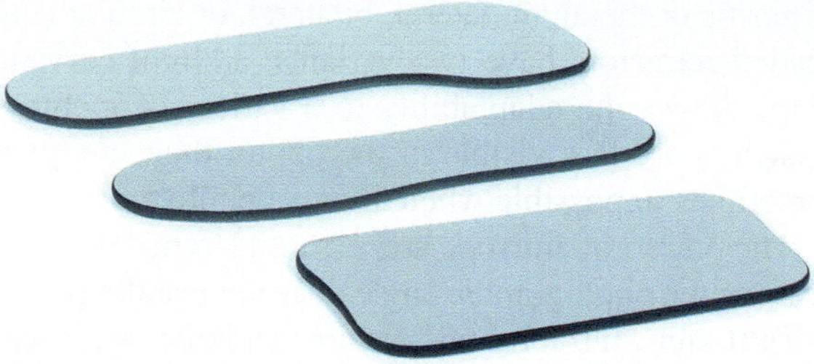

handle, in one plane or angled, and in several sizes for both occlusal and buccal photographs (Fig. 1.49). To prevent the mirror from fogging during intraoral photography, heat it or blow air on it. Pack the reflective surfaces separately, and do not mix them with other instruments to protect them from potential damage.

Dental photo contrasters are designed to give a better image of the teeth by covering the soft parts and oral mucosa. The contrasters are placed behind the teeth so that it creates a black background onto which the teeth will be projected in the photographic image (anterior contrasters) or into the vestibule, removing the lips and covering the bottom of the buccal pouch (occlusal contrasters) (Fig. 1.50).

1.1.7.8 Potential Mobile Phone Shooting Protocol

Intraoral Photography

First, we will need lip retractors to hold the lips in place and not appear in the picture. We will place them at about 45°. Disinfect the mobile phone to avoid possible infections transmitted to the patient. Next, place a straight contraster with a handle in the patient's mouth to prevent the tongue from interfering with the image and

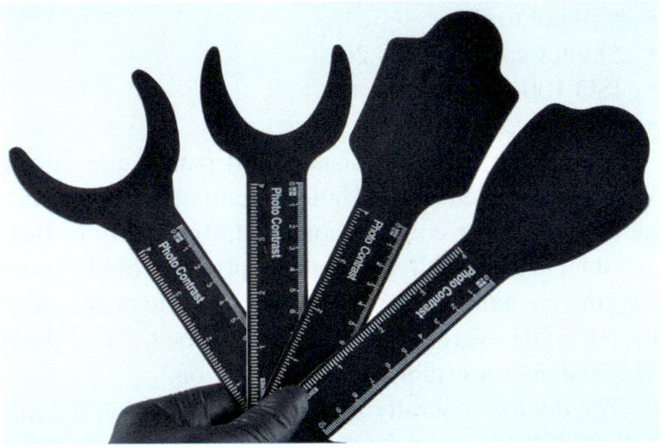

Fig. 1.50 Black metal contrasters for dental photography

creating contrast. This opaque contractor will also be used as a support to hold the smartphone, placing it at 45°.

As for lighting, use the lamp light that is built into the dental chair. It is not recommended for the light to be cast directly onto the teeth; rather, it should be diffused to reduce the intensity. One way to achieve this is to cover the light source with a textile, a sheet of paper, or a white bag, which is used as a light diffuser; when considering LED lamps that do not heat the material, space must be left between the lamp and the cover and the material should be placed in the shape of a bag. Place the lamp over the patient at about 90° to get a better image of the texture.

If the dental chair lamp is not chosen to take photos, another option is a specially designed flash for mobile phones (e.g., SmileLite MDP, Styleitaliano). Take the photos from the standard set.

Extraoral Photos

The extraoral photographs are taken as portraits. The patient needs to have a completely natural smile. The nose has to be in the center of the picture. There should be no shadows on the wall where the photo is taken, and the background should be white or black. Place the mobile phone at the patient's eye level and take the picture.

Potential Protocol for DSLR Camera Photography

Some recommendations for intraoral photography can be adjusted to the clinician's preference when the clinician already has minimal photography experience.

Set the camera to "manual" mode, and then make the proper settings depending on the DSLR camera used.

Possible settings for taking extraoral photos:

- f/8–10,
- Shutter speed 1/125–200.
- ISO 100–200.
- Magnification 1:10.

Possible settings for taking intraoral photos:

- f/20–22 to f32,
- Shutter speed 1/125–200.
- ISO 100--200.
- Magnification 1:2 or 1:3.

The doctor, dental assistant, and patient are all involved in taking the photos. Ideally, the patient should hold the unilateral retractors with his or her hands because he/she has better comfort control during traction. Before taking a photograph, the assistant will dry all the teeth involved, provide suction, and control the mirror's fogging by gently blowing the air spray over the mirror (mirrors can also be pre-heated). The mirror and contraster can be held by the patient or the dental assistant after the doctor establishes their position.

The doctor generally takes the photographs: the intraoral photos, those with the patient lying down in the dental unit, and the extraoral photos with the patient sitting in a standard chair with a uniform white or black background. A possible set of basic intraoral and extraoral photographs could be portrait (extraoral), smile, anterior, right buccal, left buccal, maxillary occlusal, and mandibular occlusal. The doctor's and patient's position in taking the photo is unique for each photo (Fig. 1.51).

Because of the tongue, taking an occlusal photograph of the mandibular arch is one of the most challenging photos to take. In most cases, the tongue can be retracted by placing the occlusal mirror under it, followed by positioning the mirror's edge distally to the second molar. As with all mirror images, it must be carefully ensured that the photograph includes only the mirror image of the teeth. In many cases, visibility can be increased if the patient tilts the chin slightly upward.

In the case of photo/video documentation, using a built-in camera or a camera attached to a dental microscope operator requires some details to be paid attention to, due to the magnification of the operating field. Thus, as the magnification steps increase, the image of the operating field becomes increasingly narrower and less illuminated. In order to maintain maximum illumination, it is possible to change some DSLR camera settings (e.g., ISO) or to increase the brightness of the microscope's variometer.

Conclusion

Taking dental photos has become increasingly affordable, with accessories available for both classic DSLR cameras and mobile phones. Their shooting protocol ranges from a minimal one allowing communication with the patient, other dentists, or dental technicians to a professional one, suitable for marketing, art, and educational purposes satisfying the demands of the photo enthusiasts. Depending on the clinical case, the minimum protocol includes only intraoral and extraoral photographs. The use of specific accessories (mirrors, viewfinders, lights, etc.), a working protocol, and the device setting are directly related to obtaining good-quality images (framing, visibility, brightness, color, contrast).

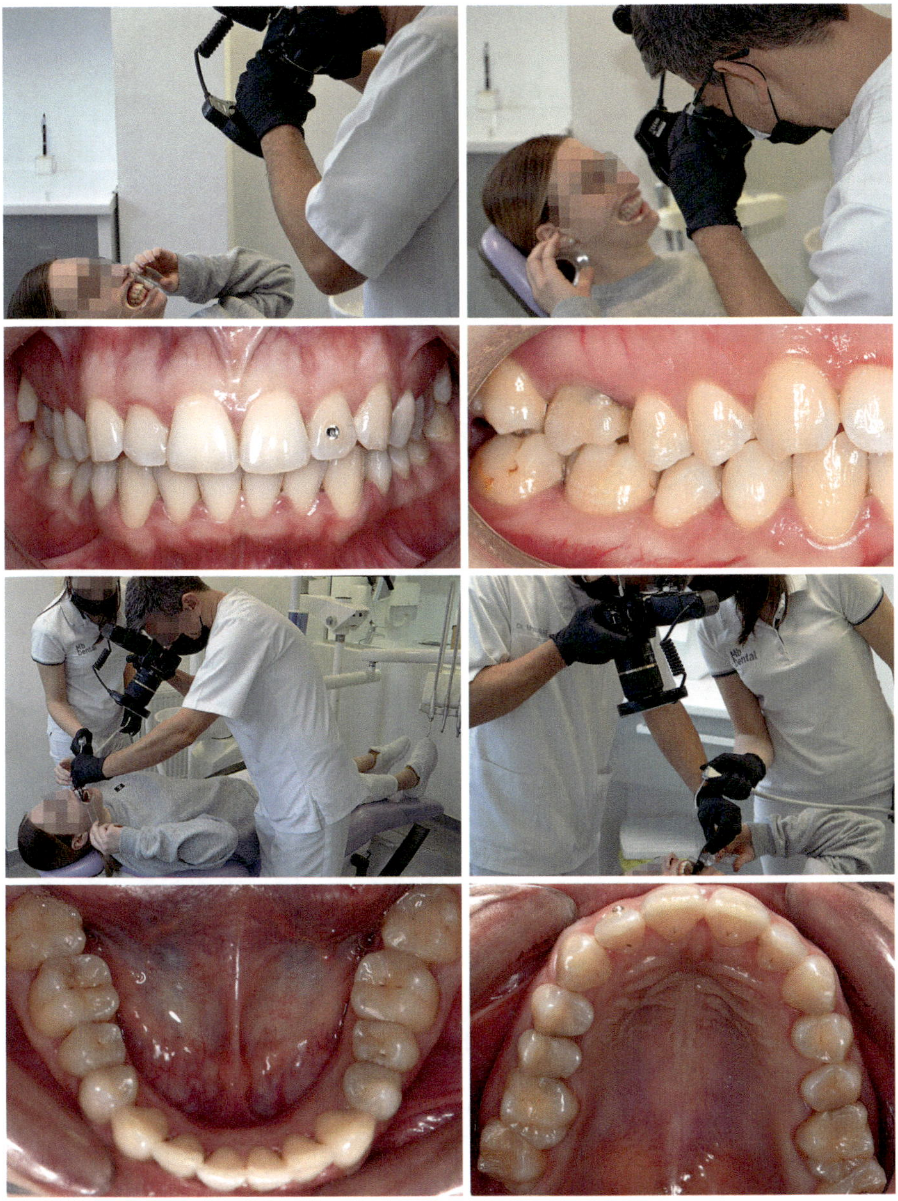

Fig. 1.51 Minimal set of photographs and the dentist's positioning

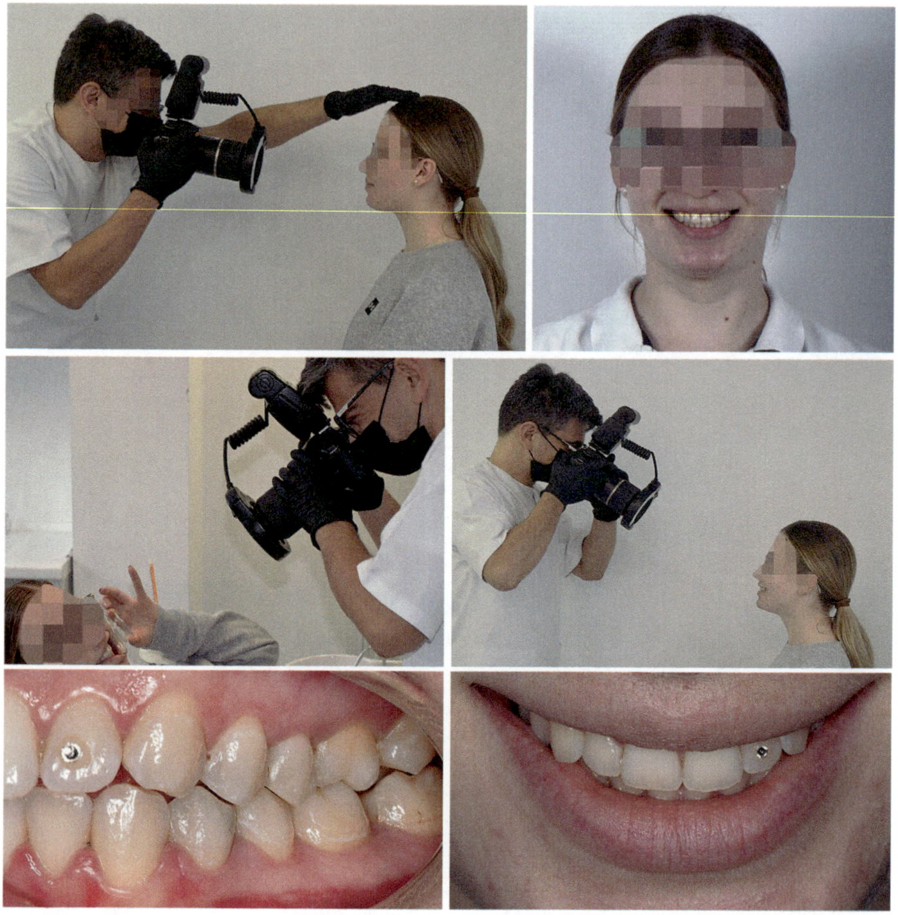

Fig. 1.51 (continued)

Review Questions

1. What are the main types of flashes that can be used for dental photography, and what are their characteristics?
2. What is a possible protocol for taking photographs with DSLR cameras?
3. What are the settings of a DSLR camera?

1.2 Dental Materials

1.2.1 Cavity Disinfection

After the cavity preparation is complete, the cavity is cleaned most commonly with water/air jet flushing to remove any remaining dentinal debris. The disinfection of the cavity is an essential step aimed at removing the remaining bacteria and decreasing the related postoperative sensitivity. The solutions commonly indicated for this purpose are chlorhexidine (CHX) or sodium hypochlorite in low concentrations. CHX can be applied into the cavity on cotton wool pellets, using a microbrush applicator or directly from a syringe.

1.2.2 Materials for Pulp Protection

Branstrom's hydrodynamic theory explains postoperative sensitivity after restorative treatments by changing the osmotic pressure in the dentinal tubules following cavity preparation and application of restorative materials [73]. This theory still stands today, although the author demonstrated a few years later that it is not the restorative materials that cause pulp inflammation but in fact the bacterial microleakage following restoration [74].

Recent studies claim that the remaining bacteria or the bacterial microleakage and their exotoxins cause postoperative sensitivity [75]. The microleakage between the restorative material and the tooth is mainly caused by adhesion defects correlated with light-curing shrinkage, allowing an influx of bacteria from the oral cavity. Thus, marginal pigmentation, postoperative sensitivity, inflammation, and pulp necrosis may occur in this area [76].

The heat transfer from the polymerization lamp to the light-curing materials placed in the vicinity of the pulp chamber (see Sect. 1.1.6), enhanced by their exothermic reaction, may be factors that lead to pulp damage.

In addition to these possible causes of dental damage, the toxicity of the remaining unpolymerized monomers in acrylic resins must also be considered, as the degree of conversion by light-curing is never complete, being around 70–80% [77] and varying from one composite to another. The unpolymerized monomers may have a possible toxic effect on the pulp and may reduce the clinical longevity of composite dental fillings and color stability. The remaining unpolymerized monomers are not the only compounds with a toxic potential—in the long term, the degradation of the composite materials may also produce harmful compounds [78].

The protection offered to the dental pulp by different materials can be passive (chemical, thermal, mechanical, electrical) or active (anti-inflammatory, disinfectant, neo-denitrifying) [79]. The recommended materials, such as liners and bases, largely overlap.

Conclusion

Considering the reliability of all the results of the published studies on pulp damage related to direct restorations, we can conclude that inflammation or necrosis of the dental pulp can be caused individually or by the accumulation of several factors, among which we mention:

- Bacterial infiltration consequent to restorations with inadequate seal (marginal sealing).
- Chemical effect of residual monomers following incomplete light-curing.
- Thermal effect of pulp overheating during light-curing of composite materials.

1.2.3 Bases and Liners

Bases and liners are two concepts whose roles and recommendations have been the subject of much debate in dentistry. Published studies are frequently contradictory in terms of their definition, protocol, and necessity [80].

The term "liner" is used to denote a material applied as a thin layer of maximum 0.5 mm thickness, according to some authors [81], or a maximum 1 mm thickness, according to others [82], in order to achieve clinical benefits related to pulp protection: fluoride release, antibacterial effect, and dentin sealing.

Currently, it is considered that there is insufficient evidence to prove a significant difference between the postoperative sensitivity [83, 84] and the longevity [85] of restorations placed with or without a liner on the cavity base.

The term "base" is used to name a material, typically cement, applied in a layer thicker than 1 mm to the base of the cavity. In 1985, a *base* was defined as an isolating material placed in certain dentin areas of a prepared cavity. Ten years later, in 1994, one of the fathers of modern restorative dentistry, James B. Summitt, defined the bases as dentin replacement materials. These can be used for mass replacement of the dentin structure to reduce the composite mass required for restoration, thus decreasing the overall light-curing shrinkage coefficient or developing undercut areas for indirect restorations [86]. However, their role in compensating or absorbing the overlying composites' polymerization stress remains questionable, with many studies showing that no such role exists [87].

This perspective regarding bases was quickly adopted, and it is still supported by many authors [88–90] and many dental schools worldwide. Some authors state that the primary differentiation criterion between the liner and the base is the thickness of the material layer, stipulating that the designation of the pulp protection layer depends on its thickness: liner (0.2–1 mm) and base (over 1 mm) [79].

The use of base materials based on classical types of cement placed under composite fillings can be seen as a continuation of the working protocols used for amalgam. Their use in combination with the composite materials has been shown to bring disadvantages in terms of:

- Poor adaptation of restorations to the internal cavity walls [91, 92].
- Increased risk of material fracture [93].

The "sandwich" restorations with CIS were the preferred way to achieve adhesion between dentin and composite resin during a time when dentin adhesives were still of inferior quality. Adhesives' later development led to a decrease in the frequency of use and even the disappearance of the sandwich technique [94]. The application of this kind of layer was considered favorable for compensating polymerization stress [95], but this concept of an elastic layer has been contested [96, 97]. The increased failure rate of restorations with a base made from a glass ionomer cement has been attributed to higher fatigue, correlating with the less mechanically resistant cement layer.

So, although there is no sufficient evidence to recommend using a conventional cement base under composite fillings, the surveys conducted among dental faculties or dentists from different countries show conflicting results. They show that there is no standard regarding liner and base application, which is directly related to the lack of consensus in the academic field. Analyzing the protocols taught in 33 dental schools in Germany, Austria, and Switzerland, Kanzow et al. [98] showed that none of the protocols indicated the use of liners in the posterior middle cavities or shallow posterior cavities. In the deep cavity case, 58% of these higher-educational institutions recommend using liners, but the rest do not.

Lynch et al. [99] also found a lack of a unified vision by analyzing the university protocols in the UK and Ireland and found that in 3 out of 18 faculties, the students are taught not to use liners even in deep cavities. Two-thirds recommend using a base made of a glass ionomer cement, even in medium cavities, while one-third of faculties indicate neither liner nor base. Dentists commonly follow the protocols learned in dental schools in clinical practice, so the responsibility for medically correct and scientifically valid protocols lies within each educational institution.

Conclusion

We can conclude that both bases and liners have been introduced into restorative protocols to protect the pulp from a possible harmful effect of the final restorative materials and decrease postoperative sensitivity [100].

Over time, the view on bases has shifted toward reducing the composite mass required for restoration, thus lowering the overall light-curing shrinkage coefficient of the composite resins used for long-term restoration and for relining retentive areas in indirect restorative preparations and less to provide pulp protection (Summitt's, McCoy).

Today, the concept of the base is becoming less and less used with the emergence of bulk composites, which are dentin substitutes. Summarizing the information presented above and considering that the composite resins are poor thermal conductors, we claim that the application of a cement base under composite resin restorations is limited to the cases where a self-curing liner, such as calcium hydroxide [101] or classical MTA (where a composite resin adhesion cannot adhere), has been applied over.

We believe we can use another composite material, such as the dentin composite used in the bilaminar technique or a bulk composite, as a base after the liner application for filling a deep cavity.

The most commonly used materials as liners are based on calcium hydroxide, glass ionomer cement, bioceramics (MTA, Biodentine), and compomers.

1. Calcium hydroxide

   The self-polymerizing calcium hydroxide variants for pulp protection (Fig. 1.52a) (e.g., Kerr Life, Calcimol, Hydrocal) are biocompatible, they have antibacterial properties, and they stimulate the formation of new dentin [102], but they have poor physical properties [103], being soluble and having poor adhesion to dentin. Their application is indicated in the smallest possible areas,

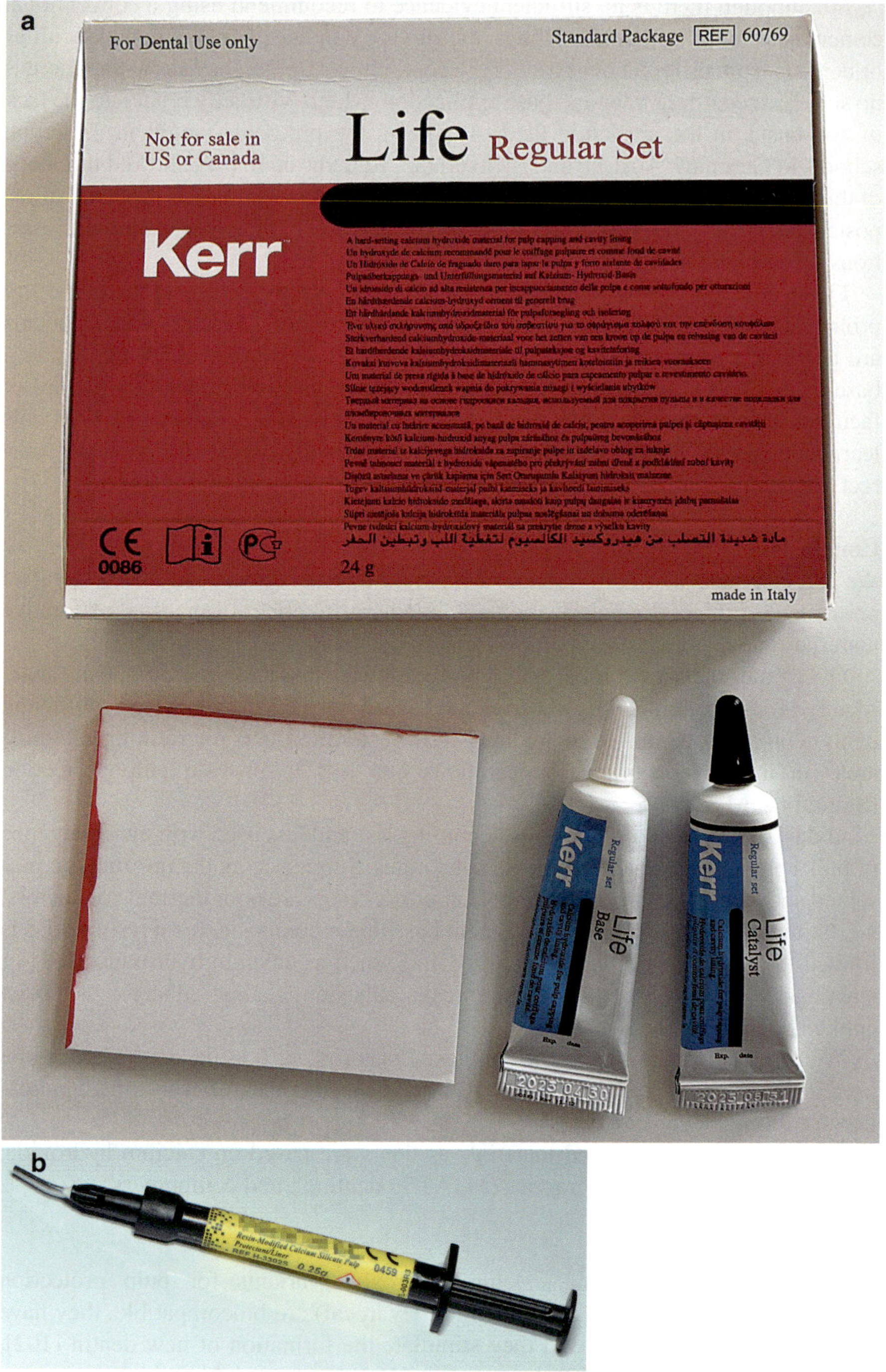

Fig. 1.52 Self-curing calcium hydroxide cement (**a**) and light-curing cement

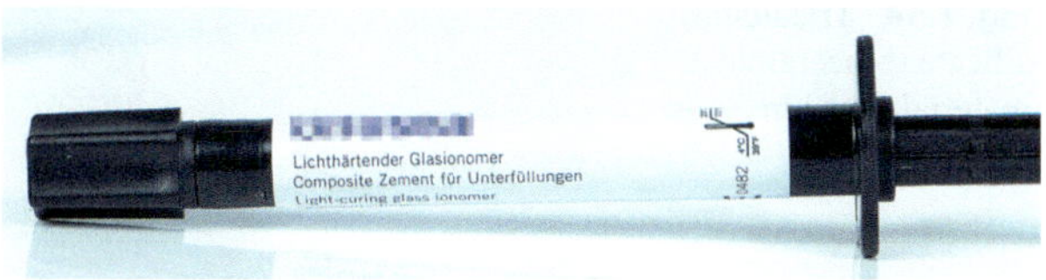

Fig. 1.53 Light-curing glass ionomer liner cement

where an imminent approach to the pulp chamber is anticipated [104]. The surface extension of the calcium hydroxide layer has no benefit for the pulp; on the contrary, it decreases the dentin surface area available for adhesion for restoration. The light-curing variants (Fig. 1.52b) that have subsequently appeared have improved these aspects (e.g., TheraCal LC, Septocal LC, Calciplus LC, Ultra-Blend plus, etc.);

2. Glass ionomer cement (GIc)

   GIc adheres well to dentin, removes fluoride, and has good physical properties in both self-curing and light-curing versions (Fig. 1.53). Resin-modified glass ionomer cement (RMGIc) is recommended for direct restoration cases when the composite is placed directly over the liner, having better mechanical strength and adhesion to dentin [105].

   Both materials in the light-curing version raise the problem of increasing the temperature of the dental pulp during their light-curing (see Sect. 1.1.6). The temperature developed during polymerization can be lowered by blowing air gently after the first few seconds when polymerization has already started in the material and when there is no risk of it being dislodged by the air jet.

   Most manufacturers indicate in their material leaflets that, like self-curing GIc materials, RMGIc is also applied after conditioning the dentin with a 10–25% polyacrylic acid.. Some published studies have shown that preconditioning with 37% orthophosphoric acid of the dentin for 10–15 s can improve the adhesion of RMGIc to dentin [106]. Furthermore, the additional use of an adhesive system may increase the adhesion by forming a hybrid layer [107] on both dentin and enamel [108, 109], but there is strong evidence that fluoride release is strongly affected in this case [110, 111]. The increasing adhesion and the decreasing microleakage provide more significant benefits than fluoride release per se [112].

3. Tricalcium silicate-based materials, also called bioceramics, have been introduced more recently in dentistry and were first used in endodontics [113]. However, as indicated by manufacturers, they have also been proven to be as effective as the liner/base materials for direct [114] and indirect capping. The most popular is MTA (mineral trioxide aggregate) which, besides its endodontic use, can be used as a liner, base, material for direct/indirect capping, and pulpotomies, according to the instructions provided by the manufacturers (e.g., MTA Plus, Prevest Denpro). It can be in powder form mixed with liquid or premixed in a syringe (Fig. 1.54a, b).

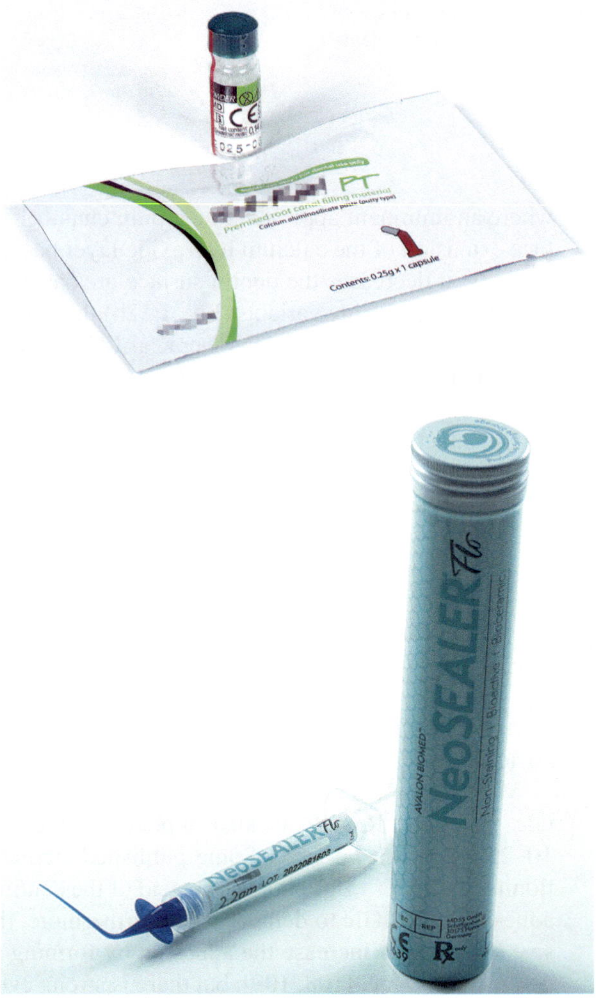

Fig. 1.54 Tricalcium silicate (bioceramics) materials used in endodontics

One of the most versatile bioceramic materials based on tricalcium silicates is biodentine (Biodentine—Septodont, France). It is indicated according to the manufacturers to be used for:

- Temporary enamel restoration.
- Permanent dentin restoration.
- Deep or extensive carious lesions.
- Deep root or cervical lesions.
- Direct tooth capping.
- Pulpotomy.
- Treatment of root perforations (furcation area).
- Internal/external resorptions.
- Apexifications and retrograde obturations.

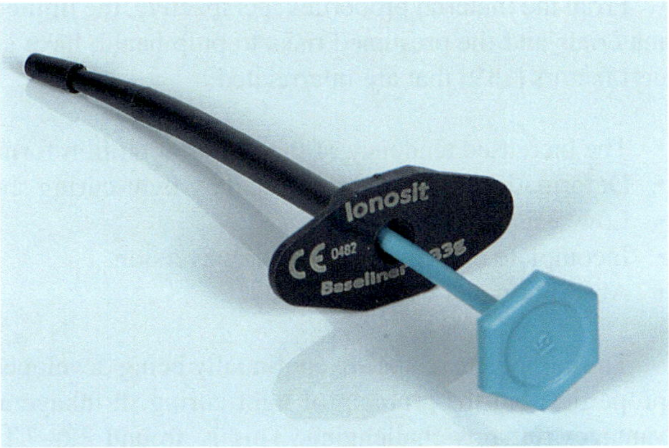

Fig. 1.55 Light-curing compomer liner: Ionosit

4. The compomers are materials with intermediate properties between a glass ionomer cement and a composite resin, which can also be indicated as liners/bases in deep cavities (e.g., Ionosite, DMG) (Fig. 1.55).

   The studies published until now have shown that for the long-term success of direct restorations, the type of liner used is not as important as the existence of proper circumferential adhesion of the filling, in order to prevent bacterial microleakage [115].

Conclusion
Due to improved properties and ease of working, the current trend is to use light-cured or premixed liners, mostly in deep cavities, as indicated by most composite manufacturers.

The pulp protection protocols vary by school and country, ranging from the most cautious to total contraindication [116].

1.2.4 Materials for Long-Term Restorations

1.2.4.1 Composite Resins

The composite resins are complex, tooth-colored filling materials that offer excellent aesthetic potential and good longevity without the need for aggressive and complicated preparation of dental cavities. They allow minimally invasive preparation, or they can sometimes even be applied without prior preparation.

The limited longevity of the direct composite material restorations due to fracture/fissuring in the material/marginal volume and secondary caries and the possible risks to pulp health are critical challenges these materials face. The failure rate of direct composite material restorations reported by studies ranges from 3% to 11% [117, 118]. Therefore, resin-based composite materials have been the subject of much clinical and basic academic research.

From the material properties' perspective, the limited longevity of the composite materials and the presumed risks to pulp health have generally been linked to several factors [119] that are interrelated:

- The increased tendency of the bacterial biofilm formation on their surface.
- Deformation and stress generated by light-curing shrinkage.
- Low resistance to fracture.
- Incomplete degree of monomer conversion.
- Absorption and water solubility.

The composite resins are continually being developed with constantly improving properties, but the problem of light-curing shrinkage associated with many disadvantages remains challenging. This is around 2.6–7.1% [120]. Thus, it has been suggested by various authors that these materials should be limited to small cavities to increase their clinical success [121]. The polymerization shrinkage can lead to marginal void formation and microleakage, debonding the restoration/tooth interface, cusp deformation, and microfractures of tooth structures [122].

1.2.4.2 Classification

Restoration materials can be exclusively diacrylic-based composite resins, or they can be hybrid materials. Most composites are methacrylate-based, but other types (ceromers, ormocers, siloranes) are also available. It is claimed that each has to offer some advantages over the methacrylate systems, but it is not yet clear whether these improvements make a significant difference in their clinical performance. However, the performance of each material must be individually assessed, and they cannot be extrapolated to other categories. We know that for the average clinician, the issues of classification and chemical structure differentiation are not always of interest, but an overview is helpful to make the right decisions for use. The main chemical properties and indications of different material classes are perishable information constantly changing as new materials with improved characteristics are brought to the market.

Some classifications consider the viscosity of materials, polymerization mode, particle size, type of organic matrix, polymerization shrinkage values, etc.

Traditionally, dental composites are classified according to filler particle size into microfilled, microhybrid filled, nanofilled, and nanohybrid composites. In general, large particle-size fillers provide increased mechanical strength, and they reduce polymerization shrinkage. On the other hand, the smaller particles are more favorable for achieving superior aesthetics and polish, plus more excellent wear resistance. The homogeneous dispersion and the complete resin wetting of nano-sized filler particles improve nano-based composites' aesthetic and mechanical properties.

When considering the benefits or limitations of nanocomposites, it is problematic that the actual amount of larger nanoparticle size is rarely disclosed by manufacturers. Certain dental adhesives are the main dental materials that can benefit from nanoparticle filling. Virtually, all restorative "nanocomposites" are, in fact, "nanohybrids" that contain much larger volumes of non-nanoparticles, micron-sized or submicron-sized [123].

In terms of viscosity, composite resins can be divided into two broad classes: flowable and packable, both of which can vary in viscosity depending on the brand or product. Packable is a more appropriate term for resins that can be applied, pressed, and molded into cavities. The term "condensable composite" is less fortunate, given that the term "condensation" means a change in density due to volume compression. This is true in the case of amalgam, but it is not applicable to composite resins that do not reduce their volume when packed in a cavity [124].

The materials can be classified into four different groups based on the nature of their matrix:

1. Methacrylates—the classical methacrylate-based composite resins (Ceram.x, Spectra-Dentsply Sirona; Tetric EvoCeram, Evetric-Ivoclar Vivadent; Gradia, Gaenial-GC; Herculite, Premise-Kerr; Estelite-Tokuyama, etc.)
2. Compomers—Dyract (Dentsply Sirona).
3. Ormocers—Admira, Voco.
4. Silorane-based—Filtek Silorane, 3 M.

Composite Resins

The best-known materials in the dental composite group are methacrylate composites. In dentistry, the combination of methacrylates with different varieties of fillers, coupled with silane, is used. The fillers are composed of quartz, silica, ceramics, and other oxides.

Giomers represent a new group of aesthetic restorative materials (glass ionomer + polymer), whose organic matrix is similar to traditional composites but with less light-curing shrinkage [125] and fluoride release. Currently, a wide range of commercial products is available on the market. A common indication for giomers is cervical restorations with poor adhesion [126], but they can be used as liners, bases, and long-lasting fillings in all cavities.

Giomers are a type of conventional composite resin generally of fluid consistency, but they also exist in conventional packable or bulk form (Fig. 1.56). Their distinctive feature is that they are partially filled with a glass ionomer cement that has been finely crushed. This causes the giomers to release fluorine moderately, but their general properties are those of conventional composite resins. There is some evidence that they release enough fluoride to be considered antibacterial. Bulk giomers (e.g., Beautifil bulk restorative giomer, Shofu Dental) are being polymerized in thick layers up to 4 mm [127] and are associated with small cuspidal deformations, statistically comparable to ormocers (Admira Fusion x-tra, Voco) [128].

Compomers

They were introduced in the late 1990s, combining the advantages of composites with GIc, which is reflected in their company name "Comp," from composites, and "Omer," from ionomer. This objective was partially achieved. Compomers are a well-defined class of restorative materials used mainly in pediatric dentistry,

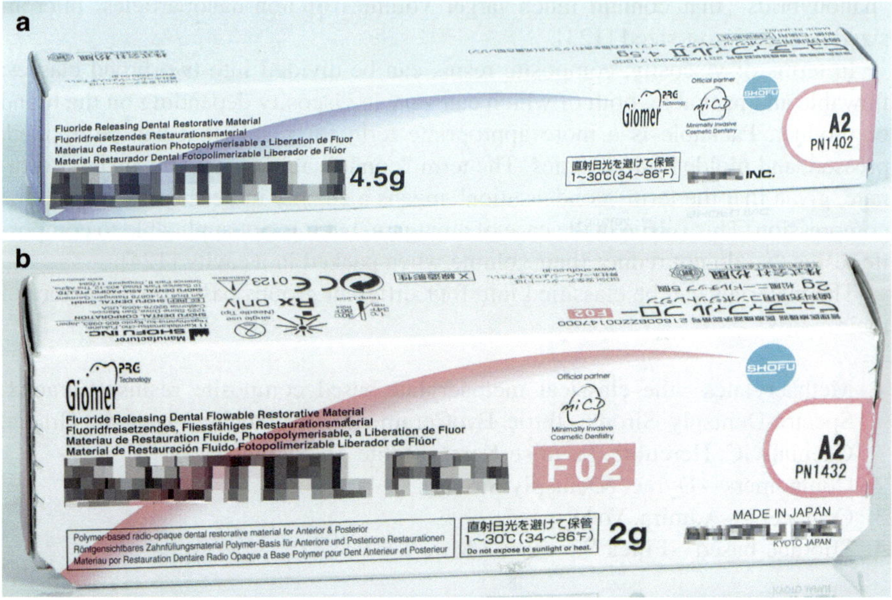

Fig. 1.56 Giomer-based restorative materials in different versions: packable (**a**); flowable (**b**)

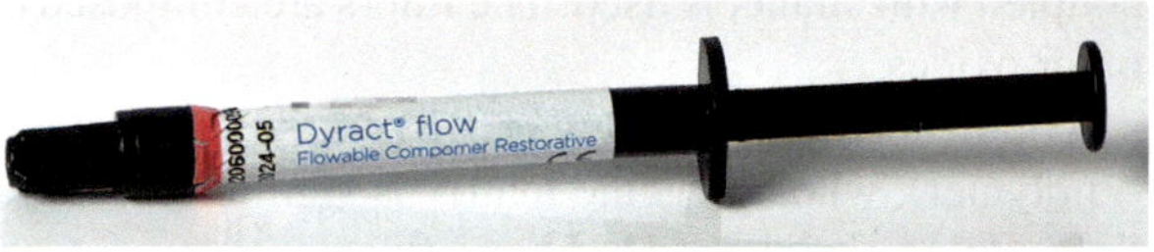

Fig. 1.57 Dyract flow compomer

especially temporary teeth, because they release fluoride and have a moderate abrasion index. Although they release fluoride, this feature is weaker than in the case of GIc (self-curing or light-curing). They are combined with adhesive systems, having increased elasticity, which is why they may be indicated in cervical areas where they perform better than RMGIc but weaker than other hybrid composites. One of widely used compomers is Dyract (Dentsply Sirona, Germany) packable or flowable resin (Fig. 1.57).

Ormocers

Ormocers were introduced into dentistry in 1998 (Admira, Voco), and they were previously used in the plastic lens industry to prevent scratching of lens surfaces. Their name is an acronym for "ORganically-MOdified-direct-CERamic." These materials have a hardness similar to a glass, which gives them increased resistance to abrasion and behave like composite resins but with improved properties. They are hydrophobic, so they do not absorb water [129]. Theoretically, the ormocers do not generate unpolymerized residual monomers, which is an advantage over the classical composites [130]. Their shrinkage coefficient is much lower compared to classical composites [131]. One of the widely used brands of ormocers is Admira Fusion (Voco, Germany)) (Fig. 1.58).

Silorane-Based Composites (Low Shrink)

The silorane-based composites are a combination of siloxanes (known for their hydrophilicity) and oxiranes (known for their low shrinkage and stability) that are classically layered in layers smaller than 2 mm. They generate low polymerization contraction [132], below 1% [133], leading to lower microleakage scores [134], improved marginal adaptation [135], and reduced cusp deflection [136]. These benefits occur while maintaining mechanical properties comparable to classical composite resins. However, the cavity wall adaptation and light-curing problems in deep cavities remain [137], which is why the use of another cavity-based material has been suggested [138]. The reduced light-curing contraction of silorane-based composites does not represent a clinically significant advantage over the classical composite resins, according to the scientific literature. Also, their physical and mechanical properties and ability to bind to dentin have been proven comparable to classical composite resins [139] by the in vitro studies. Among the most popular silorane-based composites on the market is Filtek Silorane (3 M Espe) (Fig. 1.59).

1.2.4.3 Bulk Composites

Bulk-fill composites have been designed to simplify the execution of posterior restorations, especially for obturating deep cavities filled with classical composite resins by layering with an incremental technique (overlapping the layers whose thickness is limited to 2 mm). Bulk-fill composites, currently developed, have a light-curing depth of 4–5 mm and a relatively low light-curing contraction (1.6–2% for medium viscosity materials, 2.5–4.1% for flowable materials) [140]. Bulk composites have a good marginal fit, similar to conventional composites [141]. Studies have shown a similar frequency of interface voids occurring in bulk composites when compared to conventional composites [142].

It is known that both the light-curing lamp and the light-curing chemical reaction of materials generate heat that can be transmitted to the dental pulp. A proportional relationship between temperature growth and the amount of applied composite resin

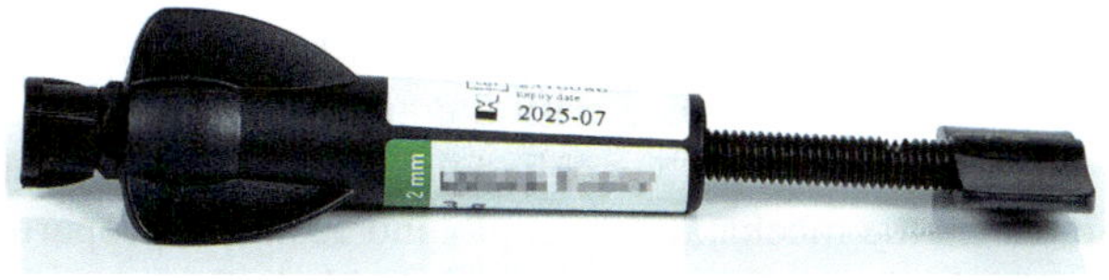

Fig. 1.58 Ormocer packable

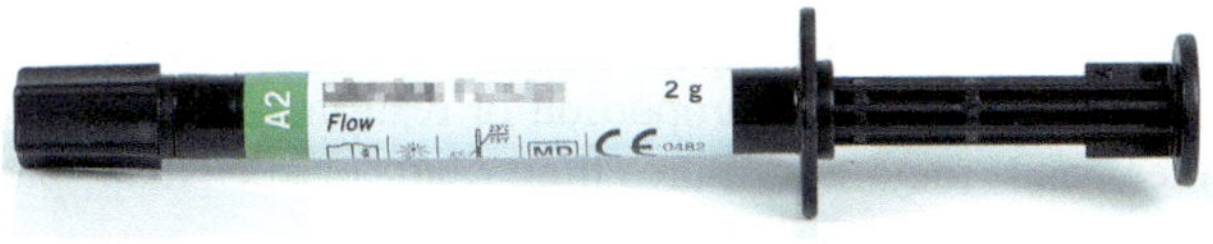

Fig. 1.59 Ormocer flowable

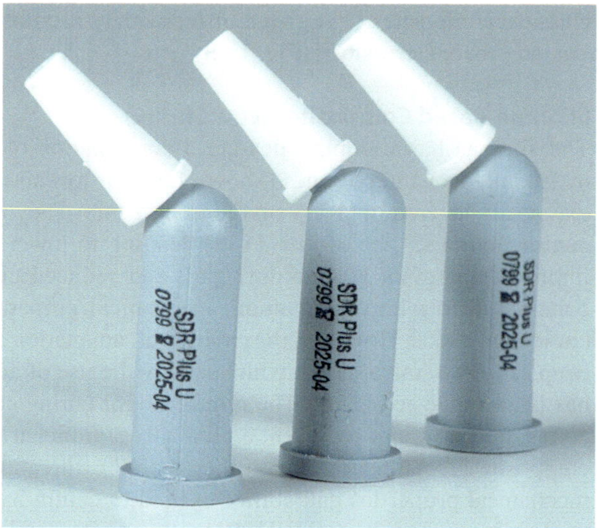

Fig. 1.60 SDR® flow bulk composite resin

has been established. It has been found that in bulk-fill composite resins and fiber-reinforced composite resins, there was a higher increase in temperature transmitted to the pulp rather compared to the conventional ones (with an upper limit of 11 °C) and a lower degree of monomer conversion in the deep layer [143]. Therefore, the possibility of pulpal inflammation caused by the temperature increase should be considered when using light-cured bulk materials in very deep cavities. In this clinical situation, it is suggested that the first composite layer applied to the cavity base should not be very thick [144–146] on the vital teeth.

Apart from packable bulk composites, the new generation of flowable bulk composites was introduced in dentistry in 2009 to compensate for the light-curing contact of the subjacent packable composites. The first bulk-fill fluid composite resin was the SureFil® SDR® bulk-fill composite resin (Dentsply Caulk) (Fig. 1.60). The flowable bulk-fill composites have a higher filler content and better mechanical properties than conventional flowable composites, and they can be recommended for more extensive posterior restorations [147]. Subsequent studies have confirmed that they allow a depth of cure of more than 4 mm, having a low light-curing shrinkage [148].

Flowable bulk composites contain less filler than packable ones, which is why they must be combined with a conventional packable/high viscosity microhybrid composite. It should be applied to the restoration surface (1.5–2 mm thick layer) to enhance the mechanical strength and aesthetic properties, sometimes compromised by the high translucency of the flowable bulk material [149].

1.2.4.4 Flowable Composites

Flowable composite resins contain less filler (60–70% by weight and 46–70% by volume) and a higher proportion of resin matrix than hybrid resins. They have less filler, and they are more fluid and elastic than packable composites. Their manufacturers, supported by scientific studies, recommend using flowable composites as liners on the cavity base and the gingival edge because they can reduce light-curing shrinkage by absorbing the general polymerization stress of the packable composite [150].

The fluid composite presence decreases the possibility of voids occurring at the cavities gingival edge level, extended up to or below the cementoenamel junction (CEJ) [151]. A survey done by the American Dental Association (ADA) shows that over 90% of dentists use fluid composites in their practice [152].

Attar et al. and Chuang et al. [153] demonstrated that the microleakage in the gingival margin area of class II cavity restorations is lower when the first layer of flowable composite is applied to the cervical margin followed by the proximal wall restoration using packable composite. Furthermore, packable composites can sometimes be difficult to be applied and compressed in inaccessible areas. This can lead to inadequate adaptation to the cavity shape and material void occurrence. The application of a flowable composite layer and its polymerization, followed by the restoration completion, has the best results compared to the technique where the flowable and packable composites are light-cured simultaneously (snow plow technique) or in which the layer is replaced by light-curing GIc [154].

There are several indications for the fluid composites' usage that we can mention:

- Minimally invasive preventive occlusal restorations in tiny cavities, especially in pediatric dentistry [155].
- Groove and fissure sealing for which this is the material of choice [156].
- Cavity liners [157].
- Minimally invasive restorations on proximal surfaces that do not involve the occlusal surface, while the marginal ridge is intact [158].
- Improved marginal sealing on the gingival edge of class II cavities or MOD cavities [159].
- Cervical non-carious cavity restoration [160].
- Minimally invasive class 3 cavity restoration [161].

The use of magnification can reduce the edge void emergence through better visual control of the material when applied in the gingival edge area [162].

1.2.4.5 Adhesive Systems

The use of adhesives is essential for all types of composite resins. Adhesion to enamel is easier to obtain and has better quality than adhesion to dentin—due to the different chemical structures between enamel and dentin.

The mechanism through which composite materials adhere to tooth structure has evolved over the many generations of adhesive systems, but the fourth generation is considered the gold standard because it provides an outstanding level of adhesion. This fourth generation was described by Nakabayashi et al., and it is produced by the resin monomer infiltration into the microretentions of enamel and dentin wall, with subsequent light-curing, constituting in this way retentive extensions. This produces a hybrid layer at the interface between the dental substrate and the composite resin, and the process is called hybridization. The quality of the tooth structure influences this whole process.

Enamel provides a mineral substrate with minimal organic matrix and no natural micromechanical retentions. The enamel can be treated with an acid that subtracts minerals and leads to microporosity formation. Experience has shown that this role is best fulfilled by the orthophosphoric acid ~37% concentration in a gel form. The acid attack ceases when the acid gel is washed away with water that fills the obtained cavities. Resin monomers are generally hydrophobic, so a hydrophilic substance must be used as a precursor to infiltration, called a primer, followed by applying the adhesive containing the unpolymerized resin. In the fourth-generation adhesive systems, each of the three components is separate: the acid, which must be washed off after application, the primer, and the adhesive.

The superficial dentin surface layer that results from the primer and adhesive impregnation is called a hybrid layer [163].

Adhesion to dentin is difficult, partly due to the moisture content, yet there are two approaches to dentin adhesion: etch-and-rinse and self-etching.

Adhesion to dentin is different because dentin contains an essential organic component, it has dentinal tubules in its structure, and it is essentially wet. The fourth generation of adhesive systems was the first to produce substantial amounts of adhesion by opening the dentinal canaliculi blocked by the dentinal smear layer obtained through cavity preparation and by preventing the collagen fibers in the structure from collapsing.

The next generations of adhesive systems have been designed to shorten working times and improve adhesion, especially to dentin. There is one classification of adhesive systems in generations (from generation 1 to generation 8) and one in the number of steps concerning the mechanism of action (one, two, and three steps). The latest adhesive generations are those that are commonly used clinically:

Generation IV: acid; primer; adhesive – separate.
Generation V: acid; primer + adhesive (together).
Generation VI: acid + primer (together); adhesive.
Generation VII: acid + primer + adhesive (all together).
Generation VIII: all together + nanofiller.

So, we now have etch-and-rinse, self-etch, and universal adhesives available. The latter can be used with both etch-and-rinse and self-etch techniques. Etch-and-rinse systems remove the smear layer, while the self-etch systems, on the contrary, integrate the smear layer.

Etch-and-rinse dental adhesives in three steps and self-etch adhesives in two steps are the most stable because they lead to more durable restorations than their simplified counterparts [164]. Despite their inferior clinical performance, simplified adhesives have become very popular because dentists tend to choose materials that are easier to use. However, clinical and laboratory research has shown a trade-off between simplifying dental adhesives and outcomes [165].

Conclusion

The evolution over time of composite resins has introduced new classes of materials (compomers, ormocers, siloranes, giomers) that have partially or totally solved some shortcomings. These have some characteristics that need improvement, so the statistical significance of clinical treatment improvements remains questionable, there are conflicting studies. The light-curing shrinkage of conventional and bulk composites has been significantly reduced in the new generations. This is directly associated with good marginal integrity of restorations and increased long-term success. The adhesive systems have become increasingly versatile, but the standard has remained the etch-and-rinse with primer (three-step) system.

Review Questions

1. What is the difference between liners and bases?
2. What are the main categories of materials used as liners, and what are their main characteristics?
3. What are the main categories of resin-based materials used for long-term restorations, and what are their main characteristics?
4. What are flowable composites, and what are their main characteristics?
5. What are bulk composites, and what are their main characteristics?
6. What are the main classes of adhesive systems?

1.3 Treatment Ergonomics Using Dental Operating Microscope: Four-Handed Dentistry

There are several prerequisites for the proper application of the working protocols and thus for obtaining accurate results when using the dental operating microscope. The use of magnification and dental operating microscope requires the application of these preconditions, which are interlinked:

- Ergonomic working posture.
- Four-handed work.
- Use of rubber dam isolation.
- Working in an indirect vision using the dental mirror.

Four-handed working is essential for microscope treatments for two significant reasons: protecting the doctor's eyes from frequent defocusing and maintaining the workflow treatment. It is necessary to establish and respect working positions that the dentist-assistant team must correctly master during four-handed work with magnification:

- The patient is horizontally positioned in the dental chair (Fig. 1.61). We recommend the patients are provided protective glasses because in this position, the patient's eyes are very close and below the instrument transfer area, and they can easily be injured or splashed with liquids or other materials in the eyes (Fig. 1.62).

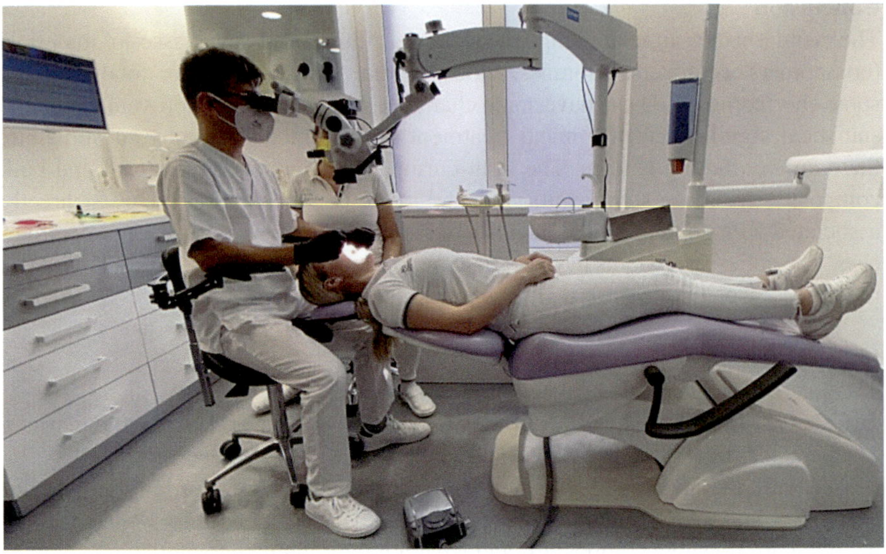

Fig. 1.61 Doctor's posture and patient's treatment positioning

Fig. 1.62 Patient with safety glasses and rubber dam isolation

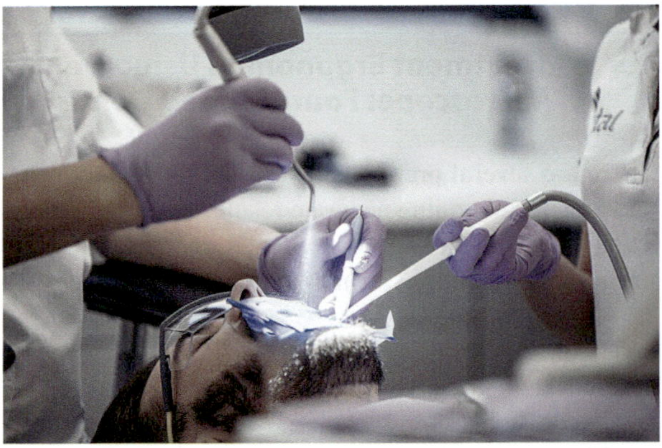

- The patient's head needs positioning (in the headrest) according to the arch that is being treated. If the procedure takes place on the mandible in direct view, the patient will hold the chin on the chest, and the doctor will adjust the headrest to help the patient achieve this position. If the procedure is taking place on the maxillary teeth in indirect view, the patient will hold the head extended, and the doctor will adjust the position of the headrest. In this way, the position of the maxillary occlusal plane will be vertical or slightly tilted toward the doctor.
- The doctor's correct posture, sitting on a dedicated chair with backrest and armrests. The positioning during work should be at around 11–12 am (Fig. 1.63).
- The doctor should not look up from the microscope to pick up instruments from the working field or terminals from racks (handpieces, spray).

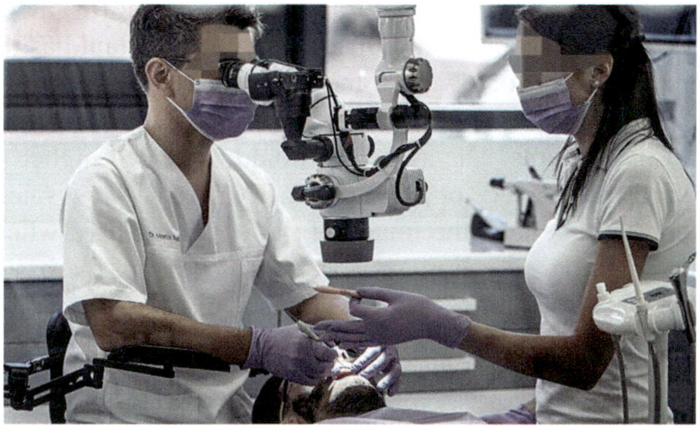

Fig. 1.63 Dentist's and dental assistant's face-to-face positioning during work

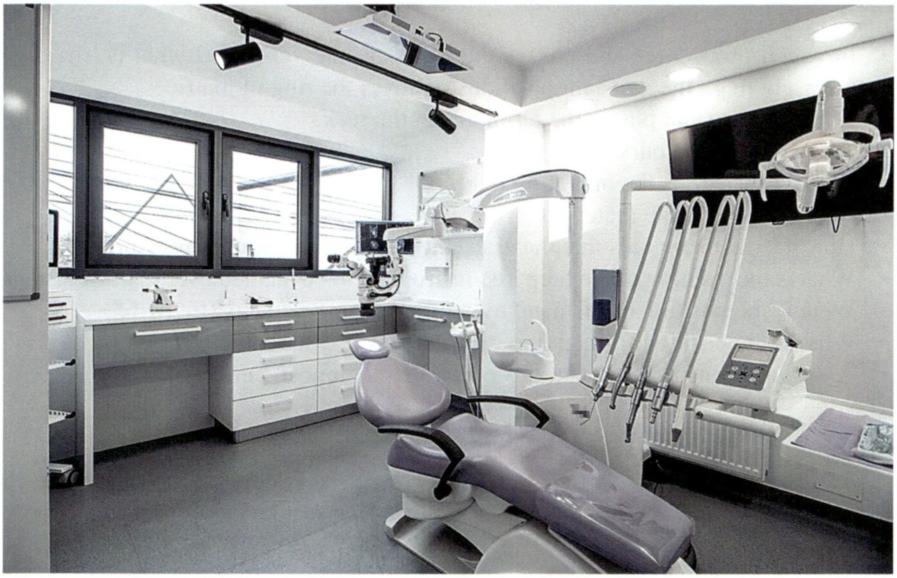

Fig. 1.64 Dental unit with retractable terminals

- Instruments or unit terminals are to be handed by the dental assistant or taken by the doctor without looking up from the microscope. This is relatively easy to do when the units with the terminals/hoses are mounted at the top and positioned above the patient's chest (Fig. 1.64). Dental units with terminals/hoses hanging from the bottom are usually mounted underneath/in front of the unit table and located on the opposite side of the nurse, so access to the terminals is difficult or impossible. In these situations, good ergonomics require that the doctor has a second assistant to handle the terminals, or the doctor handles the terminals without taking their eyes off the microscope.

Personnel's additional training is essential for microscope work. Given that the peripheral vision is minimal, the dental assistant has to transfer most of the instruments to the doctor and sometimes even guide his/her hand to the working position. The assistant should be positioned facing the operator to make an efficient exchange of instruments. The assistant should be seated higher than the operator and have a separate eyepiece or preferably a TV screen. This is necessary in order to be able to constantly check the image of the operating field where the assistant will perform the suction procedure, but at the same time, the assistant must also monitor the patient as a whole (whether he/she is making signs, whether he/she is communicating visually with the medical team, etc.).

This protocol should determine which procedures the dentist and assistant perform. The protocol should determine which technique to transfer instruments and determine which are the verbal and nonverbal signals agreed upon by the physician and assistant for handover/takeover:

- In which procedures and phases the assistant intervenes and what he/she does precisely (e.g., the assistant positions/removes the ring of matrices).
- Who picks up and places the terminals in the rack.
- Who changes the burs.
- Who washes/dries the operating field.
- Who light-cures the materials.
- How the doctor signals that the assistant can pick up the used instrument.
- What is the position of the prepared instrument to be handed over to the assistant.
- What is the position of the hand to get the new instruments (Fig. 1.65).
- What is the position for handing over the new instrument.
- A verbal coding of the quantities of required composite material.

Difficulties that may occur	Potential solutions
The assistant does not have access to the terminals	Move the unit table closer to the assistant so that he/she can take/put in the racks, or the doctor will care of this task
The patient is moving too much	The doctor explains to the patient how the magnification works and the importance of staying steady to maintain focus and image clarity
The assistant does not see the doctor's signals (nonverbal)	Heed a warning and reiterate the instructions

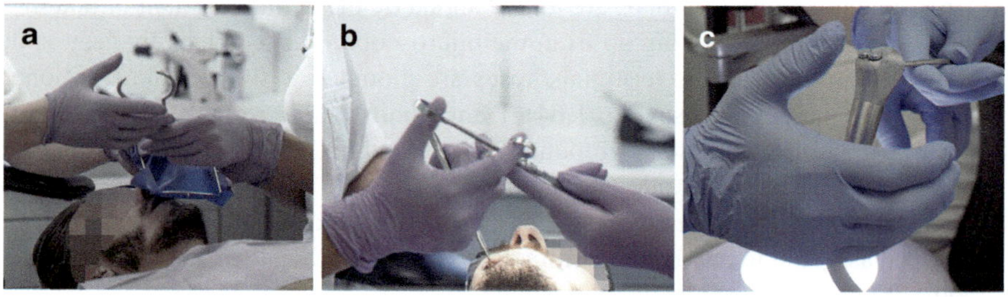

Fig. 1.65 Instruments' transfer: rubber dam clamp applicator for upper posterior teeth (**a**); atraumatic needle syringe for anesthesia (**b**); water/air-spray gun (**c**)

Conclusion

Compliance with the ergonomic principles and the assistant's training is essential for performing microscope treatments. In addition, the choice of certain types of equipment can improve ergonomics (e.g., top-mounted terminal units and doctor's chairs with armrests).

1.3.1 Transferring Instruments

The paralleling technique is the most commonly used technique for instrument transfer in four-handed working conditions, with the doctor positioned at 12 o'clock.

The paralleling technique advantages are the following:

- It prevents interference of the used/old instrument, which is taken over, with the new instrument to be handed over.
- It prevents accidents (e.g., stabbing with sharp or cutting instruments).
- It prevents the materials that are applied onto the active tips of tools from falling by crossing the tools.
- It requires only one hand from the assistant in which both the old and new instruments will be held.
- It allows the assistant to have one hand free, most commonly needed for handling the aspirator/suction or water/air spray.

1.3.1.1 Paralleling Technique Description

The new instrument can be grasped using a minimum of two fingers (thumb and index). The most stable grip of the new instrument, handed over by the assistant, is made with three fingers, between the thumb, index, and middle finger, or four fingers (Fig. 1.66), but this is adapted according to the motor abilities of each person. The position of the new instrument is the shaft along the arm, and the palm is oriented upward. To pick up the old instrument, the assistant will stretch one, two, or three fingers to grip the instrument between the fingers and the palm bridge (Fig. 1.66b, c).

The doctor will signal that the old instrument can be removed by gently removing it from the oral cavity and aligning its axis with the patient body axis without losing the fulcrum (Fig. 1.67a). The assistant reaches out, brings the new instrument close to the old one, and with one, two, or three fingers (little, ring, or middle)

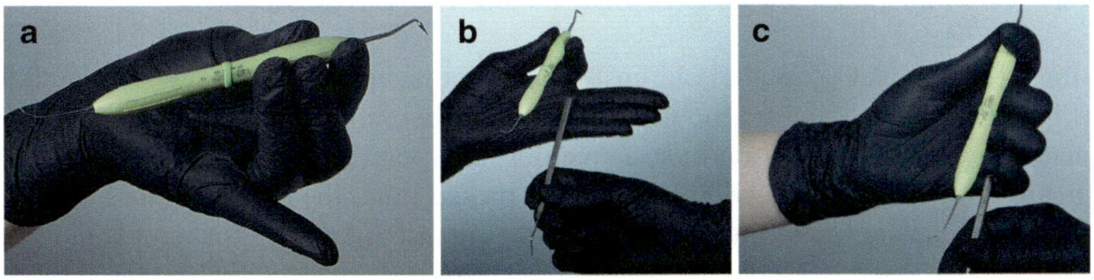

Fig. 1.66 Assistant hand positioning for instrument transfer using the paralleling technique

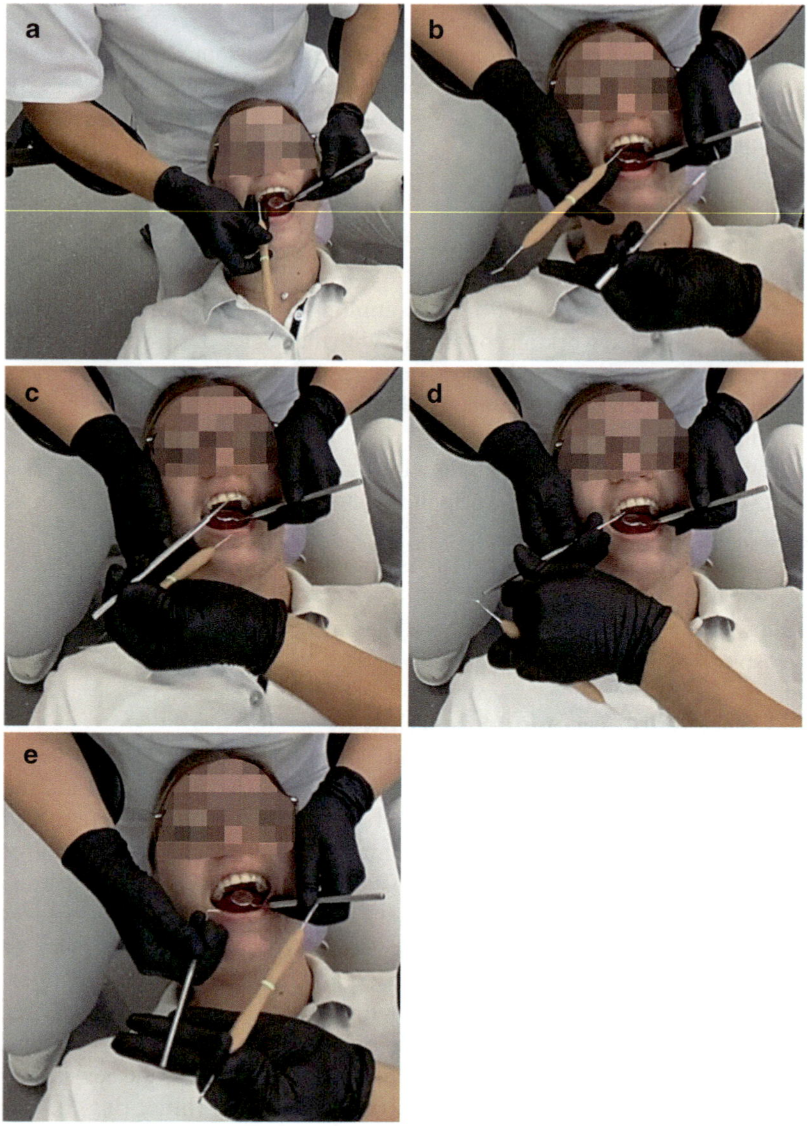

Fig. 1.67 Instrument transfer between dentist and dental assistant during treatment

(Fig. 1.67b), picks up the old instrument but keeps the instruments parallel (Fig. 1.67c). This prevents the instruments from bumping into each other, spilling materials that are carried on their active tips, and possible injuries. As soon as the doctor has grasped the new instrument and picked it up, the assistant takes the fingers off it and removes the old instrument (Fig. 1.67d). The assistant should get

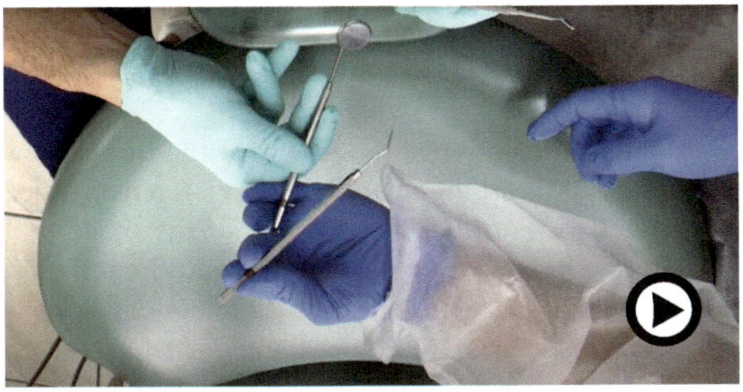

Fig. 1.68 The paralleling technique for instrument handling (▶ https://doi.org/10.1007/000-bqf)

close enough to the doctor's hand so that he or she can easily hand over and pick up the instruments. The picking and handing over of the instruments should be done gently but firmly so that the doctor, who does not have peripheral vision when looking through the microscope, can easily perceive that the assistant has grasped the instrument and can therefore release it without the risk of falling. The same firm movements are made when a new instrument is placed in the doctor's hand. Instruments are handed to the doctor in the exact position they will be used (Fig. 1.68).

The equipment that requires activation with the push of a button by the doctor (e.g., a light-curing lamp) will be handed over by sticking the button on the doctor's thumb. In this way, the doctor does not have to make other movements after grasping the handle of an instrument/device.

Difficulties that may occur	Potential solutions
The assistant handles the instruments poorly	The doctor has to refuse to receive an instrument that is not correctly handed in
Some instruments are too heavy/large to be handled using the paralleling technique (e.g., light-curing lamps, dental forceps, etc.)	The assistant will use one hand to have a good grip on the instruments and hand them over, yet use the other hand to pick up the old instrument, if necessary
The assistant does not bring the new instrument close enough to the doctor's hand, so the doctor has to bring his/her hand closer and let go of the fulcrum	The doctor's hand support should be kept on point when transferring the instruments. In this way, the doctor does not have to make any approach movements, thus forcing the assistant to bring the new instrument into the proper position

The doctor and the assistant should face each other and transfer the instruments using the paralleling technique for good ergonomics. The doctor is responsible for training the assistant and supervising the implementation of the established rules.

1.3.2 Working in Indirect Vision with a Mirror and the Position of the Patient While Using a DOM

The microscope cannot be positioned to allow work in direct view for all cases. The mirror is necessary for working in an indirect vision in most cases. Rhodium mirrors are recommended. For this, the position of the patient's head is essential. The optimum angle between the microscope and the mirror is 45°, and the doctor must achieve this angle without putting the patient in an awkward position. This angle is relatively easy to achieve for maxillary teeth. The patient's head is positioned to create a 90° angle between the maxillary occlusal plane and binocular. In this position, the mirror's position for optimal viewing will be at 45°. The mirror should be placed at a distance from the tooth worked on to allow the insertion of instruments and avoid splashing with water and debris from the turbine or spray (Fig. 1.69). Repositioning the mirror requires microscope adjustments, making the whole procedure time-consuming and tedious. The chosen magnification level is generally a small one. It is essential not to select unrealistic magnification levels for procedures that do not require fine detail (e.g., ring matrix application). Higher magnification steps should only be used occasionally, as they strongly reduce the size of the working field and the depth of view.

During work, the mirror can be kept clean in several ways that work together:

- The cleaning is done by the assistant, who will always have a tissue in hand in which he or she holds the mirror between the thumb and the other fingers, cleaning it with the thumb.
- Placing the mirror as far away as possible from the head of the water-spraying turbine head, sometimes just outside the oral cavity.
- Water and debris removal can be achieved during work by air spray.
- Treating the mirror surface with a special antifog solution.

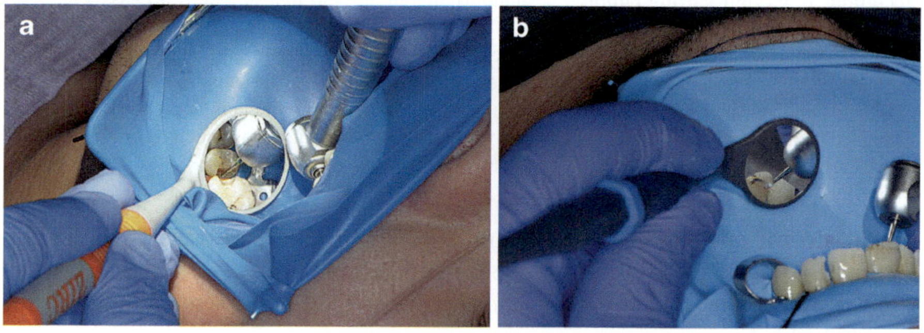

Fig. 1.69 Positioning the mirror away from the working tooth to allow turbine access (**a**) and avoid splashing water (**b**)

Difficulties that may occur	Potential solutions
The mirror remains dirty even after wiping	Change a mirror that is possibly scratched. Make sure the assistant knows how to clean the mirror properly
The mirror has no room in the oral cavity	Choose a smaller mirror size
The mirror image is covered with the turbine head/contra-angle, making it impossible to see the cavity	Mirror and turbine/contra-angle piece angulation change; choice of small-headed turbine/contra-angle pieces recommended for microscope work

Conclusion

Most procedures performed with magnification require the use of the mirror for the indirect view. Therefore, the physician must have excellent working command in indirect vision and be able to remedy possible impediments fluently.

Review Questions

1. What working positions must the doctor-assistant team correctly master for the four-handed microscope working method?
2. What are the advantages of using the parallel technique for transferring instruments between the doctor and the assistant?
3. What are the ways to keep the mirror clean during indirect vision work?

References

1. Perrin P, Jacky D, Hotz P. Das Operationsmikroskop in der zahnärztlichen praxis: minimal-invasive Füllungen. The operating microscope in dental practice: minimally invasive restorations. Schweiz Monatsschr Zahnmed. 2002;112(7):722–32.
2. Bud M, Jitaru S, Lucaciu O, et al. The advantages of the dental operative microscope in restorative dentistry. Med Pharm Rep. 2021;94(1):22–7.
3. Rubinstein RA, Kim S. Short-term observation of the results of endodontic surgery with the use of a surgical operating microscope and super-EBA as rootend filling material. J Endod. 1999;25:43–8.
4. Kinomoto Y, Takeshige F, Hayashi M, Ebisu S. Optimal positioning for a dental operating microscope during non-surgical endodontics. J Endod. 2004;30(12):860–2.
5. Bud M, Pricope R, Pop RC, Onaca R, Swerts PJ, Lucaciu O, Deleana A. Comparative analysis of 5 preclinical dental students' working postures using dental loupes and dental operating microscope. Eur J Dent Educ. 2021;25(3):516–23.
6. Bud M, Spătaru S, Pop RC, Pricope R, Lucaciu O, Câmpean S, Delean A. The ergonomic challenges students face during operative dentistry treatment. J Clin Diagn Res. 2021;15(8):ZC33–7.
7. Comes C, Vâlceanu A, Rusu D, Didilescu A, Bucur A, Anghel M, Argeşanu V, Stratul SI. A study on the ergonomical working modalities using the dental operating microscope (DOM). Part I: ergonomic principles in dental medicine. Timiş Med J. 2008;58:3–4.
8. Richman MJ. The use of ultrasonics in root canal therapy and root resection. J Dent Med Sci. 1957;12:12.
9. Mm J, Nk B, Pathak A. Minimal intervention dentistry—a new frontier in clinical dentistry. J Clin Diagn Res. 2014;8(7):ZE04–ZE8.
10. Postle HH. Ultrasonic cavity preparation. J Prosthet Dent. 1958;8(1):153–60.
11. Black RB. Airbrasive: some fundamentals. J Am Dent Assoc. 1950;41(6):701–10.

12. Christensen GJ. Air abrasion tooth cutting: state of the art 1998. J Am Dent Assoc. 1998;129(4):484–5.
13. Goldstein RE, Parkins FM. Using air-abrasive technology to diagnose and restore pit and fissure caries. J Am Dent Assoc. 1995;126(6):761–6.
14. Rodrigues Jde A, de Vita TM, Cordeiro RC. In vitro evaluation of the influence of air abrasion on detection of occlusal caries lesions in primary teeth. Pediatr Dent. 2008;30(1):15–8.
15. Antunes LA, Pedro RL, Vieira AS, Maia LC. Effectiveness of high speed instrument and air abrasion on different dental substrates. Braz Oral Res. 2008;22(3):235–41.
16. Paolinelis G, Watson TF, Banerjee A. Microhardness as a predictor of sound and carious dentine removal using alumina air abrasion. Caries Res. 2006;40(4):292–5.
17. Santos-Pinto L, Peruchi C, Marker VA, Cordeiro R. Effect of handpiece tip design on the cutting efficiency of an air abrasion system. Am J Dent. 2001;14(6):397–401.
18. Orchardson R, Gangarosa LP Sr, Holland GR, et al. Dentine hypersensitivity-into the 21st century. Arch Oral Biol. 1994;39(Suppl):113S–9S.
19. Horiguchi S, Yamada T, Inokoshi S, Tagami J. Selective caries removal with air abrasion. Oper Dent. 1998;23(5):236–43.
20. Banerjee A, Pabari H, Paolinelis G, Thompson ID, Watson TF. An in vitro evaluation of selective demineralised enamel removal using bio-active glass air abrasion. Clin Oral Investig. 2011;15(6):895–900.
21. Petersilka GJ. Subgingival air–polishing in the treatment of periodontal biofilm infections. Periodontol 2000. 2011;55(1):124–42.
22. Pelka M, Trautmann S, Petschelt A, Lohbauer U. Influence of air-polishing devices and abrasives on root dentin-an in vitro confocal laser scanning microscope study. Quintessence Int. 2010;41(7):e141–8.
23. Petersilka GJ, Steinmann D, Häberlein I, Heinecke A, Flemmig TF. Subgingival plaque removal in buccal and lingual sites using a novel low abrasive air-polishing powder. J Clin Periodontol. 2003;30(4):328–33.
24. Giacomelli L, Salerno M, Derchi G, Genovesi A, Paganin PP, Covani U. Effect of air polishing with glycine and bicarbonate powders on nanocomposite used in dental restorations: an in vitro study. Int J Periodontics Restorative Dent. 2001;31(5):e51–6.
25. Graumann SJ, Sensat ML, Stoltenberg JL. Air polishing: a review of current literature. J Dent Hyg. 2013;87(4):173–80.
26. Chimello-Sousa DT, de Souza AE, Chinelatti MA, Pécora JD, Palma-Dibb RG, Milori Corona SA. Influence of Er: YAG laser irradiation distance on the bond strength of a restorative system to enamel. J Dent. 2006;34:245–51.
27. Degrange H, Roulet JF. Minimally invasive dentistry with bonding. J Am Dent Assoc. 1998;129:484–5.
28. De Moor RJ, Delme KI. Laser-assisted cavity preparation and adhesion to erbium-lased tooth structure: part 2. Present-day adhesion to erbium-lased tooth structure in permanent teeth. J Adhes Dent. 2010;12:91–102.
29. Montedori A, Abraha I, Orso M, D'Errico PG, Pagano S, Lombardo G. Lasers for caries removal in deciduous and permanent teeth. Cochrane Database Syst Rev. 2016;9(9):CD010229.
30. Sedrez-Porto JA, Münchow EA, Cenci MS, Pereira-Cenci T. Translucency and color stability of resin composite and dental adhesives as modeling liquids—a one-year evaluation. Braz Oral Res. 2017;31:e54.
31. Sedrez-Porto JA, Münchow EA, Brondani LP, Cenci MS, Pereira-Cenci T. Effects of modeling liquid/resin and polishing on the color change of resin composite. Braz Oral Res. 2016;30(1):S1806-83242016000100275.
32. Münchow EA, Sedrez-Porto JA, Piva E, Pereira-Cenci T, Cenci MS. Use of dental adhesives as modeler liquid of resin composites. Dent Mater. 2016;32(4):570–7.
33. Bayraktar ET, Atali PY, Korkut B, Kesimli EG, Tarcin B, Turkmen C. Effect of modeling resins on microhardness of resin composites. Eur J Dent. 2021;15(3):481–7.

34. Abdulmajeed A, et al. Fatiguing and preheating effect on mechanical properties of composite resins. J Dent Res. 2019;98:1879.
35. Tauböck TT, Tarle Z, Marovic D, Attin T. Pre-heating of high-viscosity bulk-fill resin composites: effects on shrinkage force and monomer conversion. J Dent. 2015;43(11):1358–64.
36. Bauer JG, Crispin BJ. Evolution of the matrix for Class 2 restorations. Oper Dent. 1986;Suppl 4:1–37.
37. Raghu R, Srinivasan R. Optimizing tooth form with direct posterior composite restorations. J Conserv Dent. 2011;14:330–6.
38. Saber MH, Loomans BA, El Zohairy A, Dörfer CE, El-Badrawy W. Evaluation of proximal contact tightness of class II resin composite restorations. Oper Dent. 2010;35:37–43.
39. Loomans BA, Opdam NJ, Roeters FJ, Bronkhorst EM, Burgersdijk RC. Comparison of proximal contacts of class II resin composite restorations in vitro. Oper Dent. 2006;31:688–93.
40. Saber MH, El-Badrawy W, Loomans BA, Ahmed DR, Dörfer CE, El Zohairy A. Creating tight proximal contacts for MOD resin composite restorations. Oper Dent. 2011;36(3):304–10.
41. Tarnow DP, Magner AW, Fletcher P. The effect of the distance from the contact point to the crest of bone on the presence or absence of the interproximal dental papilla. J Periodontol. 1992;63(12):995–6.
42. Milicich G, Rainey JT. Clinical presentations of stress distribution in teeth and the significance in operative dentistry. Pract Periodontics Aesthet Dent. 2000;12(7):695–702.
43. Loomans BA, Roeters FJ, Opdam NJ, Kuijs RH. The effect of proximal contour on marginal ridge fracture of class II composite resin restorations. J Dent. 2008;36(10):828–32.
44. Owens BM, Phebus JG. An evidence-based review of dental matrix systems. Gen Dent. 2016;64(5):64–70.
45. Loomans BA, Opdam NJ, Roeters FJ, Bronkhorst EM, Burgersdijk RC, Dörfer CE. A randomized clinical trial on proximal contacts of posterior composites. J Dent. 2006;34(4):292–7.
46. Triodent. FAQS. https://www.triodent.com/faqs/. Accessed Feb 2021.
47. Bailey O, O'Connor C. Papilla management in sub-gingival, interproximal, direct composite restoration: a key step to success. Br Dent J. 2019;226(12):933–7.
48. Cho SD, Browning WD, Walton KS. Clinical use of a sectional matrix and ring. Oper Dent. 2010;35(5):587–91.
49. Caughman WF, Rueggeberg FA, Curtis JW Jr. Clinical guidelines for photocuring restorative resins. J Am Dent Assoc. 1995;126(9):1280–6.
50. Jung H, Friedl KH, Hiller KA, Furch H, Bernhart S, Schmalz G. Polymerization efficiency of different photocuring units through ceramic discs. Oper Dent. 2006;31:68–77.
51. Knezević A, Tarle Z, Meniga A, Sutalo J, Pichler G, Ristić M. Degree of conversion and temperature rise during polymerization of composite resin samples with blue diodes. J Oral Rehabil. 2001;28(6):586–91.
52. Leprince J, Devaux J, Mullier T, Vreven J, Leloup G. Pulpal–temperature rise and polymerization efficiency of LED curing lights. Oper Dent. 2010;35(2):220–30.
53. Gritsch K, Souvannasot S, Schembri C, Farge P, Grosgogeat B. Influence of light energy and power density on the microhardness of two nanohybrid composites. Eur J Oral Sci. 2008;116(1):77–82.
54. Rueggeberg FA, Giannini M, Arrais CAG, Price RBT. Light curing in dentistry and clinical implications: a literature review. Braz Oral Res. 2017;31(Suppl 1):e61.
55. Price RB, Dérand T, Sedarous M, Andreou P, Loney RW. Effect of distance on the power density from two light guides. J Esthet Dent. 2000;12(6):320–7.
56. Kaurani M, Bhagwat SV. Clinical evaluation of postoperative sensitivity in composite resin restorations using various liners. N Y State Dent J. 2007;73(2):23–9.
57. Sakaguchi RL. Review of the current status and challenges for dental posterior restorative composites: clinical, chemistry, and physical behavior considerations. Summary of discussion from the Portland Composites Symposium (POCOS) June 17–19, 2004, Oregon Health and Science University, Portland, Oregon. Dent Mater. 2005;21(1):3–6.

58. Palin WM, Fleming GJ, Nathwani H, Burke FJ, Randall RC. In vitro cuspal deflection and microleakage of maxillary premolars restored with novel low–shrink dental composites. Dent Mater. 2005;21(4):324–35.
59. Puckett AD, Smith R. Method to measure the polymerization shrinkage of light–cured composites. J Prosthet Dent. 1992;68(1):56–8.
60. Pashley DH, Carvalho RM. Dentine permeability and dentine adhesion. J Dent. 1997;25(5):355–72.
61. Zöllner A, Gaengler P. Pulp reactions to different preparation techniques on teeth exhibiting periodontal disease. J Oral Rehabil. 2000;27(2):93–102.
62. Mjör IA. Pulp–dentin biology in restorative dentistry. Part 7: the exposed pulp. Quintessence Int. 2002;33(2):113–35.
63. Baldissara P, Catapano S, Scotti R. Clinical and histological evaluation of thermal injury thresholds in human teeth: a preliminary study. J Oral Rehabil. 1997;24(11):791–801.
64. Danesh G, Davids H, Duda S, Kaup M, Ott K, Schäfer E. Temperature rise in the pulp chamber induced by a conventional halogen light-curing source and a plasma arc lamp. Am J Dent. 2004;17(3):203–8.
65. Daronch M, Rueggeberg FA, Hall G, De Goes MF. Effect of composite temperature on in vitro intrapulpal temperature rise. Dent Mater. 2007;23(10):1283–8.
66. Runnacles P, Arrais CA, Pochapski MT, Dos Santos FA, Coelho U, Gomes JC, De Goes MF, Gomes OM, Rueggeberg FA. In vivo temperature rise in anesthetized human pulp during exposure to a polywave LED light curing unit. Dent Mater. 2015;31(5):505–13.
67. Cantekin K, Buyuk SK, Delikan E, Pedük K, Demirbuga S. Pulp chamber temperature increase from curing light units: an in vitro study. J Dent Child (Chic). 2014;81(3):128–32.
68. Zach L, Cohen G. Pulp response to externally applied heat. Oral Surg Oral Med Oral Pathol. 1965;19:515–30.
69. Cerveira GP, Berthold TB, Souto AA, Spohr AM, Marchioro EM. Degree of conversion and hardness of an orthodontic resin cured with a light-emitting diode and a quartz-tungsten-halogen light. Eur J Orthod. 2010;32(1):83–6.
70. Ward DH. The vision of digital dental photography. Dent Today. 2007;26(5):100–5.
71. Styleitaliano. SmileLite MDP mobile dental photography by Prof. Louis Hardan. https://products.styleitaliano.org/smileline/smilelite-mdp/. Accessed 17 Jan 2022.
72. Terry DA, Snow SR, McLaren EA. Contemporary dental photography: selection and application. Compend Contin Educ Dent. 2008;29:432–49.
73. Brannstrom M. The hydrodynamic theory of dentinal pain: sensation in preparations, caries, and the dentinal crack syndrome. J Endod. 1986;12(10):453–7.
74. Brännström M, Mattsson B, Torstenson B. Materials techniques for lining composite resin restorations: a critical approach. J Dent. 1991;19(2):71–9.
75. Camps J, Déjou J, Rémusat M, About I. Factors influencing pulpal response to cavity restorations. Dent Mater. 2000;16(6):432–40.
76. Murray PE, About I, Franquin JC, Remusat M, Smith AJ. Restorative pulpal and repair responses. J Am Dent Assoc. 2001;132:482–91. Erratum in: *J Am Dent Assoc* 2001;132:1095.
77. Peutzfeldt A. Resin composites in dentistry: the monomer systems. Eur J Oral Sci. 1997;105:97–116.
78. Moldovan M, Balazsi R, Soanca A, et al. Evaluation of the degree of conversion, residual monomers and mechanical properties of some light-cured dental resin composites. Materials (Basel). 2019;12(13):2109.
79. Manual pentru rezidentiat stomatologie. ISBN 978-606-011-168-9. Editura Universitara "Carol Davila" Bucuresti, 2021, p. 73.
80. Hilton TJ. Keys to clinical success with pulp capping: a review of the literature. Oper Dent. 2009;34(5):615–25.
81. McCoy RB. Bases, liners and varnishes update. Oper Dent. 1995;20:2016.
82. Gomes Torres CR. Modern operative dentistry. Cham: Springer; 2019.
83. Burrow MF, Banomyong D, Harnirattisai C, Messer HH. Effect of glass-ionomer cement lining on postoperative sensitivity in occlusal cavities restored with resin composite—a randomized clinical trial. Oper Dent. 2009;34(6):648–55.

84. Strober B, Veitz-Keenan A, Barna JA, et al. Effectiveness of a resin-modified glass ionomer liner in reducing hypersensitivity in posterior restorations: a study from the practitioners engaged in applied research and learning network. J Am Dent Assoc. 2013;144(8):886–97.
85. Schenkel AB, Peltz I, Veitz-Keenan A. Dental cavity liners for class I and class II resin-based composite restorations. Cochrane Database Syst Rev. 2016;2016:10.
86. Summitt JB. On bases, liners, and varnishes. Oper Dent. 1994;19(35):35.
87. Oliveira LCA, Duarte S, Araujo CA, Abrahão A. Effect of low-elastic modulus liner and base as stress-absorbing layer in composite resin restorations. Dent Mater. 2010;26(3):159–69.
88. McCoy RB. On liners, bases, and varnishes update. Oper Dent. 1995;20(5):216.
89. Hilton TJ. Cavity sealers, liners, and bases: current philosophies and indications for use. Oper Dent. 1996;21(4):134–46.
90. van Noort R, Barbour M. Introduction to dental materials. Edinburgh: Mosby; 2010.
91. Peliz MIL, Duarte S, Dinelli W. Scanning electron microscope analysis of internal adaptation of materials used for pulp protection under composite resin restorations. J Esthet Restor Dent. 2005;17(2):118–28.
92. Chailert O, Banomyong D, Vongphan N, Ekworapoj P, Birrow M. Internal adaptation of resin composite restorations with different thicknesses of glass ionomer cement lining. J Investig Clin Dent. 2018;9(2):e12308.
93. Opdam NJM, Bronkhorst EM, Roeters JM, Loomans BAC. Longevity and reasons for failure of sandwich and total-etch posterior composite resin restorations. J Adhes Dent. 2007;9(5):469–75.
94. Opdam NJ, van de Sande FH, Bronkhorst E, et al. Longevity of posterior composite restorations: a systematic review and meta-analysis. J Dent Res. 2014;93(10):943–9.
95. Perdigão J, Lambrechts P, Van Meerbeek B, et al. The interaction of adhesive systems with human dentin. Am J Dent. 1996;9(4):167–73.
96. De Munck J, Van Landuyt KL, Coutinho E, et al. Fatigue resistance of dentin/composite interfaces with an additional intermediate elastic layer. Eur J Oral Sci. 2005;113(1):77–82.
97. van Dijken JW. Durability of resin composite restorations in high C-factor cavities: a 12-year follow-up. J Dent. 2010;38(6):469–74.
98. Kanzow P, Büttcher AF, Wilson NHF, Lynch CD, Blum IR. Contemporary teaching of posterior composites at dental schools in Austria, Germany, and Switzerland. J Dent. 2020;96:103321.
99. Lynch CD, Blum IR, McConnell RJ, Frazier KB, Brunton PA, Wilson NHF. Teaching posterior resin composites in UK and Ireland dental schools: do current teaching programmes match the expectation of clinical practice arrangements? Br Dent J. 2018;224(12):967–72.
100. Weiner R. Liners and bases in general dentistry. Aust Dent J. 2011;56(Suppl 1):11–22.
101. Blum IR, Wilson NHF. Consequences of no more linings under composite restorations. Br Dent J. 2019;226(10):749–52.
102. Stanley HR. Human pulp response to Restorative dental procedures. Gainesville: Sorter; 1981.
103. Craig RG. Restorative dental materials. 8th ed. St Louis: Mosby; 1989.
104. Bayne SC, Heymann HO, Swift EJ Jr. Update on dental composite restorations. J Am Dent Assoc. 1994;125(6):687–701.
105. Hilton TJ, Ferracane JL, Broome JC, Santos JD, Summitt JB. Summitt's fundamentals of operative. A contemporany approach. 4th ed. Hanover Park: Quintessence Pub Co.; 2013.
106. Di Nicolo R, Shintome LK, Myaki SI, Nagayassu MP. Bond strength of resin modified glass ionomer cement to primary dentin after cutting with different bur types and dentin conditioning. J Appl Oral Sci. 2007;15(5):459–64.
107. Besnault C, Attal JP, Ruse D, Degrange M. Self-etching adhesives improve the shear bond strength of a resin-modified glass-ionomer cement to dentin. J Adhes Dent. 2004;6(1):55–9.
108. Khoroushi M, Karvandi TM, Kamali B, Mazaheri H. Marginal microleakage of resin-modified glass-ionomer and composite resin restorations: effect of using etch-and-rinse and self-etch adhesives. Indian J Dent Res. 2012;23(3):378–83.
109. Imbery TA, Namboodiri A, Duncan A, Amos R, Best AM, Moon PC. Evaluating dentin surface treatments for resin-modified glass ionomer restorative materials. Oper Dent. 2013;38(4):429–38.

110. Mazzaoui SA, Burrow MF, Tyas MJ. Fluoride release from glass ionomer cements and resin composites coated with a dentin adhesive. Dent Mater. 2000;16(3):166–71.
111. Burgess J, Norling B, Summit J. Resin ionomer restorative materials: the new generation. J Esthe Dent. 1994;6:207–15.
112. Miranda LA, Weidlich P, Samuel SM, Maltz M. Fluoride release from restorative materials coated with an adhesive. Braz Dent J. 2002;13(1):39–43.
113. Jitaru S, Hodişan I, Timiş L, Lucian A, Bud M. The use of bioceramics in endodontics—literature review. Clujul Med. 2016;89(4):470–3.
114. Alex G. Direct and indirect pulp capping: a brief history, material innovations, and clinical case report. Compend Contin Educ Dent. 2018;39(3):182–9.
115. Maltz M, de Oliveira EF, Fontanella V, Bianchi R. A clinical, microbiologic, and radiographic study of deep caries lesions after incomplete caries removal. Quintessence Int. 2002;33(2):151–9.
116. Arandi NZ, Rabi T. Cavity bases revisited. Clin Cosmet Investig Dent. 2020;12:305–12.
117. Demarco FF, Corrêa MB, Cenci MS, Moraes RR, Opdam NJ. Longevity of posterior composite restorations: not only a matter of materials. Dent Mater. 2012;28(1):87–101.
118. Demarco FF, Collares K, Coelho-de-Souza FH, et al. Anterior composite restorations: a systematic review on long-term survival and reasons for failure. Dent Mater. 2015;31(10):1214–24.
119. Aminoroaya A, Esmaeely Neisiany R, Khorasani SN, Panahi P, Das O, Madry H, Cucchiarini M, Ramakrishna S. A review of dental composites: challenges, chemistry aspects, filler influences, and future insights. Compos Part B. 2021;216:108852.
120. Feilzer AJ, De Gee AJ, Davidson CL. Curing contraction of composites and glass-ionomer cements. J Prosthet Dent. 1988;59(3):297–300.
121. Gemalmaz D, Kukrer D. In vivo and in vitro evaluation of marginal fit of class II ceromer inlays. J Oral Rehabil. 2006;33:436–42.
122. Cho NY, Ferracane JL, Lee IB. Acoustic emission analysis of tooth-composite interfacial debonding. J Dent Res. 2013;92(1):76–81.
123. Jandt KD, Watts DC. Nanotechnology in dentistry: present and future perspectives on dental nanomaterials. Dent Mater. 2020;36(11):1365–78.
124. Choi KK, Ferracane JL, Hilton TJ, Charlton D. Properties of packable dental composites. J Esthet Dent. 2000;12(4):216–26.
125. Naoum S, Martin E, Ellakwa A. Long-term fluoride exchanges at restoration surfaces and effects on surface mechanical properties. ISRN Dent. 2013;2013:579039.
126. Rusnac ME, Gasparik C, Irimie AI, Grecu AG, Mesaroş AŞ, Dudea D. Giomers in dentistry—at the boundary between dental composites and glass-ionomers. Med Pharm Rep. 2019;92(2):123–8.
127. Finan L, Palin WM, Moskwa N, McGinley EL, Fleming GJ. The influence of irradiation potential on the degree of conversion and mechanical properties of two bulk-fill flowable RBC base materials. Dent Mater. 2013;29(8):906–12.
128. Ilie N. High viscosity bulk-fill giomer and ormocer-based resin composites: an in-vitro comparison of their mechanical behaviour. Stoma Edu J. 2016;3(1–2):54–62.
129. Krishna AR. Restorative materials: composite resins. In: Dental materials science. New Delhi: Jaypee Brothers Medical Publishers (P) Ltd; 2013. p. 130–48.
130. Nicholson J, Czarnecka B. Composite resins. In: Materials for the direct restoration of teeth. Sawston: Woodhead Publishing; 2016. p. 37–67.
131. Lavnya D, Divya B, Mantena SR, Madhu Varma K, Bheemalingeswara Rao D, Chandrappa V. Recent advances in dental composites: an overview. Int J Dent Mater. 2019;1(2):48–54.
132. Ilie N, Hickel R. Silorane-based dental composite: behavior and abilities. Dent Mater J. 2006;25(3):445–54.
133. Weinmann W, Thalacker C, Guggenberger R. Siloranes in dental composites. Dent Mater. 2005;21(1):68–74.

134. Kusgoz A, Ulker M, Yesilyurt C, Yoldas OH, Ozil M, Tanriver M. Silorane-based composite: depth of cure, surface hardness, degree of conversion, and cervical microleakage in class II cavities. J Esthet Restor Dent. 2001;23(5):324–35.
135. Papadogiannis D, Kakaboura A, Palaghias G, Eliades G. Setting characteristics and cavity adaptation of low-shrinking resin composites. Dent Mater. 2009;25(12):1509–16.
136. Kwon Y, Ferracane J, Lee IB. Effect of layering methods, composite type, and flowable liner on the polymerization shrinkage stress of light cured composites. Dent Mater. 2012;28(7):801–9.
137. Van Ende A, De Munck J, Mine A, Lambrechts P, Van Meerbeek B. Does a low-shrinking composite induce less stress at the adhesive interface? Dent Mater. 2010;26(3):215–22.
138. Babannavar R, Shenoy A. Evaluation of shear bond strength of silorane resin to conventional, resin-modified glass ionomers and nano-ionomer cements. J Investig Clin Dent. 2014;5(4):295–300.
139. Alzraikat H, Burrow MF, Maghaireh GA, Taha NA. Nanofilled resin composite properties and clinical performance: a review. Oper Dent. 2018;43(4):E173–90.
140. Chaput F, Faure AC. Dental composites. Techniques de l'Ingénieur. Technologies Biomédicales. 2021;23
141. Garcia D, Yaman P, Dennison J, Neiva G. Polymerization shrinkage and depth of cure of bulk fill flowable composite resins. Oper Dent. 2014;39(4):441–8.
142. Alrahlah A, Silikas N, Watts DC. Post-cure depth of cure of bulk fill dental resin-composites. Dent Mater. 2014;30(2):149–54.
143. Lempel E, Őri Z, Kincses D, Lovász BV, Kunsági-Máté S, Szalma J. Degree of conversion and in vitro temperature rise of pulp chamber during polymerization of flowable and sculptable conventional, bulk-fill and short-fibre reinforced resin composites. Dent Mater. 2021;37(6):983–97.
144. Kim RJ, Lee IB, Yoo JY, et al. Real-time analysis of temperature changes in composite increments and pulp chamber during photopolymerization. Biomed Res Int. 2015;2015:923808.
145. Uhl A, Volpel A, Sigusch BW. Influence of heat from light curing units and dental composite polymerization on cells in vitro. J Dent. 2006;34:298–306.
146. Weerrakoon AT, Meyers IA, Symons AL, Walsh LJ. Pulpal heat changes with newly developed resin photopolymerization systems. Aust Endod J. 2002;28:108–11.
147. Ikeda I, Otsuki M, Sadr A, Nomura T, Kishikawa R, Tagami J. Effect of filler content of flowable composites on resin-cavity interface. Dent Mater J. 2009;28(6):679–85.
148. Campodonico CE, Tantbirojn D, Olin PS, Versluis A. Cuspal deflection and depth of cure in resin-based composite restorations filled by using bulk, incremental and transtooth-illumination techniques. J Am Dent Assoc. 2011;142(10):1176–82.
149. Manhart J, et al. The face—a vascular perspective. a literature review. Swiss Dent J. 2014;124:29–37.
150. Schneider LF, Cavalcante LM, Silikas N. Shrinkage stresses generated during resin-composite applications: a review. J Dent Biomech. 2010;2010:131630.
151. Unterbrink GL, Liebenberg WH. Flowable resin composites as "filled adhesives": literature review and clinical recommendations. Quintessence Int. 1999;30(4):249–57.
152. Flowable Composites. ADA Professional Product Review. Spring. 2009;4(2).
153. Chuang SF, Jin YT, Lin TS, Chang CH, García-Godoy F. Effects of lining materials on microleakage and internal voids of class II resin-based composite restorations. Am J Dent. 2003;16(2):84–90.
154. Bore Gowda V, Sreenivasa Murthy BV, Hegde S, Venkataramanaswamy SD, Pai VS, Krishna R. Evaluation of gingival microleakage in class II composite restorations with different lining techniques: an in vitro study. Scientifica (Cairo). 2015;2015:896507.
155. Savage B, McWhorter AG, Kerins CA. Preventive resin restorations: practice and billing patterns of pediatric dentists. Pediatr Dent. 2009;31:210–5.
156. Beauchamp J, Caufield PW, Crall JJ, Donly K, Feigal R, Gooch B, et al. Evidence-based clinical recommendations for the use of pit-and-fissure sealants. J Am Dent Assoc. 2008;139:257–67.

157. Payne JH. The marginal seal of class ii restorations: flowable composite resin compared to injectable glass ionomer. J Clin Pediatr Dent. 1999;23:123–30.
158. Strassler HE. Predicatable and successful posterior packable class II composite resins. Am Dent Inst Continuing Educ. 2001;75:15–23.
159. Leevailoj C. Microleakage of posterior packable resin composites with and without flowable liners. Oper Dent. 2001;26:302–7.
160. Perez CR. Alternative technique for class V resin composite restorations with minimum finishing/polishing procedures. Oper Dent. 2010;35(3):375–9.
161. Fortin D, Vargas M. The Spectrum of composites: new techniques and materials. J Am Dent Assoc. 2000;131:26–30.
162. Reddy P, Jain V, Kaushik M, et al. Assessment of marginal integrity of proximal composite resin restorations performed with or without magnification. J Clin Diagn Res. 2017;11(12):ZC01–4.
163. Söderholm KJ. Dental adhesives how it all started and later evolved. J Adhes Dent. 2007;9(2):227–30.
164. Peumans M, De Munck J, Mine A, Van Meerbeek B. Clinical effectiveness of contemporary adhesives for the restoration of non-carious cervical lesions. A systematic review. Dent Mater. 2014;30:1089–103.
165. Perdigão J, Araujo E, Ramos RQ, Gomes G, Pizzolotto L. Adhesive dentistry: current concepts and clinical considerations. J Esthet Restor Dent. 2021;33(1):51–68.

2 Diagnosis, Planning, and Working Protocols

Although the prevalence of dental caries has declined in recent years, dental caries remain the most common condition worldwide [1]. More than 90% of adults, 20% of people from all age groups in the United States, and a third of people from all age groups worldwide have been diagnosed with dental caries [2]. According to a review by Eltahlah et al. [3], in 2018, 44% of dental restorations were made of composite resins, 40.9% made of amalgam, and 13.4% made of GIc or RMGIc.

The dentist must conduct a thorough and appropriate examination of the patient to assess the condition of the patient's dental, oral, and perioral tissues. This information should be correlated with the subjective aspects reported by the patient. The clinician identifies the dental, medical, and hereditary factors that are likely to be relevant for the present condition and its previous management if considered necessary. This way, an appropriate diagnosis of the condition is established by combining the information provided by history, anamnesis, and paraclinical investigations.

The examination aims to evaluate the anatomy and physiology of normal and abnormal intra- and extraoral structures and tissues and the existing treatments. The most common complementary examinations are retroalveolar radiography, bitewing radiography, panoramic radiography, CBCT scans, vitality tests, and hematological and microbiological tests.

This chapter will be focusing on anamnesis, examination, complementary investigations, diagnosis, treatment plan, clinical steps, and working protocol for direct restorations.

Supplementary Information The online version contains supplementary material available at https://doi.org/10.1007/978-3-031-55899-3_2. The videos can be accessed individually by clicking the DOI link in the accompanying figure caption or by scanning this link with the SN More Media App.

© The Author(s), under exclusive license to Springer Nature Switzerland AG 2024

M. Bud, *Direct Restorations*, https://doi.org/10.1007/978-3-031-55899-3_2

2.1 Anamnesis, Examination, Complementary Investigations, and Diagnosis

A detailed examination of the head and neck is carried out, trying simultaneously to pinpoint the signs and symptoms of systemic diseases. After that, a comprehensive examination of the oral cavity, teeth, and adjacent periodontal tissues is performed, distinguishing between the physiological and pathological conditions and processes.

The patient's oral health status is assessed using suitable clinical indices (hygiene, bleeding, abrasion, degree of mobility, etc.).

2.1.1 Exooral

The inspection is performed visually, and the preservation of facial symmetry and certain deformities that may appear are considered.

The palpation is performed with the hands, the occurrence of pain in particular areas of interest is assessed, any tooth sensitivity is assessed, and the identification and evaluation of lymph node sensitivity and the examination of normal or indurated tissue consistency are ultimately assessed.

2.1.2 Intraoral

2.1.2.1 Anamnesis: Subjective Tooth Examination

The preliminary information related to the history of a dental lesion is obtained from the patient. Thus, the doctor will find out from the patient whether there has been or there is painful symptomatology of the examined tooth and what its characteristics are: spontaneous or provoked, radiating or localized, and conditions of exacerbation and remission. Furthermore, the patient can report any previous treatments and details (possible accidents; complications; personal, functional, and aesthetic satisfaction; and previous radiographs that the patient might have).

The intraoral clinical examination for the restorative treatment of a tooth will include a subjective and objective dental examination and a periodontal and occlusal examination.

2.1.2.2 Objective Tooth Examination

This examination is always carried out under optimal visibility and lighting conditions, using a combination of direct and indirect vision (using the mirror). The essential condition for a reliable pit and fissure analysis is that the tooth surface must be clean to be accurately assessed. After a careful *airflow* cleaning with bicarbonate or glycine, examining the tooth surfaces with a magnification system (dental loupes or microscope) is always recommended. The possibility of misdiagnosis must be taken into account.

The dental surfaces should be air-dried for a minimum of 5 s to correctly assess the texture and to identify any existing restorations more efficiently, as well as the type of material used for them. The examination will include inspection, the use on an explorer, axial and lateral percussion, and mobility assessment.

During the inspection, the following things are going to be assessed: any lack of substance and its location, the existence of pigmentations in pits and fissures, the existence of tooth discolorations, and the existence of previous restorations on the tooth. For these restorations, the position, the extent, and the material will be identified, and the restorations will be checked for appropriate marginal sealing, morphology, and aesthetics.

The cracks and fractures discovered during the inspection may significantly impact the later treatment decision. Although inspection is one of the most common methods of caries diagnosis [4, 5], it is not necessarily very effective.

Identifying proximal caries through direct visual examination is tricky, but studies carried out with several observers have shown a high degree of disagreement among each other [6]. Visual inspection can only be done on visible tooth surfaces. Many tooth surfaces cannot be examined this way, and possible carious lesions can be missed. Dentists cannot always determine the slight visual and tactile differences between the active and inactive enamel lesions by performing a single clinical examination [7].

When using an explorer, the depth of a cavity or missing substance can be pinpointed and the sensitivity to touch or pressure.

When the percussion test is performed with the metal handle of an instrument, in the tooth axis, it is possible to evaluate whether there is an inflammation of the periapical periodontium. When the percussion is performed laterally, perpendicular to the tooth axis, the inflammation of the marginal periodontium can be assessed. The presence of sensitivity or pain indicates a positive percussion test.

When assessing tooth mobility, the doctor will assess whether there is an excellent, medium to long-term prognosis for the examined tooth. This way, they will make the most appropriate restorative decision to maintain the tooth.

The doctor will make the teeth chart based on the objective dental examination information. The chart includes listing the existing treatments and the lesions observed by the doctor during examination: carious lesions, previously prepared cavities, non-carious wear lesions, cracks, fractures, etc.

The doctor can use several classifications to categorize caries, prepared cavities, or wear lesions. These are the following:

1. Carious lesions are mainly classified using ICDAS and FDI indices.
2. Prepared cavities after the removal of carious processes can be classified using the system proposed by Black (classes I–VI), Mount and Hume (also called SiSta, acronym of Site and Stage) [8], etc.
3. Non-carious lesions and wear lesions can be classified using the indices proposed by Smith and Knight.

The most commonly used carious lesion classification system is ICDAS [9] (International Caries Detection and Assessment System).

The ICDAS I and II criteria incorporate concepts from research by Ekstrand et al. [10, 11] and other caries detection systems described by Ismail [12].

ICDAS II codes:

Code 0—Healthy tooth surface: no signs of caries after 5 s of air drying.
Code 1—First visual change in enamel: opacity or discoloration (white or brown), is visible at the entrance to the pit or fissure seen after prolonged air drying.
Code 2—Distinct visual change in enamel when it is wet; the lesion must be visible when dry.
Code 3—Localized enamel breakdown (without clinical visual signs of dentinal involvement) seen when wet and after prolonged drying.
Code 4—Underlying dark shadow from dentine.
Code 5—Distinct cavity with visible dentine.
Code 6—Extensive (more than half the surface) distinct cavity with visible dentine.

However, in daily clinical practice, the most commonly used classification method of carious lesions is based on the location and estimated depth of the cavities (e.g., superficial occlusal caries, deep mesio-occlusal caries, etc.).

Black or Mount and Hume (SiSta) described the most commonly used classifications for prepared cavities, and they bear their names.

Classes of caries in Black's classification:

Class I—Cavities involving pits and fissures on the occlusal surfaces of molars and premolars, occlusal two-thirds of buccal surfaces of molars and premolars and oral surfaces of anterior upper teeth
Class II—Cavities involving proximal surfaces of molars and premolars
Class III—Cavities involving proximal surfaces of central incisors, lateral incisors, and canines without involving incisal angles
Class IV—Cavities involving proximal surfaces including incisal angles of anterior teeth
Class V—Cavities involving gingival one-third of buccal or lingual surfaces of anterior or posterior teeth
Class VI—Cavities involving cusp tips of molars, premolars, and canines

Non-carious dental lesions are mainly represented by tooth wear:

- Attrition—physiological wear
- Erosion—chemical wear
- Abrasion—wear due to an interposed object
- Abfraction—wear at a distance due to occlusal trauma

The most commonly used classification system for non-carious lesions is the one proposed by Smith and Knight [13]:

Code 0—No loss of enamel surface characteristics. No change in contour
Code 1—Loss of enamel characteristics. Minimal loss of contour

Code 2—Loss of enamel exposing dentine for less than one-third of the surface, loss of enamel just exposing dentine, and defects less than 1 mm deep

Code 3—Loss of enamel exposing dentine for more than one-third of the surface. Loss of enamel and substantial loss of dentine, but not exposing the pulp of secondary dentine. Defect 1–2 mm deep

Code 4—Complete loss of enamel, pulp exposure, or exposure of secondary dentine. Defect more than 2 mm deep

2.1.3 Periodontal Examination

The periodontal examination aims to identify the clinical signs of the periodontal disease that concern the clinician who performs the direct restorations:

- Inflammation in the marginal periodontium or in the interdental papilla where the bleeding is favored by inflammation, and that could negatively affect the isolation required for direct restorations, especially in the bonding and layering phase
- Gingival recession
- Periodontal pockets
- Secondary migration
- Dental mobility

The presence of calculus and pigmentation prevents optimal restorations, which is why they must be removed before treatment.

In the case of subgingival damage, the doctor must assess the presence or violation of the biological height. This is the height of the gingival tissue attached to the tooth above the bone crest, with an average value of 2.04 mm [14]. Therefore, the distance between the dental limit of the marginal threshold of a proximal cavity and the bone level (bone sounding) should be evaluated. This can be done with a periodontal probe after the installation of anesthesia (it is recommended in the absence of gingival inflammation or on radiographs).

If the measured size is less than 2 mm, then the biological space is invaded, and a crown lengthening with partial resection of the bone septum may be performed to ensure the appropriate biological space. Placing a restoration too deeply, subgingivally, will maintain the constant inflammation of the interdental papilla [15]. This leads to qualitative and quantitative changes in microflora, increased plaque index, gingival recession, and periodontal pockets [16]. Nevins and Skurow recommend limiting the subgingival extension to 0.5–1.0 mm because it is impossible for the clinician to detect where the sulcus epithelium ends and where the junctional epithelium begins [17].

2.1.4 Occlusion Examination

Occlusion examination is very important for future direct restorations. The clinician needs to know the initial occlusal relationships because after cavity preparation, certain morphological elements (fissures, marginal edges, etc.)—which contribute

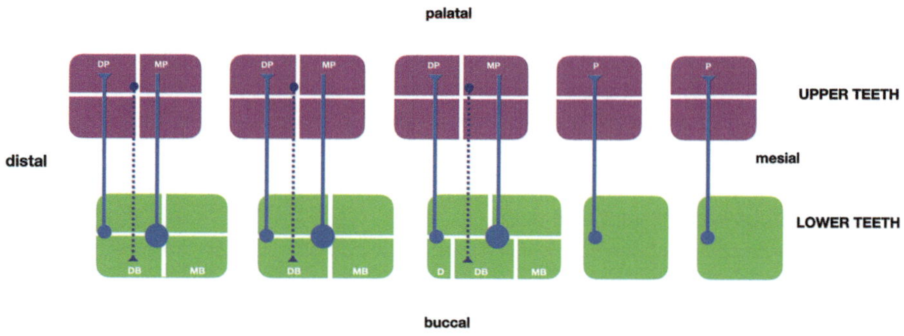

Fig. 2.1 The occlusal contacts of posterior teeth diagram: class I stops and class III stops

to occlusal stops—may disappear. In these cases, direct composite resin restorations are designed to restore these occlusal stops:

1. **Class I stops**: the buccal cusps of the mandibular posterior teeth come into contact with the mesial marginal ridge of the counterpart and the distal ridge of the tooth situated mesially to it. The distobuccal cusps of the lower M2 and M3, plus the distobuccal cusp of the lower M1, come into a three-point contact with the central fossa of the superiors (Fig. 2.1—indicated with purple dotted lines). Thus, the marginal ridge are anatomical elements of utmost importance that absorb the occlusal forces, which is why their restoration must be done in an anatomical way and with appropriate contact with the antagonists.
2. **Class II stops**: the incisal edges of the mandibular incisors come into contact with the palatal surfaces of the upper supra-cingular frontal teeth.
3. **Class III stops**: the palatal cusps of the premolars and the distopalatal cusps of the upper molars come into contact with the distal fossae of the lower counterparts. The mesio-palatal cusps of the upper molars come into contact with the antagonistic central fossa (Fig. 2.1—indicated by blue lines).

2.1.5 Complementary Examinations

The complementary examinations most commonly used in clinical practice for direct restorations are:

- Classical vitality tests using vitality spray
- Cold sensitivity tests with water/air spray
- Imaging examinations

Proximal caries can be missed on visual examination as they are not visible to the eye (Fig. 2.2). They can be detected on periapical or bitewing radiographs (Fig. 2.3). Bitewing radiographs are the best choice for proximal caries diagnosis, providing the most accurate radiological image of the proximal areas.

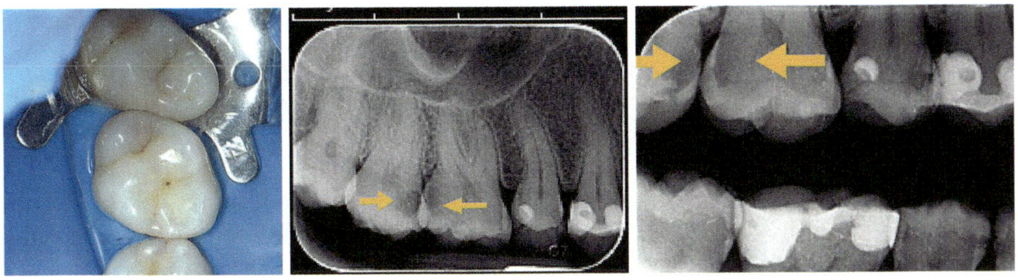

Fig. 2.2 Proximal caries on 16–17: intraoral occlusal photo

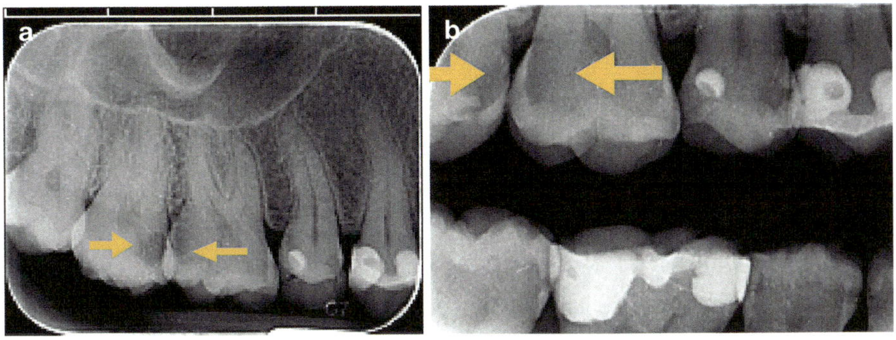

Fig. 2.3 Periapical radiography (**a**); bitewing radiography (**b**)

Besides these types of X-rays, panoramic X-rays and CBCT scans are also widely used; usually, for other purposes, the doctor can use them in order to avoid additional exposures.

The decision to conduct a radiological examination is made per the principles of ALARA (as low as reasonably achievable). Whether a radiological examination could provide more information to influence the treatment decision or help achieve it is always considered.

It is recommended to be done reliably and effectively, and the relevant imaging techniques will be accurately interpreted and documented. Interpretation of radiological images should aim to identify radiolucencies that can be correlated with lack of hard dental substance: carious processes, cavities where fillings have been dislodged, fractures of teeth or restorative materials, voids in restorative materials, interface voids, or marginal sealing deficiency.

The relationship of these radiolucency areas with the pulp chamber reveals the therapeutic approach that needs to be followed: capping, liners, etc.

2.1.6 Other Complementary Examinations

Noninvasive examination methods can be based on fluorescence, transillumination, OCT (optical coherence tomography), flossing, etc.

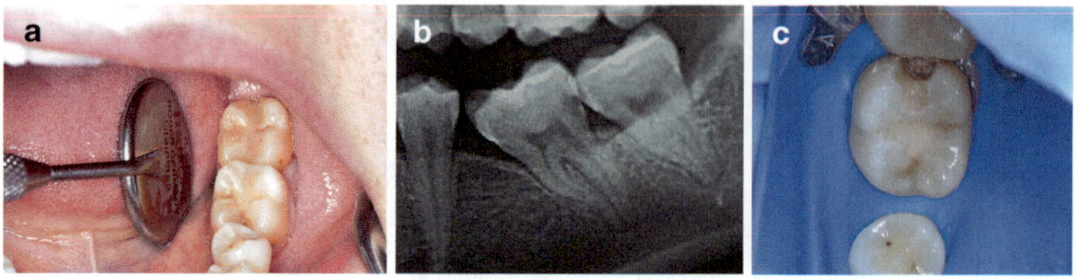

Fig. 2.4 Distal caries on tooth 37: visual inspection (**a**); radiological examination (**b**); aspect with rubber dam in place; after removal of the distal marginal ridge (**c**)

The doctor makes a diagnosis given the information gathered from the anamnesis and examination. Possible common diagnoses:

- A carious lesion, where the location and depth are specified
- Marginal secondary caries, where the location is indicated
- Recurrent caries
- Coronal fracture of the hard dental substance or restorative material
- Dislocated filling

For a present restoration, it is recommended to mention the material and the location, if the restoration is adequate in terms of marginal sealing, morphology, and aesthetics.

Following this examination sheet, the doctor can design a simplified presentation case, focusing only on the tooth or teeth targeted for treatment. These simplified case presentations help the communication between the doctor and students develop a structured and detailed thinking style about the case they are treating (Fig. 2.4).

2.2 Generating and Communicating a Treatment Plan

2.2.1 Generating the Treatment Plan

The patient has to be involved in the decision-making process for the treatment plan. For this to be practical, the patient needs to understand their dental health status; associated problems; treatment options; including the benefits and limitations of each option; and the prognosis and long-term impact of expected clinical outcomes. The treatment options will be prioritized according to the patient's complaints and symptoms, and an effective personalized treatment plan will be outlined. This plan is designed to achieve or maintain oral health and help preserve teeth and oral health by considering the patient's expectations, ability to accept different interventions, and level of cooperation.

The patient will be involved in all decision-making processes. The patient should be counseled on the proposed options, advantages, disadvantages, and risks, including biological and iatrogenic conditions and the consequences of refusing the proposed treatments. The physician must estimate and justify the prognosis of treatment options.

Treatment planning should always start with stabilization and prevention measures. After each phase of the treatment, the progress and the following steps should be reviewed and, where clinically indicated, changed with the patient's consent. Restorative treatment plan options may include:

- Direct restorations of different materials (fillings, direct veneers, direct onlays)
- Indirect restorations (inlays, onlays)
- Ceramic crowns or veneers, etc.

The suggested treatment plan should end with a review of these options, including the timeline of various steps, after which the patient accepted and signed should confirm it.

If a specific case is beyond his or her capabilities, the general dentist will decide when it is necessary to refer the patient to a more experienced colleague or a specialist (orthodontist, surgeon, periodontist, endodontist, pedodontist, or prosthodontist). We recommend writing a medical letter or a referral form where details about the case are clearly stated and what is expected from the colleague to whom the patient is referred.

2.2.2 Communicating the Treatment Plan

No matter how much a dentist believes it is medically necessary to perform a treatment, it is 100% up to the patient if they accept or refuse it. Medical ethics oblige us to present in an obvious and convincing way, with plausible arguments, the need for the patient's treatment. Even if it seems unlikely, there are situations when the effort to educate and inform the patient about the danger of not carrying out a treatment/retreatment is greater than that of carrying out the treatment itself. To explain the treatment plan, the doctor has all the documented material collected during the clinical examination stage (e.g., intraoral and extraoral photographs) (Fig. 2.5) and the complementary investigation stage (e.g., radiological investigations.) The doctor can pinpoint similar cases previously treated or can present educational models (e.g., molding, similar real prosthetic works, etc.). At the same time, the clinician should not suggest more treatments than necessary, exploiting the patient's lack of information or their unjustified wishes.

A possible list of recommendations for dealing with the patient and validating an appropriate and realistic treatment plan is as follows:

1. Learning, mastering, and applying communication skills
2. Paying more attention to nonverbal communication (posture during conversations, looks, gestures)
3. Identifying the patient's personality type to find the proper communication channels

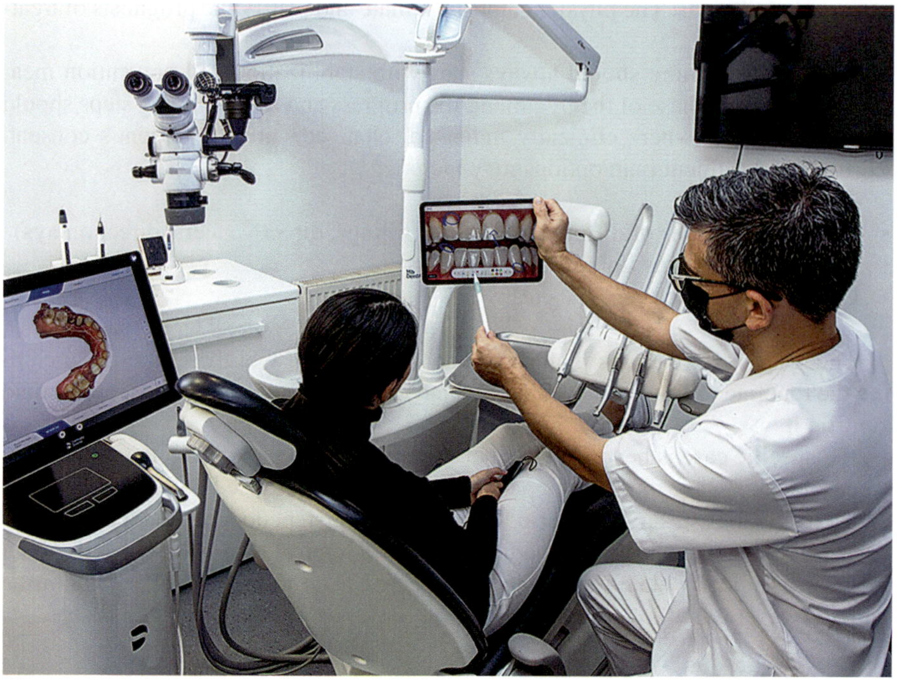

Fig. 2.5 Discussion with the patient, presentation of similar cases, or a particular digital design

4. Good management of the first visit (telephone contact, reception, contact with the doctor, consultation, treatment plan and payment estimate, final discussion)
5. Documentation of the clinical case (radiological imaging, photographs, video recordings, specialized records: endodontic, restorative, periodontal, orthodontic, aesthetic)
6. Informing the patient about the evolution and the postoperative recommendations at the patient's level of comprehension
7. Making a treatment plan by considering the skills of other doctors who could be involved
8. Making a treatment plan that satisfies both the dentist's medical vision and the patient's needs and preferences
9. Informing and explaining the need to follow the proposed treatment plan, the evolution of the conditions if the plan is not followed, implementation, and monitoring costs.
10. Informing about the need to work in a team with other colleagues to carry out the agreed, accepted, and signed plan by the patient

2.3 Clinical Steps to Perform a Direct Restoration: Working Protocol

The crown restoration can be achieved, in most cases, by following one of the four main approaches [18]:

1. Direct: one clinical session (preparation + restoration); two clinical sessions by indirect pulp capping or two clinical sessions, one restoration, and one finishing session (especially in frontal restorations)
2. Semi-direct: one clinical session + laboratory stage carried out in the dental practice (preparation, impression, final restoration, cementation)
3. Semi-indirect: two clinical sessions + one laboratory stage in the dental practice (preparation, impression, provisional restoration, final restoration, cementation)
4. Indirect: two clinical sessions + one laboratory stage carried out by the technician in the laboratory (preparation, impressions, provisional restoration, final restoration, cementation); or indirectly in one session (preparation, digital impressions, CAD/CAM milling in the dental cabinet, cementation).

The significant steps to perform a direct restoration in the posterior area that is generally valid:

(A) **Initial analysis:**
  1. Identifying the intermaxillary occlusal relationships and extension in surface and depth and evaluating the oblique ridge characteristics on the antagonist tooth
  2. Preliminary assessment of remaining occlusal contacts with articulating paper and virtually designing the future preparation/restoration contour
  3. Evaluation of the marginal ridge correlated with the neighboring tooth
  4. Choosing the color

(B) **Pre-restoration procedure:**

If necessary at this stage, duplication procedures (occlusal key, palatal key, individualized ring for matrices) (see Sect. 3.1) and supragingival cavity margin acquisition techniques (see Sect. 3.2) are performed.

The following steps are taken prior to the actual direct restoration in a clinical sequence:
  1. Pre-restoration duplication procedures (stamp technique, custom ring) (Sect. 3.1)
  2. Subgingival margin acquisition procedures (deep margin elevation, gingivectomy, crown lengthening) (Sect. 3.2)
  3. Anesthesia and rubber dam isolation (Sect. 3.3).
  4. Pre-separation and protection of neighboring teeth (prewedging, wedgeguarding) (Sect. 3.4)
  5. Cavity design and preparation (Sect. 3.5)
  6. Cavity completion: cavity detector check, beveling, and disinfection (Sect. 3.6)

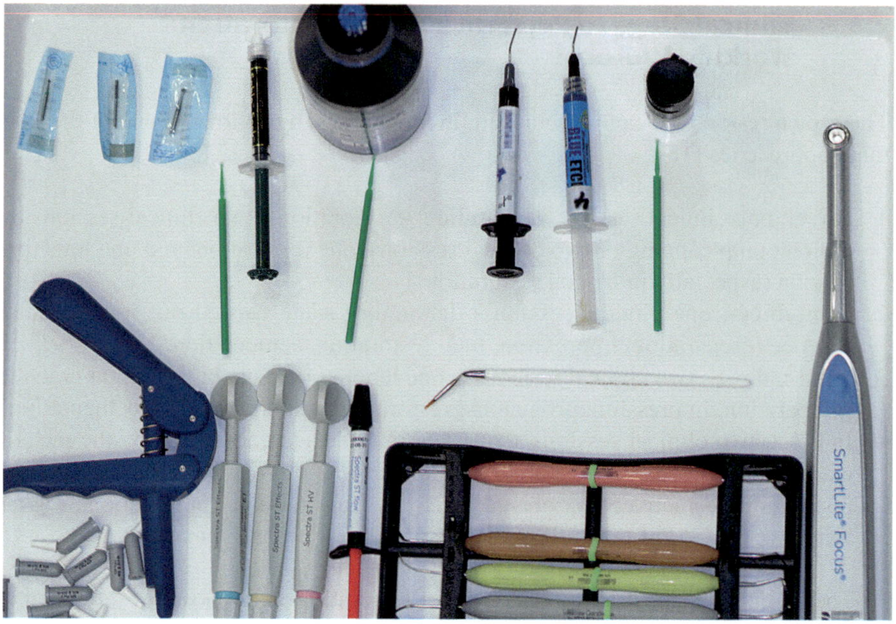

Fig. 2.6 Basic instruments and materials set up for direct restoration

7. Pulp protection or limitation of preparation and expectation: direct capping and indirect capping (Sect. 3.7)

   In order to perform a cavity preparation and the direct restoration (in the case of a cavity that does not require any duplication technique, nor does it require contact with the subgingival limits), the necessary instruments and materials are made ready (Fig. 2.6), starting with anesthesia.

(C) **Direct composite restoration:**

1. Matrix Selection and Application (Chap. 4)
2. Transformation into class I cavity using different wall restoration techniques (Sects. 4.1, 4.2, and 4.3)
3. Filling the cavity with composite layering or bulk and then achieving occlusal morphology (Chap. 5)
4. Finishing, occlusal adjustments, and polishing (Chap. 6)
5. Postoperative indications for the patient, follow-up scheduling, and failure of management (Chap. 10)

Briefly, the preparation of a medium or deep cavity is followed by disinfection, liner application, etch conditioning (Fig. 2.7), adhesive application, application of fluid or bulk composite, filling the cavity with composite, achieving occlusal

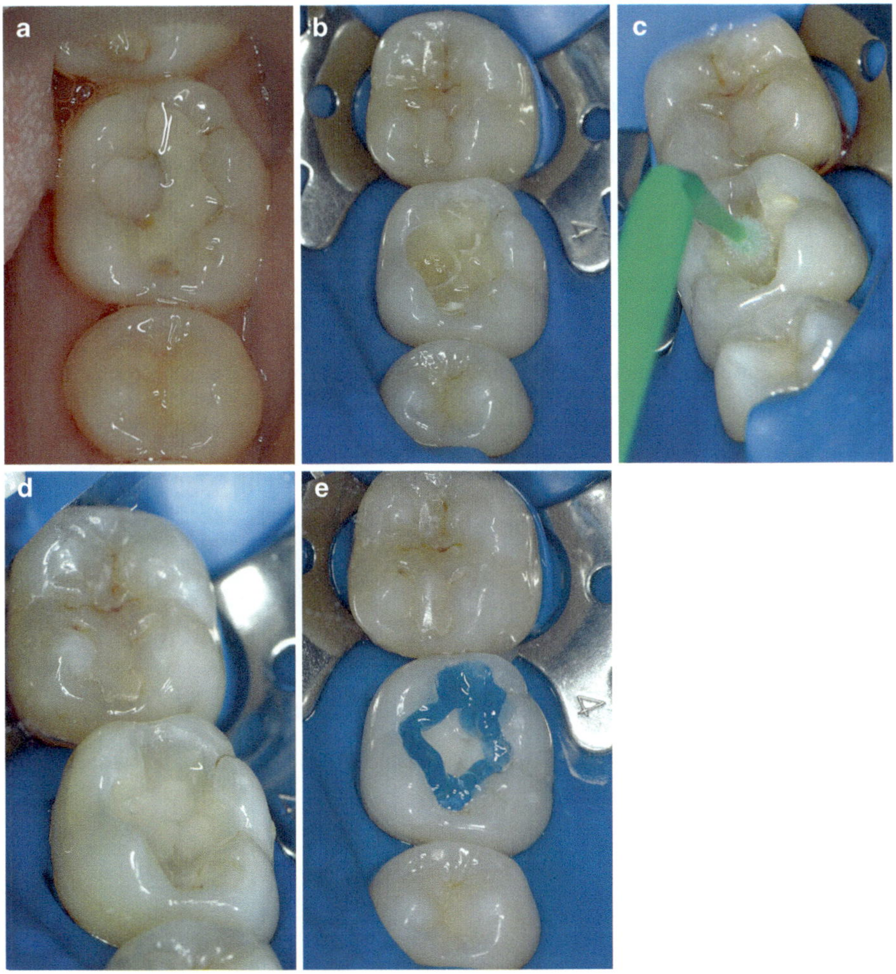

Fig. 2.7 Initial aspect of an improper composite resin occlusal restoration on tooth 36 (**a**); aspect after the removal of the old filling (**b**); disinfection of the cavity with CHX (**c**); aspect after liner application (**d**); enamel demineralization (**e**)

morphology (Fig. 2.8), occlusal check, occlusal adjustments, finishing, and polishing (Figs. 2.9 and 2.10).

A direct restoration sheet can be added to the patient's file record, containing the examination outlined above and a summary of the working protocol (Fig. 2.11). This has didactic value for students and clinical and forensic value, so it provides more details about the progress of a case.

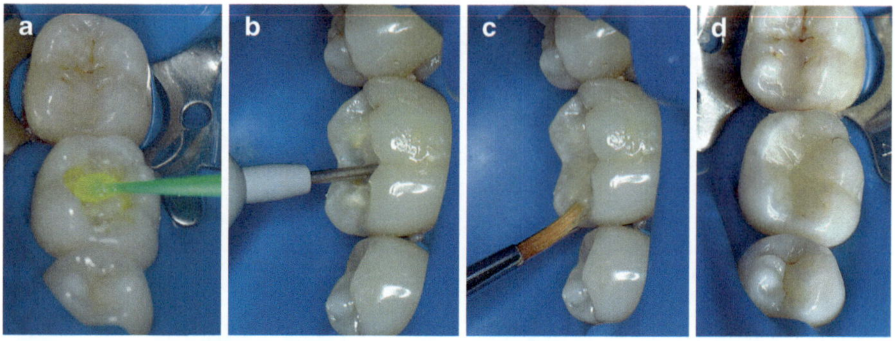

Fig. 2.8 Adhesive application (**a**); filling the cavity with bulk flowable composite resin (SDR) up to 1.5 mm to the occlusal surface (**b**); application of superficial packable composite layer and shaping the occlusal morphology by successive cusps technique (**c**); final aspect before occlusal adjustments, finishing, and polishing (**d**)

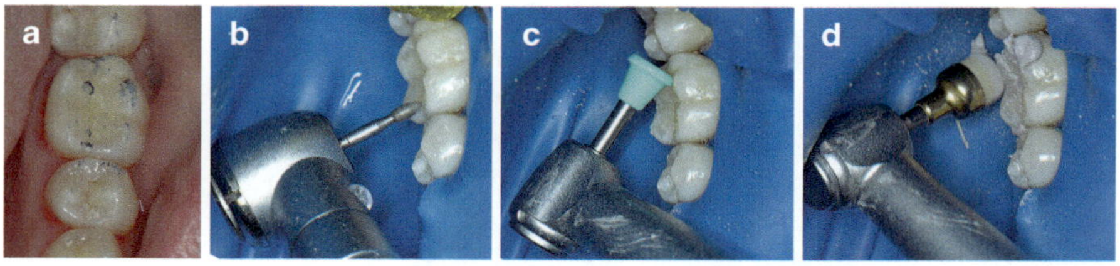

Fig. 2.9 Checking the restoration and static and dynamic occlusion (**a**); occlusal adjustments (**b**); finishing (**c**); polishing (**d**)

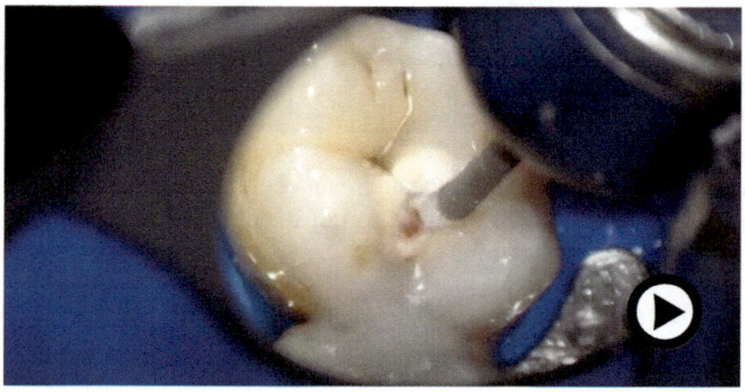

Fig. 2.10 Preparation of an occlusal cavity on the molar, steps to achieve direct composite resin restoration (▶ https://doi.org/10.1007/000-bqh)

2.3.1 Restoration Perspective

The increasing standardization level of a procedure implies increasing the work ergonomics, decreasing execution time, and obtaining predictable results. Standardizing all proximal/MOD cavities, which are easily attainable, such as the

WORKING PROTOCOL	□ ultrasonic scaling, professional brushing, airflow	
Anesthesia	□ No; Yes: □ buccal infiltration; □ block; □ intraligamentary	
Isolation	□ rubber dam; □ dental floss ligatures on teeth............................□ cotton rolls	
Cavity preparation (class) :	□ carie indicator; □ burrs □ US diamond tips; □ excavator	
Filling	□ Direct pulp capping	□ saline solution.; □ MTA; □ Ca(OH)2; ; □ GiC
Matrix used:	□ Indirect pulp capping	□ saline solution; □ CHX; □ Ca(OH)2; □ GiC; □
□ Palodent;	□ Composite resin	Color: dentin: ..../.......enamel:............ Brand:........................
□ TOR-VM;	- cavity disinfection	□ CHX; □ .....
□ Polidentia **Other**	- liner	□ Ca(OH)2; □ GiC; □ .....
	- adhesiv system	
	Layering technique □ oblique; □ bulk; □	
	Ocusal morphology modelling technique □ succesive cusps □ essential lines [?] stamp □ ...	
Finishing & Polishing		
Postoperative recommendations		

Fig. 2.11 Example of a possible restoration chart for the techniques, materials, and tools used

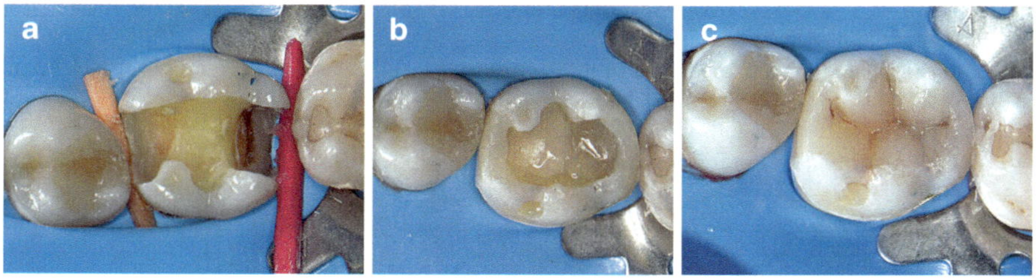

Fig. 2.12 Aspect of a MOD cavity (**a**); aspect after proximal wall restoration (**b**); filling the cavity and application of the last layer of composite with the restoration of the occlusal morphology (**c**)

medium depth class I cavity or shallow cavity, helps the overall restoration procedure, and we strongly recommend doing so.

Therefore, in order to simplify the management of composite resin restorations in class II or MOD cavities, we propose to separate the procedure into three distinct stages (Fig. 2.12a–c) due to clinical workflow, predictability, and phase control considerations:

1. Conversion of all proximal cavities to class I cavities through the initial restoration of the proximal walls/marginal ridges, according to the centripetal technique described in the literature [19]
2. Filling the cavity by layering or bulk, up to 1.5 mm from the occlusal surface
3. Performing occlusal morphology

Conclusion

The analysis, diagnosis, and treatment plan stage can be summarized as the anamnesis and the accurate examination of the patient, developing a realistic treatment plan that satisfies both medical rigor and the patient's wishes, and the doctor's practical capabilities, communicating and agreeing on the treatment plan and implementing the treatment plan.

Review Questions

1. What is anamnesis, and what is oral examination?
2. What are the most common and essential diagnoses for restorative dentistry?
3. What is the initial analysis stage for a restorative treatment?
4. What is the stage of the pre-restorative procedure for a restorative treatment?
5. What are the steps of a direct restoration?
6. What are three possible distinct stages of direct restoration which ensure good workflow and predictable results?

References

1. Marcenes W, Kassebaum NJ, Bernabé E, Flaxman A, Naghavi M, Lopez A, Murray CJ. Global burden of oral conditions in 1990–2010: a systematic analysis. J Dent Res. 2013;92(7):592–7.
2. Dye BA, Li X, Beltran-Aguilar ED. Selected oral health indicators in the United States, 2005–2008. NCHS Data Brief. 2012;96:1–8.
3. Eltahlah D, Lynch CD, Chadwick BL, Blum IR, Wilson NHF. An update on the reasons for placement and replacement of direct restorations. J Dent. 2018;72:1–7.
4. Gomez J. Detection and diagnosis of the early caries lesion. BMC Oral Health. 2015;15 Suppl 1(Suppl 1):S3.
5. Diniz MB, Eckert GJ, González-Cabezas C, Cordeiro Rde C, Ferreira-Zandona AG. Caries detection around restorations using ICDAS and optical devices. J Esthet Restor Dent. 2016;28(2):110–21.
6. Hintze H, Wenzel A, Danielsen B, Nyvad B. Reliability of visual examination, fibre-optic transillumination, and bite-wing radiography, and reproducibility of direct visual examination following tooth separation for the identification of cavitated carious lesions in contacting approximal surfaces. Caries Res. 1998;32(3):204–9.
7. Ekstrand KR, Ricketts DN, Longbottom C, Pitts NB. Visual and tactile assessment of arrested initial enamel carious lesions: an in vivo pilot study. Caries Res. 2005;39(3):173–7.
8. Mount GJ, Tyas JM, Duke ES, Hume WR, Lasfargues JJ, Kaleka R. A proposal for a new classification of lesions of exposed tooth surfaces. Int Dent J. 2006;56(2):82–91.
9. Gugnani N, Pandit IK, Srivastava N, Gupta M, Sharma M. International caries detection and assessment system (ICDAS): a new concept. Int J Clin Pediatr Dent. 2011;4(2):93–100.
10. Ekstrand KR, Ricketts DN, Kidd EA. Reproducibility and accuracy of three methods for assessment of demineralization depth of the occlusal surface: an in vitro examination. Caries Res. 1997;31(3):224–31.
11. Ekstrand KR, Kuzmina I, Bjorndal L, Thyrlstrup A. Relationship between external and histologic features of progressive stages of caries in the occlusal fossa. Caries Res. 1995;29(4):243–50.
12. Ismail AI. Visual and visuo-tactile detection of dental caries. J Dent Res. 2004;83:C56–66.
13. Smith BG, Knight JK. An index for measuring the wear of teeth. Br Dent J. 1984;156:435–8.
14. Gargiulo AW, Wentz FM, Orban B. Dimensions and relations of the dentogingival junction in humans. J Periodontol. 1961;32:261–7.
15. Waerhaug J. Healing of the dento-epithelial junction following subgingival plaque control. II: as observed on extracted teeth. J Periodontol. 1978;49:119–34.

16. Newman MG, Takei H, Klokkevold PR, Carranza FA. Carranza's clinical periodontology. 10th ed. Philadelphia: Saunders; 2006.
17. Nevins M, Skurow HM. The intracrevicular restorative margin, the biologic width, and the maintenance of the gingival margin. Int J Periodont Restor Dent. 1984;4:30–49.
18. Magne P. Non-invasive bilaminar CAD/CAM composite resin veneers: a semi-(in)direct approach. Int J Esthet Dent. 2017;12(2):134–54.
19. Bichacho N. The centripetal build-up for composite resin posterior restorations. Pract Periodontics Aesthet Dent. 1994;6(3):17–24.

Pre-restoration Procedures That Are Carried Out Before Direct Restoration

3

In all cases, some pre-restoration procedures are needed. If necessary, for some cases, duplication procedures (occlusal key, palatal key, individualized ring for matrices) or supragingival cavity margin acquisition techniques (deep margin elevation, gingivectomy, crown lengthening) may be performed. Rubber dam isolation is mandatory for a direct restoration. For class two cavities, pre-separation and protection of neighboring teeth (prewedging, wedgeguarding) **may be very helpful.** This chapter will be focusing on all these topics.

3.1 Techniques for Copying Preexisting Morphology

3.1.1 Impression of the Occlusal Surface to Produce an Occlusal Key/"Stamp Technique"

Main idea: The occlusal morphology of a direct restoration can be achieved by using an occlusal key. This can be accomplished by copying the original occlusal morphology with a light-curing flowable material.

This method can be successfully used in the case of occlusal caries with a minimal lack of substance, which has kept relatively intact the occlusal morphology. Most commonly, occlusal keys are made of liquid rubber dam.

Supplementary Information The online version contains supplementary material available at https://doi.org/10.1007/978-3-031-55899-3_3. The videos can be accessed individually by clicking the DOI link in the accompanying figure caption or by scanning this link with the SN More Media App.

© The Author(s), under exclusive license to Springer Nature Switzerland AG 2024

M. Bud, *Direct Restorations*, https://doi.org/10.1007/978-3-031-55899-3_3

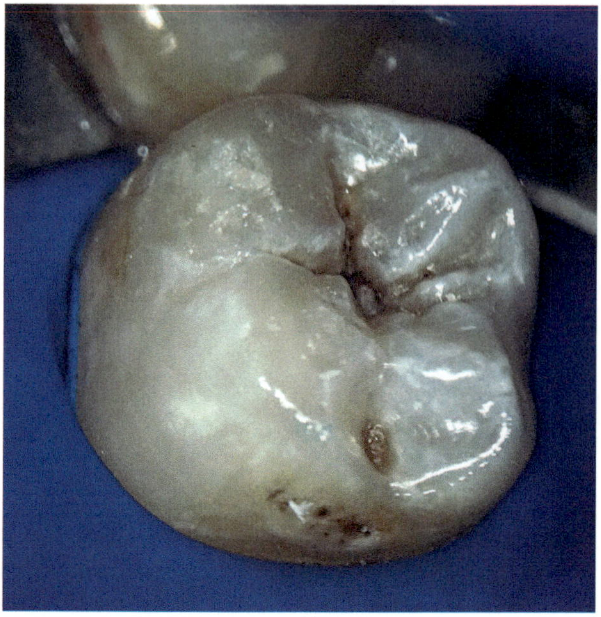

Fig. 3.1 Occlusal caries on the molar after rubber dam isolation, with the occlusal anatomy relatively preserved

The steps to make an occlusal key using a liquid rubber dam are as follows:

1. Occlusal surface examination. If there are small cavities, a temporary material can be applied before the impression to avoid the impression material penetrating the cavity. All the procedures should be performed after the rubber dam isolation (Fig. 3.1).
2. Lubricate the occlusal surface so the liquid dam does not stick to the tooth. This can be done with glycerine gel or an oily liquid from the dentist's cabinet. In most cases, simple wetting is enough to prevent the liquid dam from adhering to the occlusal surface.
3. Apply a layer of rubber liquid dam over the entire occlusal surface, no more than 1 mm thick, position the tip of the microbrush centrally, and cover it with the liquid dam (Fig. 3.2). The applicator's handle will act as a guide for positioning the key during the obturation phase, which is why it is recommended to maintain its position. The entire mass of the liquid dam is light-cured, and then the occlusal key can be removed (Fig. 3.3). If it is difficult to remove it, a dental explorer can be used to remove it. Obturators or other instruments may be used instead of the microbrush. Silicone-based impression materials (transparent or opaque) may be used to make the key, besides the diacrylic composite resins. In case of using opaque impression materials, their disadvantage may show up during light-curing the final restoration.
4. Cavity preparation, cavity checking and disinfection, application of the adhesive system, application of the composite and its polymerization so that 1.5 mm remains accessible to the occlusal surface, and the space required for the

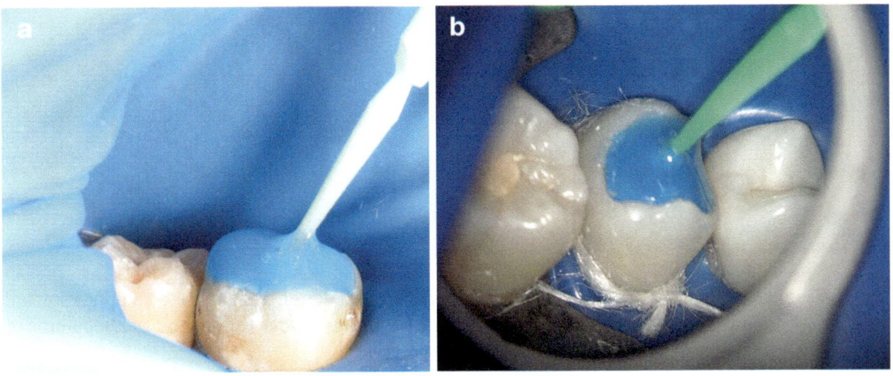

Fig. 3.2 Making a liquid dam occlusal key in which a microbrush was fixed to the molar (**a**) and premolar (**b**)

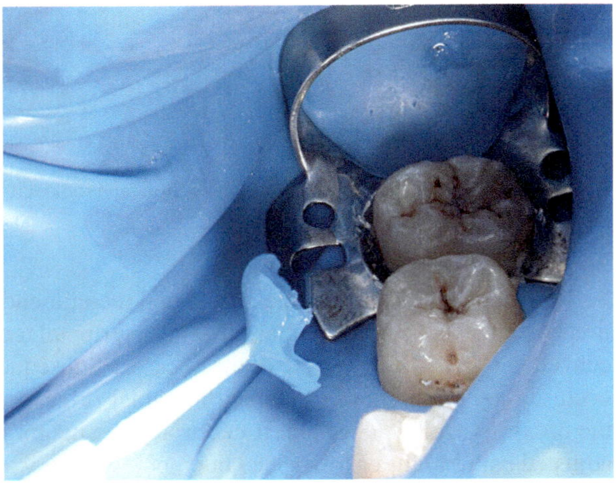

Fig. 3.3 The liquid dam occlusal key aspect after light-curing the material and removal from the occlusal surface

application of the last composite layer that is going to be conformed to the occlusal key.

5. Applying and shaping the last layer of composite, applying a PTFE (Teflon) tape as a separator between the unpolymerized composite and the occlusal key, and pressing it to engrave the initially copied morphology (Fig. 3.4).
6. A short light-curing session of a maximum of 5 s is done through the occlusal key, after which the key and PTFE tape are removed (Fig. 3.5). The excess composite resulting from pressing the occlusal key shall be removed with a hand tool (e.g., an explorer), and the composite light-curing will be continued according to the manufacturer's instructions.
7. Finishing and polishing the restoration follows the usual working protocol.

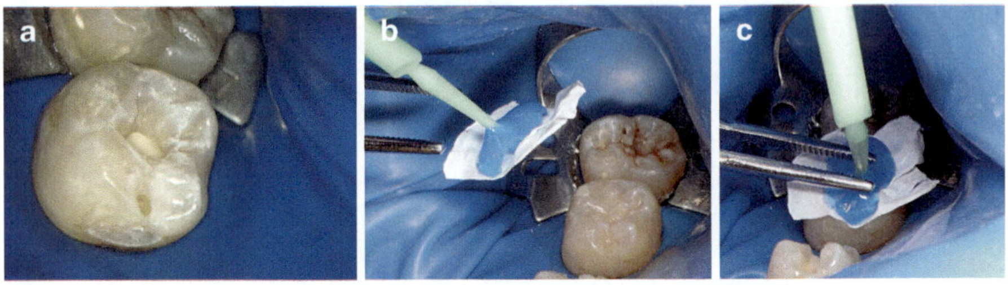

Fig. 3.4 Prepared occlusal cavity after liner application and demineralization (**a**); application and superficial shaping of the composite resin (**b**), the occlusal key, and a Teflon tape as a separator (**c**)

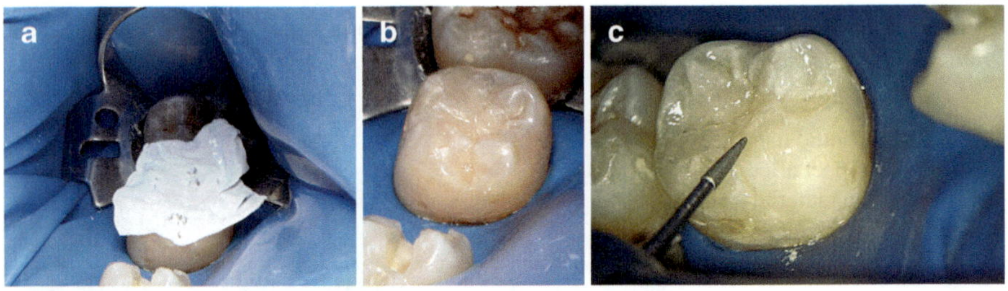

Fig. 3.5 Occlusal key removed (**a**) and the Teflon tape removed (**b**), excess removal, and occlusal adjustment and finishing (**c**)

This method was initially described and recommended for class I cavity restoration but can also be used for class II. The centripetal technique is always chosen for conversion to class I cavities in these cases. Subsequently, the positioning of the occlusal key on the newly obtained marginal ridge, which has been restored from the proximal wall, is checked. If necessary, the height of the marginal ridge can be adjusted using high- or low-speed burs, but without water. The resulting composite powder is air-blown, and a new layer of adhesive is applied, after which obturation can continue.

Difficulties that may occur	Potential solutions
Occlusal key fracture due to pressure	It can be repaired by adding a liquid rubber dam to its exterior. If this is impossible to be done, stop using it and continue with manual shaping the morphology
Impossibility of placing the key over the last composite layer, in the same position, as the time of impression. The key does not fit tightly	Careful inspection of the occlusal surface. Most likely, there is an excess of composite placed and light-cured by mistake on the occlusal surface, outside the cavity, and in the previous filling phases. This excess must be removed
The excess composite, which resulted after the initial polymerization and removal of the occlusal key, cannot be easily removed with the explorer	Perhaps the initial light-curing session was too long, or the lamp power was too high. In this case, continue with the final light-curing phase and remove the excess with burs

Conclusion

The "occlusal key" technique is easy to perform; it provides speed in execution by eliminating the occlusal shaping of the composite by the clinician and shortens the occlusal adjustment time. Although it does not meet the C-factor shrinkage objective (because all walls are linked with the same mass of composite), the technique provides an excellent marginal seal due to the efficient compaction of the composite by the pressure that is applied on the occlusal key.

3.1.2 Impression of the Palatal Surface of the Frontal/"Palatal Silicone Key"

Main idea: The palatal silicone key is required to provide physical support on which the composite is layered when performing the direct restoration of frontal teeth cavities, which involve the palatal surface and the angle or incisal edge (partially or fully).

The impression should make this palatal key of a preexisting coronal morphology. This is possible in the following situations:

- When there is an old filling that is being imprinted before being removed and replaced.
- When a wax-up is performed by the technician based on the initial impression of the clinical situation, especially in cases of fractures with large dislocated tooth fragments.
- When a provisional direct restoration is made to make a silicone impression for the palatal key, then the provisional restoration is removed.

As a quick and efficient working protocol, the palatal key can be made by making the initial impression of the case, regardless of the clinical situation, even when the crown is a missing substance (old dislocated filling, caries, fracture). In these cases, the occlusal key will be morphologically shaped using a dental turbine bur or a scalpel blade and removing the excess impression material.

The following are the steps to perform a direct frontal restoration using a palatal silicone key conformed for a consecutive direct restoration of a coronal fracture:

1. Objective visual examination of the tooth and deciding whether making a silicone palatal key for a direct restoration is possible and appropriate (vitality testing and pulp status). In the case presented below, the patient suffered trauma to tooth 21 without recovery of the fractured fragment, the fracture line did not involve the pulp chamber, and the vitality test was positive (Fig. 3.6). We recommend that the treatment be performed after anesthesia and choosing the enamel composite and dentin color before tooth dehydration and rubber dam isolation.

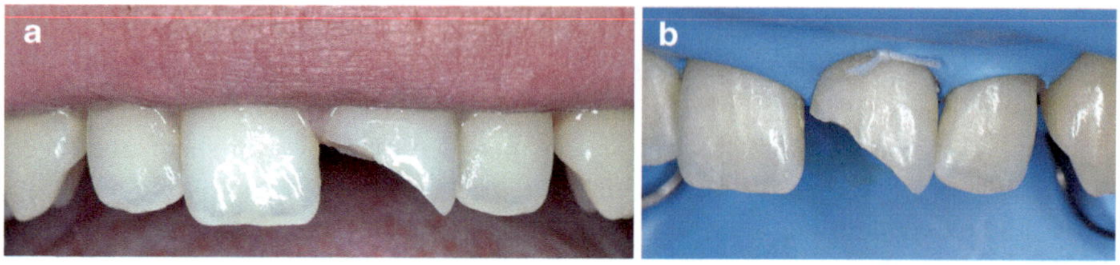

Fig. 3.6 Incisal fracture of an upper central incisor before (**a**) and after rubber dam isolation (**b**) of the frontal group

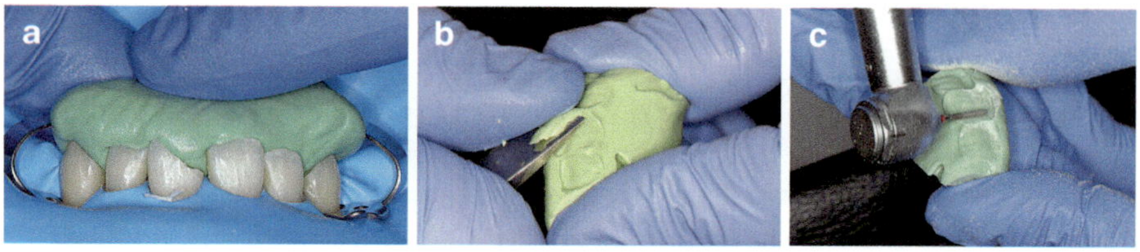

Fig. 3.7 Making the palatal silicone key by impressing the initial situation with the fracture (**a**) followed by removing the excess silicone from the fractured area with a scalpel blade (**b**) or using a diamond turbine burr (**c**)

2. Making the silicone key with silicone impression material. After mixing and applying the silicone on the palatal surface of the frontal group, the material is held with the fingers until the silicone hardens, avoiding its extension on the buccal surface (the incisal edge has to be visible). A very low volume of material is used for the impression. Excess material is cut away with a scalpel blade or a burr, following the existing anatomical contour (Fig. 3.7).
3. Finishing the tooth preparation and performing the beveling.
4. Disinfection and application of the adhesive system.
5. Restoration of the enamel palatal wall by applying a thin enamel composite layer to the area marked on the silicone key. For the application to be performed easily, the silicone key can be held in hand to apply the palatal enamel layer, and then the key can be attached to the tooth. After attachment, the enamel composite is checked for tightness on the palatal surface and is light-cured according to the manufacturer's instructions (Fig. 3.8).
6. The proximal wall restoration shall be made of enamel composite after applying a pre-curved sectional matrix for posterior teeth, vertically placed, or any other type of pre-curved sectional matrix. These can be fixed gingivally with an interdental wedge, and the incisal part can be held with the fingers to personalize the matrix's position relative to the neighboring tooth (Fig. 3.9). Thus, it can be decided to make a tight contact point or a diastema (interdental space) if the clinical situation requires it (Fig. 3.10).

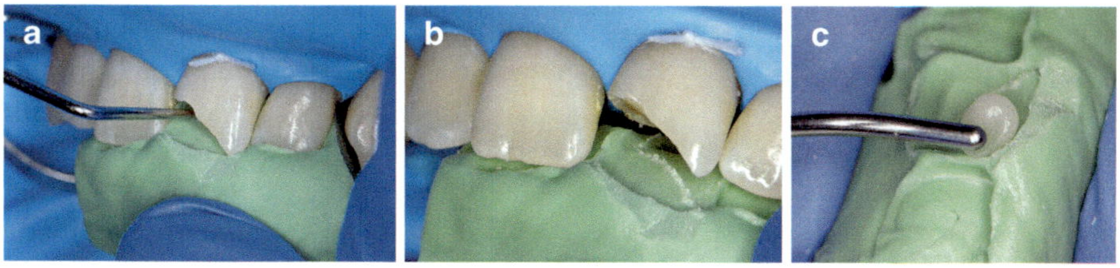

Fig. 3.8 Tracing the cavity margins on silicone with an explorer (**a, b**) and the extraoral composite application on the key for palatal wall restoration (**c**)

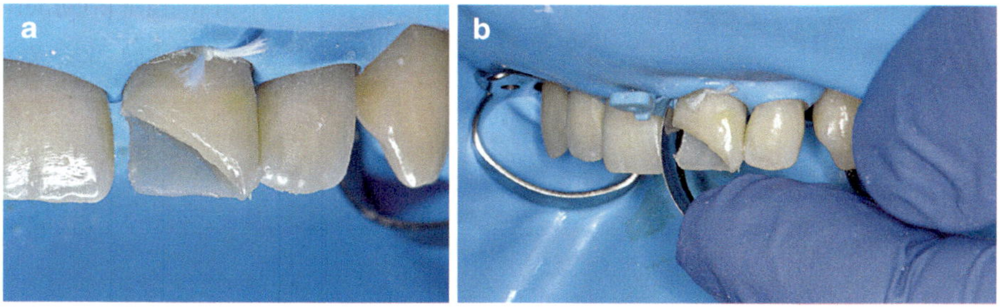

Fig. 3.9 Palatal wall after light-curing the composite and removing silicone key (**a**); mounting a metal sectional matrix in a vertical position for proximal wall restoration (**b**)

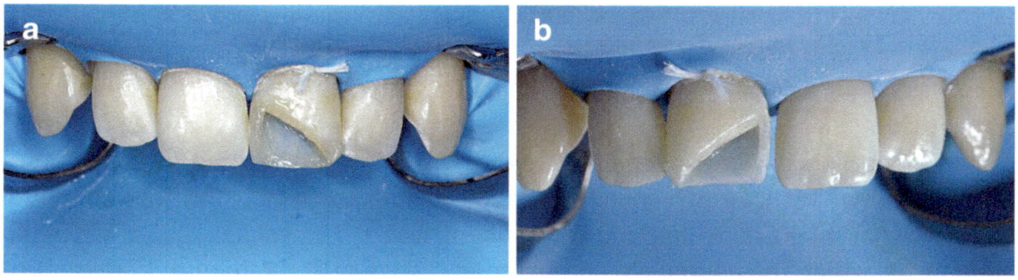

Fig. 3.10 Restored proximal wall with (**a**) or without interdental contact (**b**) with the adjacent tooth

7. Add the dentin composite shades according to the biomimetic layering technique (e.g., described by Vanini [1]) or any other simplified technique (see Sect. 5.3).
8. Application of the buccal enamel layer.
9. Checking the excess proximal material, making macro- and microtexture elements, and finishing and polishing the restoration (Fig. 3.11).

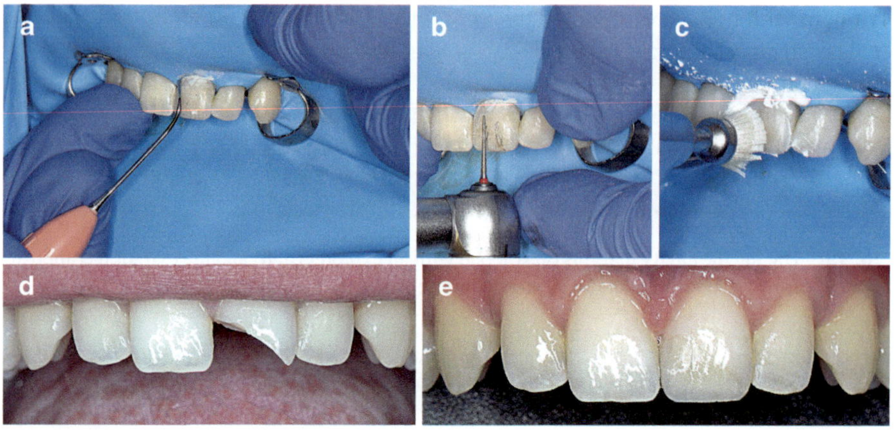

Fig. 3.11 Removal of excess composite (**a**); secondary anatomy (**b**), polishing (**c**); before and after image (**d**)

Difficulties that may occur	Potential solutions
Difficulties in removing the silicone key after material adhesion if the impression is made after the rubber dam insolation and the silicone interferes with the rubber dam clamps	This can be avoided by using a minimum amount of silicone so that the material does not reach the clamps, removing the excess material from the clamp proximity before the material sticks (to the tooth), or making the key before the rubber dam isolation
The composite resin layer is palatally applied over the key in order to displace itself when the palatal key is removed	Restoration of the palatal wall and the firmer attachment of tooth enamel in the junction area

Conclusion

The "silicone palatal key" technique is quick and easy, providing the clinician a substrate on which layering can be performed appropriately (whether a biomimetic, simplified, or monoshade layering technique is used). The palatal key provides the support on which the composite can be compressed with the required pressure to achieve a good tooth structure sealing and reduce the risk of marginal infiltration.

3.1.3 Impression of Buccal and Oral Embrasures with Classic Matrix Ring/"Custom Ring"

Main idea: When possible, the custom ring is made by adapting a classic metal matrix ring using light-curing resins/liquid rubber dam. The obtained ring can lead to increased sectional matrix adaptation on the tooth, without needing other helpful adaptation methods, with PTFE or rubber liquid dam.

The sectional matrices are adapted and fixed to the teeth using matrix rings. The main purpose of this ring is to keep the matrix in a fixed position, bonded to the tooth during the proximal wall restoration stages, and prevent the extrusion of composite materials from the cavity. There are situations where obtaining the standard matrix ring stability and adaptation is difficult or impossible due to teeth anatomy. In these situations, a *custom ring* may be fabricated. This consists of imprinting the buccal and oral embrasures with a liquid rubber dam, a material in which the metal ring tines will also be fixed [2].

The main advantage of the technique is that this ring can perfectly adapt the sectional matrix on the tooth since it was obtained by making an impression of the proximal embrasures. Clinically, this means eliminating the possibility of getting excess material, which in some situations can remain undetected and, therefore, unremoved and can cause gum inflammation and food retention.

This technique can only be applied if proximal caries does not destroy the proximal wall, and the proximal embrasure can be impressed. The ring is made before the proximal cavity is prepared. If there were an analogy, we could say that the "custom ring" technique is the "occlusal stamp technique" for the proximal embrasures.

The following tools and materials are required to make a custom ring: dental wedge (wood or plastic), classic sectional matrix metal ring (e.g., Palodent, Garrison, TOR-VM), and liquid rubber dam. The custom ring is made before cavity preparation (Fig. 3.12a, b), and it is then used to fix the sectional matrix during the restoration stage (Fig. 3.12c).

Manufacturing and handling custom ring steps:

1. Objective visual examination of the tooth and decision that making a custom ring is possible and appropriate. In the clinical case presented below, medium to deep proximal caries was diagnosed on the distal surface of the upper second premolar. Since the cavity buccal-oral opening (diameter) is small, the proximal wall was relatively preserved (Fig. 3.13), so it was possible to copy it to make a custom ring.
2. Placement of an interdental wedge to achieve pre-distancing. Its placement is crucial because the copying of proximal embrasures must be performed under

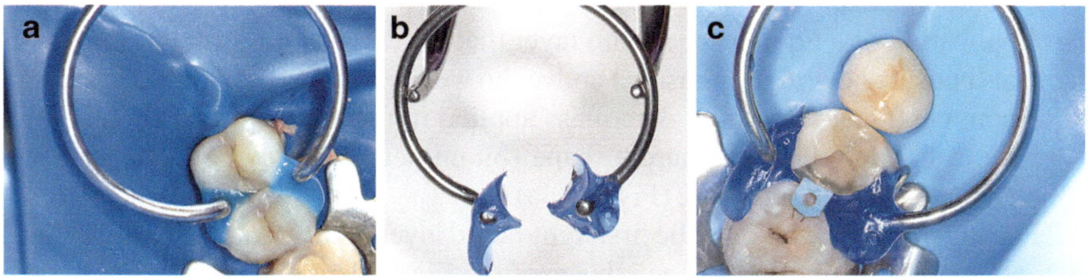

Fig. 3.12 Application of rubber liquid dam and metal ring prior to cavity preparation (**a**); aspect of a custom ring removed from teeth (**b**); custom ring mounted for fixing a sectional matrix after cavity preparation (**c**)

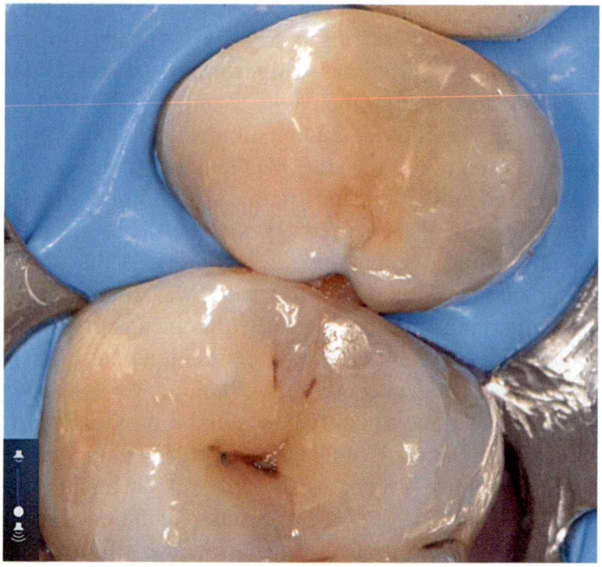

Fig. 3.13 Proximal caries with buccal and oral embrasures relatively preserved so that they can be impressed to make a custom ring

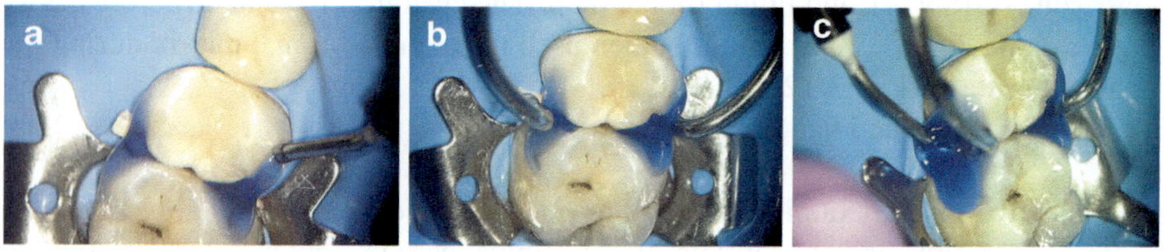

Fig. 3.14 Clinical steps for a custom ring: application and light-curing of the first layer of the liquid rubber dam (**a**); metal ring application; (**b**) coating with a new layer of the liquid rubber dam (**c**)

pre-distancing conditions. This wedge will also be used during the matrix installation (in the obturation phase). Changing the wedge to a larger size or with a different model may impede the correct positioning of the custom ring in the obturation stage.

3. Application of a liquid rubber dam layer that covers the entire area of the proximal (buccal and oral) embrasures above the wedge, followed by light-curing. We recommend that the rubber dam mass applied in this first layer be slightly concave, following the embrasure's shape (biomimetic) to provide a stable placement area for the metal ring (Fig. 3.14a).
4. Placing the metal ring over the first light-cured layer of the liquid dam (Fig. 3.14b) and then covering it with a new layer of the liquid dam that will be light-cured (Fig. 3.14c).
5. Removing the custom ring and checking it. The ring's metal tines must be fixed and stable inside the liquid dam mass. After removal, the ring is kept until the matrix application phase.

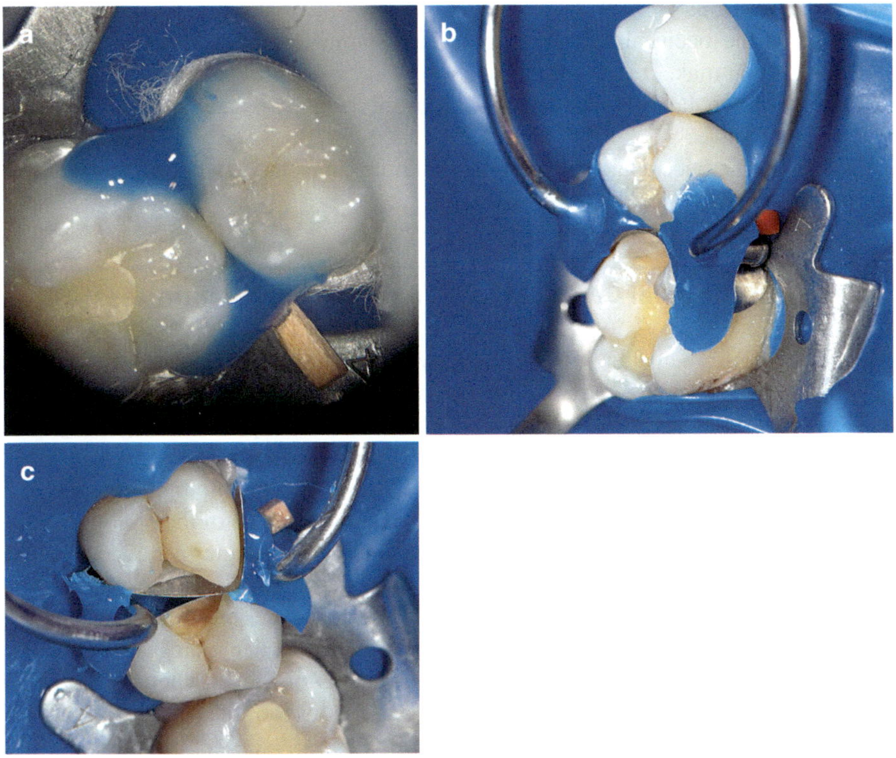

Fig. 3.15 Concave aspect of the first applied liquid dam layer (**a**); custom ring placed in a different position than the original one (**b**); custom ring fractured (**c**)

Difficulties that may appear	Potential solutions
The ring lacks stability when applied to the first layer of the light-cured liquid dam	Positioning the liquid dam in a slightly concave manner in the interdental space creates a space for positioning the ring (Fig. 3.15a)
Positioning the custom ring over the sectional matrix in a different position from the original one (Fig. 3.15b)	Keeping the same used interdental wedges when the ring was made and the same positioning
Fracture of the rubber liquid dam during the unilateral or bilateral application (Fig. 3.15c)	Adding the rubber liquid dam or the ring can be used without the fractured part. A possible cause could be the thin layer of liquid dam applied on the tooth or over the ring

Conclusion

The "custom ring" technique is rarely used by practitioners, probably because of the time for making it is discouraging. The time decreases with experience in using the technique. However, the technique can be beneficial when the practitioner does not have professional matrix systems whose rings fit the metal matrix sufficiently well on the tooth.

Review Questions

1. What is the occlusal surface impression/"stamp technique"/occlusal key, and how do you make it?
2. What is the palatal surface impression of the frontal/"palatal silicone key," and how is it made?
3. What are the buccal and oral embrasure impressions made with the custom ring, and how are they made?

3.2 Subgingival Cavity Margin Acquisition Techniques

Proximal caries are challenging to detect by direct clinical examination [3], so they may be identified and treated at later stages of development. This can be avoided by performing complementary radiological examinations that provide a high degree of cavity carious lesion detection at this level [4]. Often, they indicate the preparation of the juxta- or subgingival cavities that may interfere with the biological width. The placement of restorative margin in the sulcus, with the invasion of the biologic width, may result in sensitivity, persistent gingival inflammation, or gingival recession [5]. Studies show these problems are self-limiting after a long period [6].

After completing the proximal cavity preparation, assessing the ratio between the cavity margin and the level of interdental papilla is necessary. Thus, we can distinguish the following clinical situations depending on the ratio between the level of the proximal cavity edge/gingival margin and the level of the interdental papilla:

1. Supra- and juxtagingival—these do not require additional procedures after cavity preparation in order to make the direct restoration.
2. Subgingivally, when the distance between the proximal cavity gingival margin and the alveolar bone crest is greater or equal to 3 mm. In these cases, a gingivectomy is recommended to respect the biological width.
3. Subgingivally, the biological width is invaded when the distance between the proximal cavity gingival margin and the alveolar bone crest is less than 3 mm. Clinical crown lengthening is recommended in these cases to restore the biological width.
4. The subgingival destruction is extensive on more than one or two proximal walls and indicates a partial (surgical or orthodontic) extrusion.

The signs of invasion of biological width are [7]:

- Chronic progressive gingival inflammation at the level of gingival restoration limit
- Bleeding on probing
- Localized gingival hyperplasia, with minimal bone loss
- Gingival recession
- Periodontal pocket development
- Clinical loss of gingival attachment and alveolar bone loss

The rubber dam sheet application and its fixation with ligatures on the tooth being worked on will ensure an apical relocation of the gingival papilla level (beneficial for preparation and restoration of extensive juxta- or subgingival proximal destructions). Furthermore, dental wedges in the preparation phase (pre-distancing the teeth) can help highlight the cavity margin.

Proper proximal cavity restoration can only be achieved when there is the possibility of positioning the matrix and interdental wedge below the cavity edge/margin. This is necessary for several reasons:

1. The wedge helps the achievement of good sealing at the gingival margin level by improving the matrix seal tightness on the tooth, preventing the infiltration of liquids from the salivary environment (regardless of the isolation form: rubber dam, cotton rolls) in order to achieve material adhesion. The wedge pushes the matrix toward the tooth.
2. Placement of an interdental wedge to achieve pre-distancing.
3. The wedge's presence, which fits the matrix on the tooth, prevents the extrusion of restorative materials.

3.2.1 Deep Margin Evelation

Main idea: The edges of juxta- or slightly subgingival, enlarged cavities can be relocated in the first phase to continue the restoration through direct or indirect techniques.

The procedure is recommended for proximal subgingival destructions to relocate the cavity's gingival margin coronally. This relocation is essential in cases where an indirect restoration is going to be performed, which means that the adhesive cementation require supragingival placement of the cavity limits. This technique is recommended in cases where rubber dam isolation can be achieved. Otherwise, it is impossible to obtain good adhesion in the subgingival area [8]. The reconstruction is done up to a level that allows easy fitting of a rubber dam sheet for isolation and a pre-curved sectional matrix or the optical or classical impression for an indirect restoration (Figs. 3.16 and 3.17).

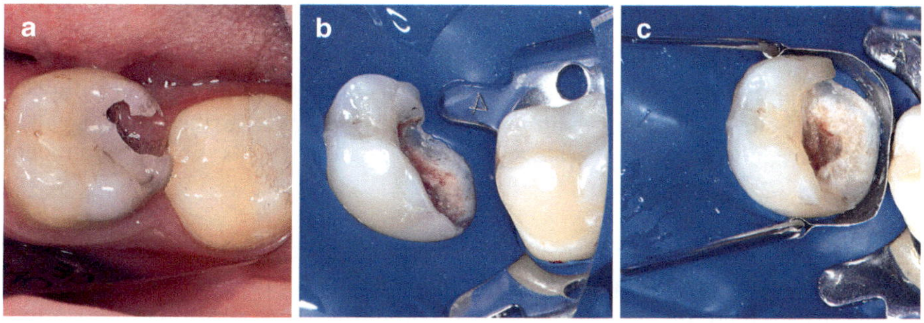

Fig. 3.16 Slightly subgingivally proximal cavity (**a**); rubber dam isolation and preparation for deep margin elevation (**b**); mounting a saddle matrix (**c**)

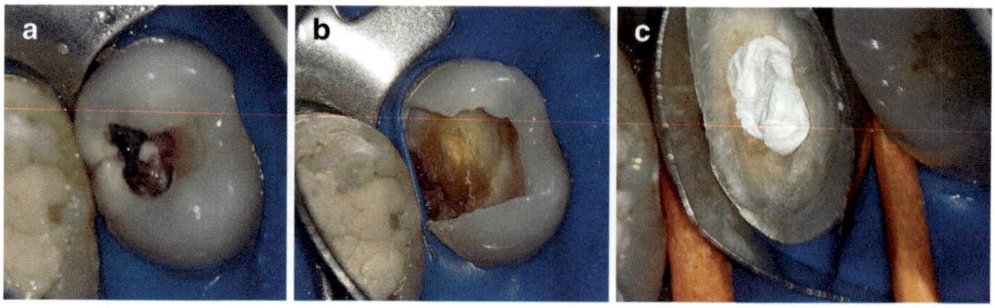

Fig. 3.17 Deep occlusal cavity (**a**) extended proximally (**b**); initially and (**c**) after cavity preparation and sectional matrix fitting (**c**)

The supragingival edge relocation is done using the following tools and materials:

- Composite resins or derivatives (e.g., giomers)
- A curved metal matrix or "banana shape," with a width of 2–3 mm
- Tofflemire matrix that allows a tight sealing in the cervical area

Although the technique initially described by Pascal Magne uses a narrowed circular matrix mounted in a Tofflemire matrix holder, other types of matrices (classic sectional, saddle, etc.) can also be used. In the case of subgingival destructions that have a greater depth, the "matrix-in-matrix" technique can be used—by fixing a piece of the sectional matrix and tightening it with a circular matrix.

Difficulties that may occur	Potential solutions
Impossibility of rubber dam isolation	Supplementing the isolation with auxiliary methods (Teflon tape, liquid rubber dam)
Gingival bleeding	Hemostasis, temporization

Conclusion

The supragingival elevation of the cavity margin is a separate essential phase that precedes an indirect or direct restoration, with juxta- or subgingival edges.

3.2.2 Gingivectomy

Main idea: When the interdental wedge is inserted, if its base does not descend below the level of the proximal cavity/gingival edge, then a gingivectomy is required.

Gingivectomy can be performed with scalpels, diamond burs installed on rotating devices, ceramic burs, periodontal burs, periodontal tips, and lasers. The most commonly used are fine turbine burs, used without water to perform cauterization,

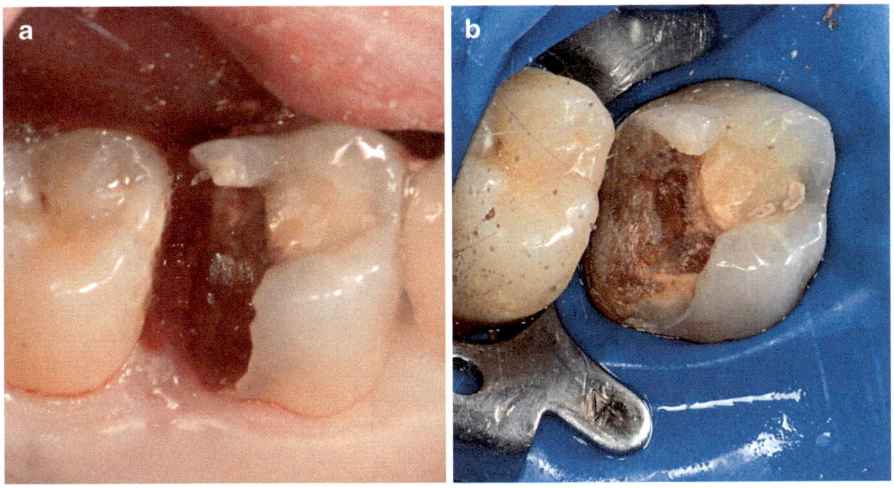

Fig. 3.18 Gingivectomy and hemostasis (**a**); rubber dam isolation for restoration (**b**)

such as Thermacut Bur (Dentsply Sirona, USA). Their use reduces bleeding to an easily controlled level with hemostatic solutions. The rubber dam isolation, after this procedure, is essential to adhesively restore the proximal wall under conditions of good salivary and blood infiltration control (Fig. 3.18a, b).

Partial gingivectomy is often sufficient to achieve supragingival exposure of the cavity edges. Gingivectomy can be performed when the distance between the alveolar bone crest and the gingival margin of the proximal cavity is greater than or equal to 3 mm. This distance can be estimated using bitewing radiography and measured with the help of periodontal probing (bone sounding) [5]. If the distance exceeds 3 mm, it is unlikely to violate the biological width [9]. Even if the size is less than 3 mm, the invasion of the biological width does not necessarily exclude the possibility of performing the gingivectomy. This can happen when the doctor does not possess the knowledge and necessary experience to perform a crown lengthening, and it is impossible to recommend the patient to a periodontist.

Moreover, the size of the biological width can be variable [10], and its size can become uncertain when associated with the subgingivally located proximal caries [11]. These cases require compromises that must be clearly explained to patients to set their expectations accordingly.

Difficulties that may occur	Potential solutions
Bleeding	Hemostatic
Bone exposure	The initial measurement of the distance between the cavity edge and the alveolar crest was not correctly performed. It is recommended to proceed with the gingivectomy with crown lengthening
Papilla does not regenerate itself, and the "black triangle" appears	This happens if the distance between the bone crest and the contact point is too large, meaning that the contact point has been set too high toward the occlusal (more than 5 mm, Denis Tarnow's law)

Conclusion
Gingivectomy is a commonly required procedure to allow teeth's direct restoration. The purpose is to obtain cavity edges that are supragingivally located. This procedure must consider the existence of/respect the biological width and the subsequent possibility of rubber dam isolation.

3.2.3 Crown Lengthening

Main idea: Crown lengthening aims to extend the exposure of the tooth's coronal portion so that this will be available for a future proper restoration. After this procedure, the limits of a cavity need to be brought supragingivally so that they allow a direct or indirect restoration or to obtain a ferrule effect for prosthetic purposes (refers to the need to have ~2 mm of sound tooth structure forming a band that excircles the external dimension of residual tooth structure for the junction with a future prosthetic crown).

This procedure should be implemented when the clinician estimates that direct restoration of a proximal subgingival cavity (with gingival margin at 1–2 mm from the alveolar bone crest) may interfere with the biological width [9]. The crown lengthening with an apically repositioned flap involves the bone recontouring [12, 13] to supragingivally expose the cavity margins that were initially located subgingivally, violating the biological width. This method was described in the 1960s by Friedman J.W., and the procedure is widely used in periodontal practice. The procedure involves sessions, additional costs, and professional skills [14]. Most frequently, these procedures are performed by periodontist specialists (Fig. 3.19).

The crown lengthening procedure involves incisions exposing the bone to reduce its level, followed by suturing. Thus, the gingival level will be relocated according to the final bone level after the removal of a portion of the bone. Wall restoration can be performed in the same session as the elongation procedure after suturing with rubber dam isolation (Fig. 3.20).

There are situations when crown lengthening is not recommended [15]:

- Deep subgingival caries that force excessive bone removal
- If the gingival level obtained after elongation affects the patient's aesthetics
- Inadequate root/crown ratio (ideally 2:1)
- Unrestorable teeth
- Increased furcation exposure risk
- Severe damage to adjacent alveolar bone support

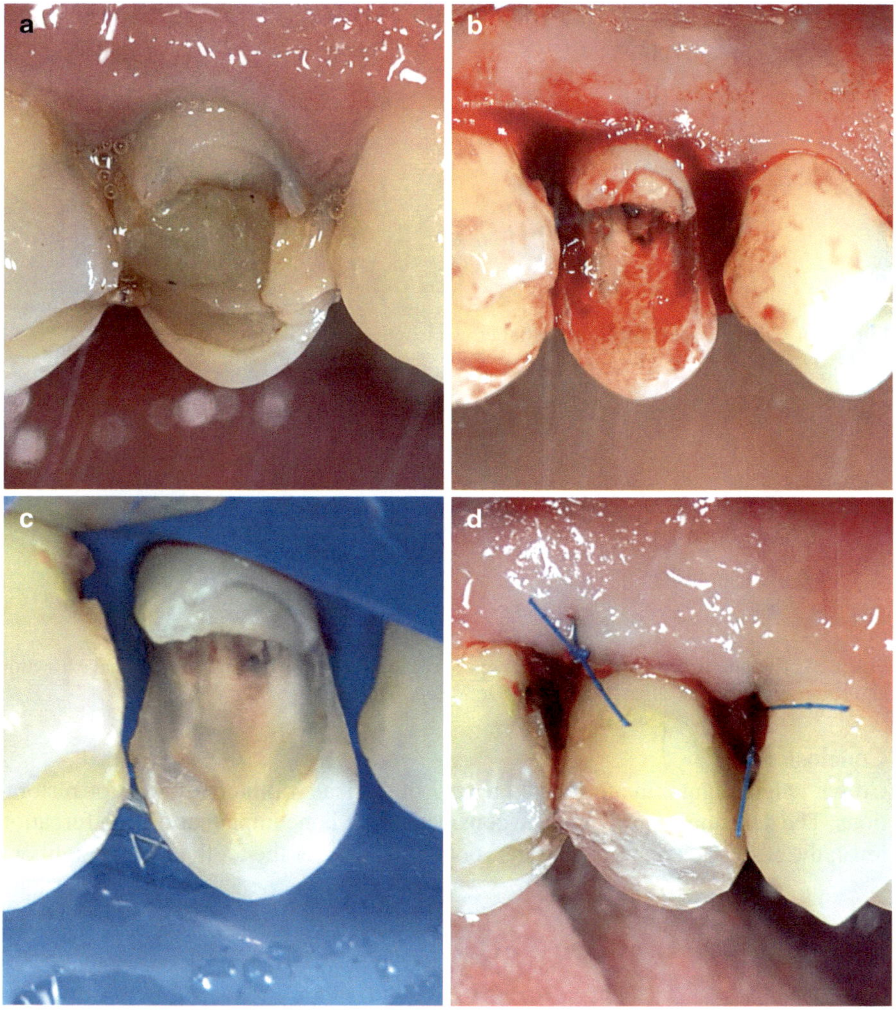

Fig. 3.19 Initial image of an improper direct restoration, extensive mesial and distal subgingival infiltration (**a**); incision, bone resection, and suture (**b**); rubber dam isolation (**c**); final result after crown lengthening (**d**)

Difficulties that may occur	Potential solutions
Emergence of black triangles	Periodontal surgery. Sealing the triangles with composite resins
Occurrence of dentinal hypersensitivity through the exposure of the radicular surface	Periodontal surgery and the use of desensitizing substances
Occurrence of radicular resorption	Avoiding the traumatic touch with the burr during bone resection
Temporary tooth mobility	Immobilization

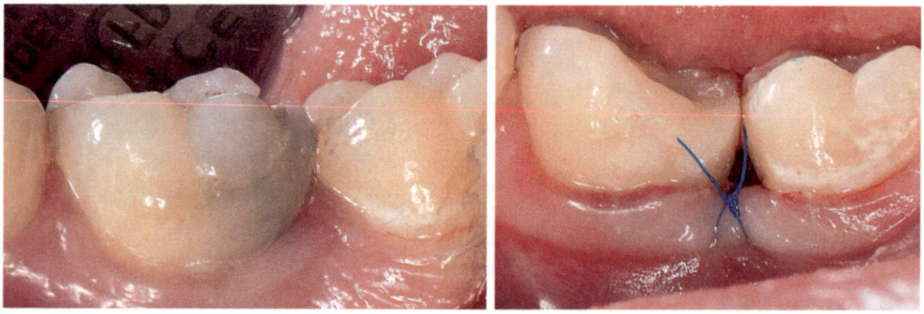

Fig. 3.20 Clinical aspect before and after crown lengthening (Dr. Mircea Muresan)

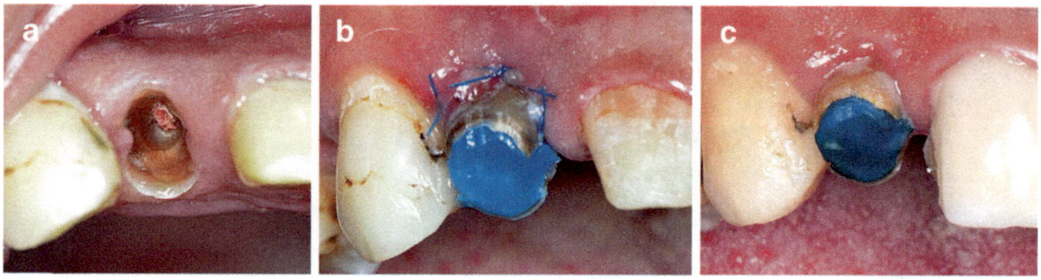

Fig. 3.21 Subgingivally restant root of a superior lateral incisor (**a**); image after partial extraction and suturing (**b**); image after 14 days (**c**) (Dr. Mircea Muresan)

Conclusion
Crown lengthening aims to create optimal biological width conditions for restorations. The decision should be made considering the bone implantation, the furcation level, the aesthetic outcome, and the root denudation of the tooth and its neighbor.

3.2.4 Surgical Extrusion (PET)

Main idea: Surgical extrusion is an alternative to the extraction of teeth with juxta- or subgingival destructions. The tooth surgical extrusion involves the tooth relocation coronally to expose supragingivally dental hard tissue that creates an encircling effect (ferrule) for prosthetic crown while respecting the biological width.

Surgical extrusion means the remaining tooth structure is repositioned coronally/ supragingivally (Fig. 3.21) in the same dental alveolus where the tooth was initially located [16].

The procedure is recommended for monoradicular teeth that are or will be devitalized. Afterward, they will be removed from the occlusion during the healing period [17]. A successful outcome means periodontal healing shows no root resorption or tooth ankylosis and no significant marginal bone loss or tooth mobility [18].

This procedure can be successfully performed when the subgingival limits of the destruction are extensive and when a crown lengthening would not help. Although we do not have extensive studies analyzing the technique, the success, and the follow-up of cases, the individual or multiple patient case presentations published so far allow us to point out this procedure as an effective and safe method [19] for the supragingival restoration of cavity margins. However, the cases that could benefit from this procedure should be carefully evaluated regarding their future ability to be restored. Orthodontic treatment involving these teeth should be postponed 6 months after the procedure [20].

Difficulties that may occur	Potential solutions
Avoiding an orthodontic treatment that could apply additional forces on the tooth with PET	Postponing the application of orthodontic forces for 6 months
Permanent loss of tooth fixation or avulsion	Suggesting tooth extraction and rethinking the treatment plan
Impossibility of atraumatic tooth luxation	Tooth extraction and rethinking the treatment plan

Conclusion

Partial surgical extrusion is suitable for monoradicular teeth, in a critical situation, that will usually be restored later with prosthetic crowns and less with direct restorations. The latter can be done temporarily (by layering or injection) during healing, but they must be removed from the occlusion.

3.2.5 Orthodontic Extrusion

Main idea: Orthodontic tooth extrusion is a slow process involving the movement in a coronal direction through the action of orthodontic forces applied to the tooth.

Although there is no consensus on this procedure [21], the results are certain and frequently applied in the current practice. It can be performed either with a segmental appliance or fixed prosthetic bridge and magnets. Extrusion reported in the literature ranges from 1 mm per month to 1 mm per week [22].

Orthodontic extrusion is a safe, minimally invasive, and highly predictable treatment, rarely associated with complications [23, 24]. It has several advantages compared to surgical crown lengthening because it preserves dento-periodontal support. The combination of orthodontic extrusion and fiberotomy can be particularly advantageous in areas of aesthetic significance, where surgical crown lengthening of a single tooth could lead to an unsatisfactory aesthetic result [25]. Furthermore, a relatively simple tooth movement is required to perform the orthodontic extrusion, which is considered one of the easiest orthodontic movements because it simulates physiological tooth eruption.

The main disadvantage of orthodontic extrusion is the time required for treatment, with an average of 4–6 weeks [22]. In addition, it may take 4–6 weeks or months for the result to stabilize. For this reason, clinicians and patients may not choose this option as their first option. If fiberotomy is performed weekly, a good patient compliance is required. Like all orthodontic treatments, it can also cause oral hygiene problems and aesthetic problems.

Difficulties that may occur	Potential solutions
Aesthetic damage and difficulty in maintaining oral hygiene	The patient must receive oral hygiene instructions and be motivated because this is a short-term orthodontic treatment
Lack of extrusion results	Most likely, there is tooth ankylosis, and the treatment plan needs to be revised

Conclusion

Although simple and with many advantages, this technique is less used by physicians and less preferred by patients because it is slow and requires a period for contention and the aesthetics and hygiene achievement are poor during this period.

Review Questions

1. What are the clinical signs of the biological width invasion to be taken into account in restorative treatments?
2. Why is it necessary to position the matrix and interdental wedge below the cavity edge?
3. What is deep margin elevation, and how is it performed?
4. What periodontal, surgical, and orthodontic techniques allow the supragingival relocation of cavity margins for restoration and how are they performed?

3.3 Operating Field Isolation

3.3.1 Rubber Dam Isolation

Main idea: Cavity preparation and filling must be carried out under optimal access and visibility conditions, without the saliva (which contains bacteria) that enters the cavity, which can cause further infection of the dentinal wound and compromise the material adhesion to the dental substrate. By isolating the operating field, neighboring anatomical elements (tongue, lips, cheeks) are kept at a distance so that they do not interfere with the operating field, thus providing better visibility for the dentist. In dentistry, two main isolation methods are widely used: Rubber dam (isolating method) and cotton rolls (absorption method).

Rubber dam isolation involves using latex foils or non-latex elastic materials stretched over a frame and secured to the teeth with metal or plastic clamps. The rubber dam sheets are perforated, the number of perforations is identical to the number of teeth that will pass through the sheet, and the teeth become isolated from the oral environment.

The rubber dam isolation is preferable for direct and indirect restorations or veneer bonding and is more effective than any other isolation method. Studies show that direct composite restorations made with the rubber dam have a higher long-term success rate [26].

The main advantages of using rubber dam isolation for direct and indirect restorations are the following:

- Effective humidity control during the treatment necessary for material adhesion.
- Prevention of contamination with bacteria from saliva, thus reducing the postoperative sensitivity.
- Improving the operating field visibility and facilitating the dentist's access to the operating field by retracting the surrounding soft tissues (tongue, lips, cheeks).
- Protection of the oral mucosa against accidents during treatment: impregnation with amalgam particles when removing amalgam and touching the mucosa with manual or rotary instruments, metal strips, matrices, etc.
- Preventing the spread of the aerosols or droplets generated by oral fluids, being a preventive measure in the spread of respiratory viruses.
- Preventing the swallowing of small, sharp instruments (needles, burs), of materials dropped from instruments (composite, cement, etc.), or of small prosthetic pieces (onlay, inlay, veneer, crown, etc.).
- Preventing the substances with an unpleasant taste and harmful action from reaching the mucosa and causing burns (e.g., sodium hypochlorite).
- Discouraging the agitated patients from requesting frequent rinses with water and spitting into the sink too often; very talkative patients are hindered from interrupting the dentist too often.
- Feeling of safety and protection for patients because the instruments, materials, liquids, and unpleasant tastes are not in direct contact with the mucosa.

In addition to the advantages mentioned above, the use of the dental operating microscope requires rubber dam isolation in order to prevent the mirror from fogging up due to patient breathing, to keep the operating field stable and visible, and to prevent the patients' movements (rinsing, spitting, or talking). Blue or green rubber dam sheets may be used to absorb the light reflected from the microscope light source and to enhance the contrast.

All these things offer the doctor the peace of mind that helps to focus on the treatment and lowers the stress levels. This ultimately contributes to the treatment quality.

The rubber dam isolation kit includes:

- Rubber dam sheets
- Clamps

- Frame
- Hole punch plier
- Rubber dam clamp forceps
- Rubber dam template for hole punching

Rubber dam isolation main steps:

1. Choosing the sheet and making the perforations
2. Choosing, checking, and placing the clamp
3. Applying the sheet on the operating field
4. Checking the clamp stability and the sealing and inversion in the gingival sulcus
5. Additional means of fixation: ligatures, liquid rubber dam, PTFE, elastic cords, etc.

3.3.1.1 Choosing the Rubber Dam Sheet and Making Perforations

The rubber dam sheets are produced in several variations of thickness, size, elasticity, texture, and color (Fig. 3.22a). The most common size for adult patients is 6 × 6 inches. A sheet is chosen by the dentist depending on the case particularities (e.g., tight or loose contact points, etc.) and subjective personal preferences (e.g., ease of fitting, color contrast).

Marking the Perforation Positions

To make the perforations, mark the positions of the future perforations on the sheet with a marker using the template. Do not mark or punch holes in edentulous space. If the teeth are malpositioned, it is recommended to stretch the sheet over them by hand and mark the perforation points in the middle of the occlusal surfaces and incisal edges. This way, the perforations can be obtained in the most suitable positions for the case.

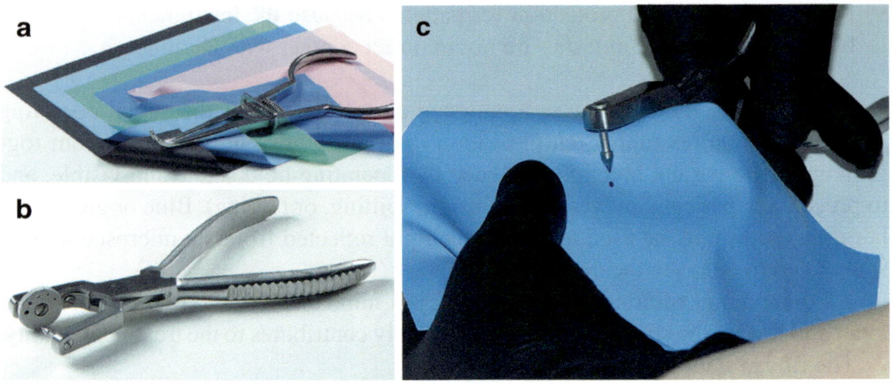

Fig. 3.22 Different rubber dam sheet thickness (**a**); rubber dam perforator (**b**); perforating a rubber dam sheet with the rubber dam punch at the marked point (**c**)

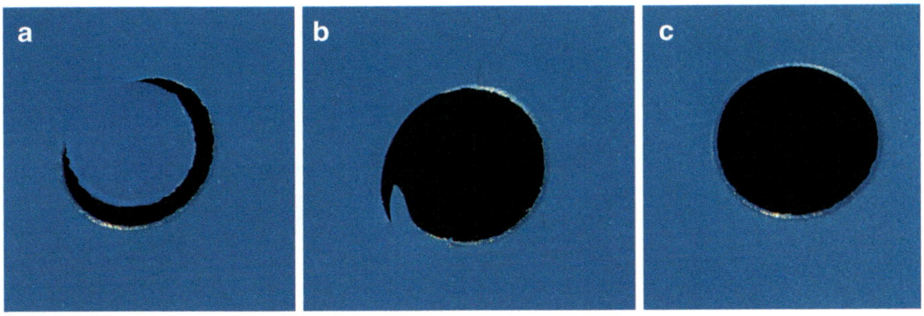

Fig. 3.23 Perforation in the rubber dam sheet: incomplete (**a**); crack in the contour (**b**); correct perforation (**c**)

Perforations

The rubber dam sheet perforation is done with a hole punch plier (Fig. 3.22b), by selecting the perforation diameter from the forceps' ring to be the same or usually having a smaller diameter than the tooth's. Hold the sheet in one hand and the puncher plier in the other, fixing the tip of the sharp pin on the marked points (Fig. 3.22c). If the cut is not complete along the entire contour of the circle, removing the incompletely cut piece by pulling will produce fissures that favor the sheet ripping when stretching and inserting the clamp (Fig. 3.23). The perforations must be cut entirely on the contour line. They can be lubricated to slide more easily on the teeth. The lubrication can also spread to the labial angle to facilitate the rubber dam sheet sliding, which exerts maximum tension at this level.

3.3.1.2 Choosing and Checking the Clamp

The rubber dam clamps can be made of stainless steel or plastic, shiny or matt. They have a memory shape, are elastic, and can be autoclaved. Winged clamps also help fix the rubber dam sheet to the tooth. Wingless clamps are marked with the initials W (wingless). Each clamp has a code that is stamped on the clamp to be easily identified. There are clamps for lateral teeth (premolars and molars) (Fig. 3.24a) and clamps for anterior teeth (Fig. 3.24b). The clamps may have the tooth-supporting tines located in a straight plane for a supragingival insertion (Fig. 3.25a, b) or in a concave plane for a subgingival insertion (Fig. 3.25c).

The B1–B6 clamps represent a particular category. They are wingless and small-sized, and they can easily be applied at the gingival level to produce gingival retraction, which is why they are also called tissue retractors or Brinker clamps (Fig. 3.26).

These are:

- Dam clamp No. B1—for lower molars.
- Dam clamp No. B2—for left upper molars.
- Dam clamp No. B3—for right lower molars.

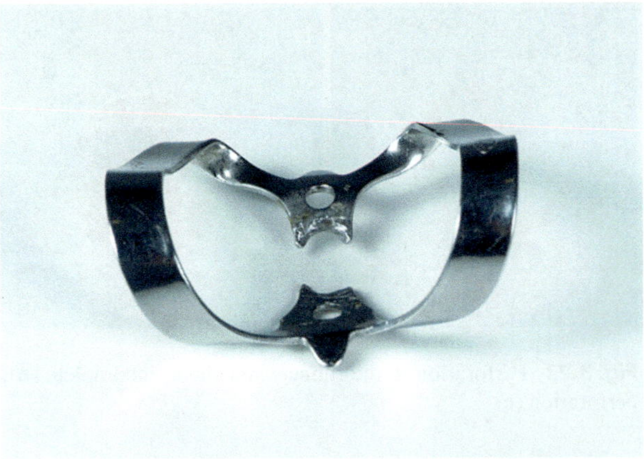

Fig. 3.24 Rubber dam clamps for anterior teeth

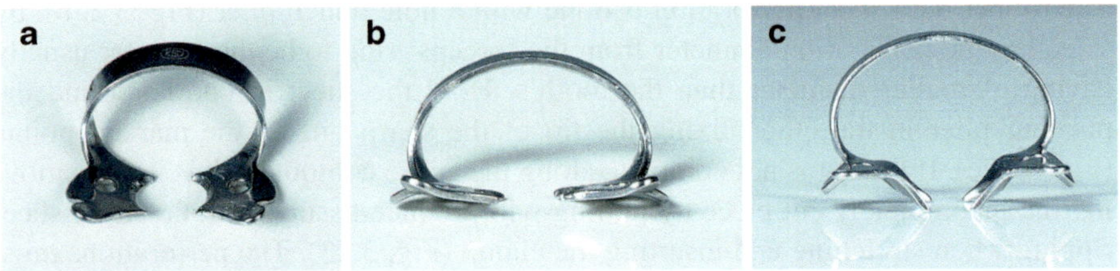

Fig. 3.25 Clamps with supragingival tines for premolars (**a**), for molars (**b**), and clamps with subgingival tines for molars (**c**)

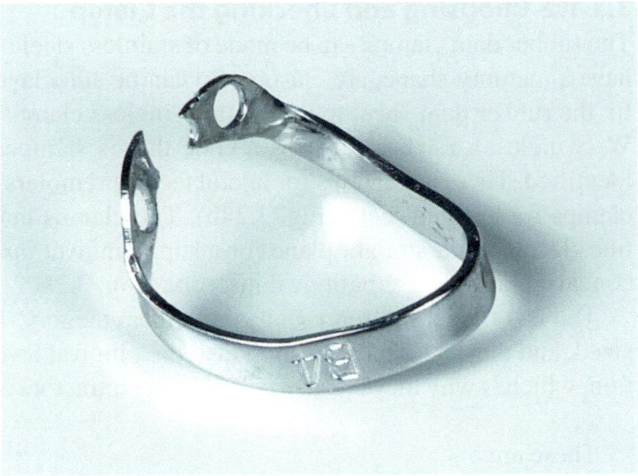

Fig. 3.26 Gingival retractor (Brinker)

- Dam clamp No. B4—for canines and anterior incisors.
- Dam clamp No. B5—for class V restorations, with narrow butterfly "jaws."
- Dam clamp No. B6—upper and lower anterior teeth have wide butterfly "jaws."

The clamp is chosen according to the type, position, and tooth size. Once the clamp is chosen, check its fit on the tooth by positioning it with the rubber dam clamp forceps (Fig. 3.27a). Since there is a risk of dropping or breaking when tensioning and detaching from the rubber dam clamp forceps, it is recommended to secure the clamp with dental floss. This may prevent the risk of swallowing. The clamp must be inserted on the tooth in four points, i.e., all four tines must be in firm contact with the tooth surface. Check the clamp stability by rocking the clamp with the fingers or forceps.

3.3.1.3 Applying the Rubber Dam Sheet to the Operating Field

There are several ways to apply the clamps, the sheet, and the frame. We will refer below to the mounting of the winged clamps:

- After choosing it, the winged clamp can be applied to the dam sheet (Fig. 3.28) and then fixed to the teeth. Afterward, the frame is applied. The disadvantage of this technique is that it requires the help of the dental assistant to fix the edges of the rubber dam sheet, which may hinder visibility during installation (Fig. 3.29a).
- The winged clamps can be applied to the rubber dam sheet and the sheet applied to the frame. All the components will fit together (Fig. 3.29b). In doing so, the help of a dental assistant is less essential at this stage; the doctor holds the frame with the sheet attached to it with one hand and the rubber dam clamp forceps

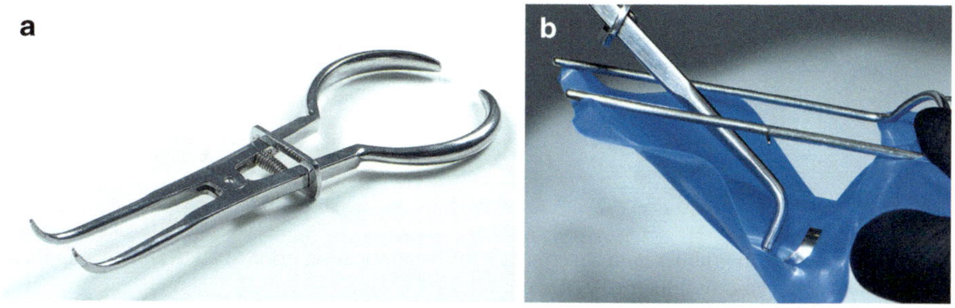

Fig. 3.27 Rubber dam clamp forceps (**a**) and how it is inserted into the clamp (**b**)

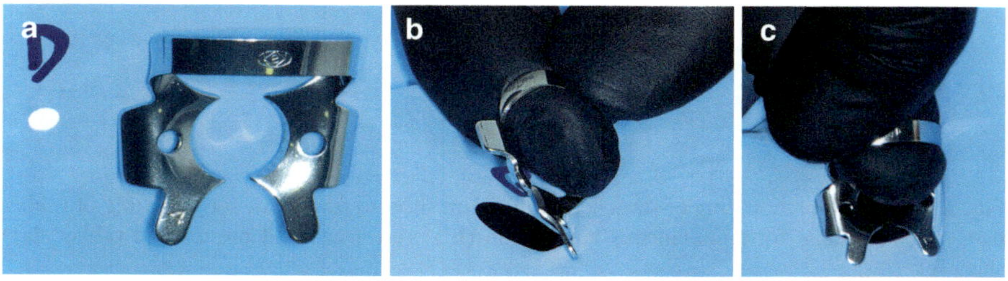

Fig. 3.28 Positioning the clamp with the spring toward distal (**a**); finger grip on the clamp (**b**) to position the clamp on the rubber dam sheet (**c**)

with the other (Fig. 3.29c). When fixing the sheet to the frame, it should not be stretched before application to the tooth (Fig. 3.30a) because it has to allow the clamp to move backward on the dental arch (Fig. 3.30b). There are also pre-formed sheets that do not require perforation with the hole punch but instead cutting it with scissors at the level of each tooth (Fig. 3.30c). Although easy to use, this type of sheet is difficult to adapt to particular cases, as it is impossible to choose the position of the perforations, which can only be made in standard positions.

3.3.1.4 Check the Stability of the Clamp and Inversion

After applying the clamp to the tooth, the following procedures are carried out:

- Check the stability of the clamp by rocking with the fingers or with a forceps. If not applied gingivally, during balancing, the clamp will slide toward the cervical area, so it will be positioned more gingivally.
- Reposition the rubber dam sheet under the clamp wings with an explorer, a spatula, or even a gloved finger and placing it below the clamp. The rubber dam sheet should reach the tooth to mold to the tooth and achieve a tight seal. If the clamp

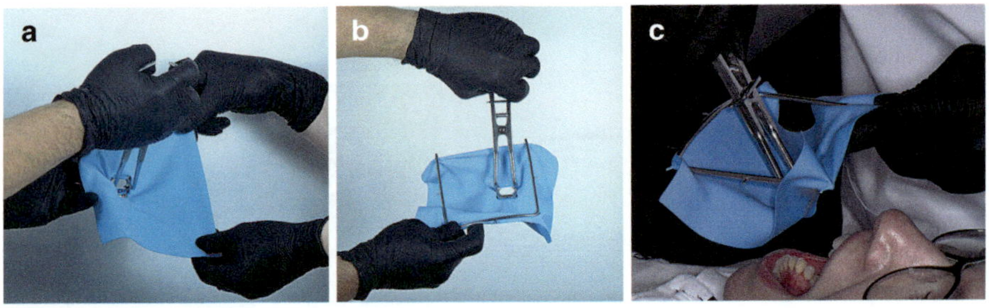

Fig. 3.29 Holding the rubber dam sheet in case of its application prior to the frame (**a**); application of sheet and frame simultaneously (**b**, **c**)

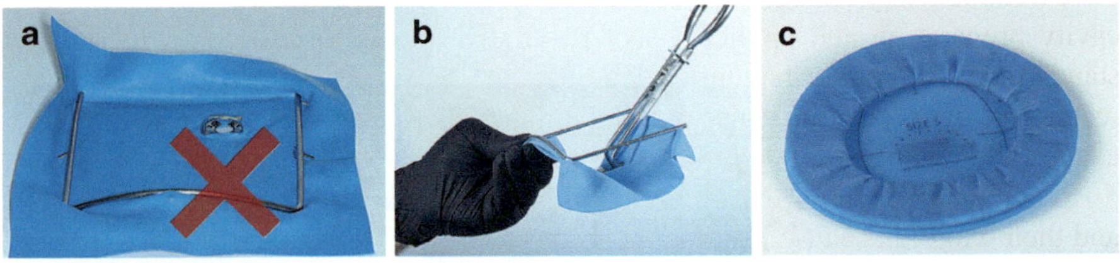

Fig. 3.30 Incorrect mounting of stretched rubber dam sheet to frame (**a**); correct fitting of rubber dam sheet to frame for simultaneous application (**b**); pre-formed and pre-marked rubber dam sheet (**c**)

tines prevent the dam from touching the tooth, then it is recommended to reposition the clamp.

- Repositioning the clamp is frequently necessary, and it consists of a slight movement of the clamp and its removal from the tooth with the rubber dam clamp forceps to allow the rubber dam sheet to reach the point and fit tightly to the tooth (Fig. 3.31).
- The sheet placement under the interdental contact points is carried out with dental floss wrapped around the fingers in sawlike movements. In the case of tight contact points, several successive loads are required after passing the floss under the contact point, which is pulled toward the buccal/oral to repeat the procedure as many times as necessary.
- The inversion of the rubber dam sheet in the sulcus is necessary to obtain a good seal on the tooth and to prevent salivary infiltration. When the perforation edges of the sheet climb onto the tooth crown, a sharp angle is formed between it and the inner face of the rubber dam sheet (Fig. 3.32a). This angle favors the infiltration and saliva "leakage" between the tooth and the sheet, affecting the good

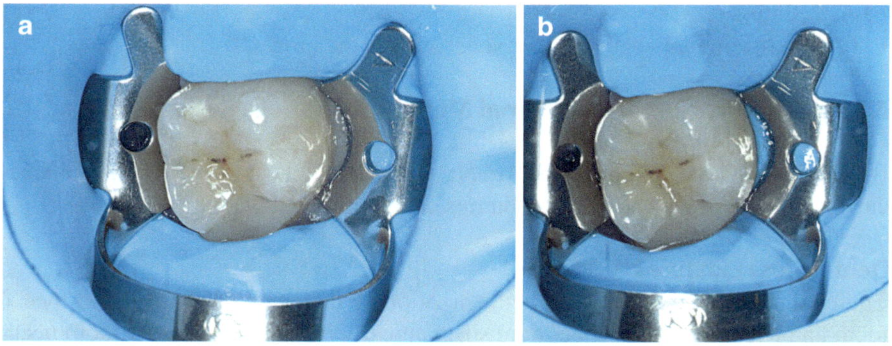

Fig. 3.31 Rubber dam sheet that does not seal the tooth (**a**); image after the clamp reposition that allows the sheet to come into circumferential contact with the tooth (**b**)

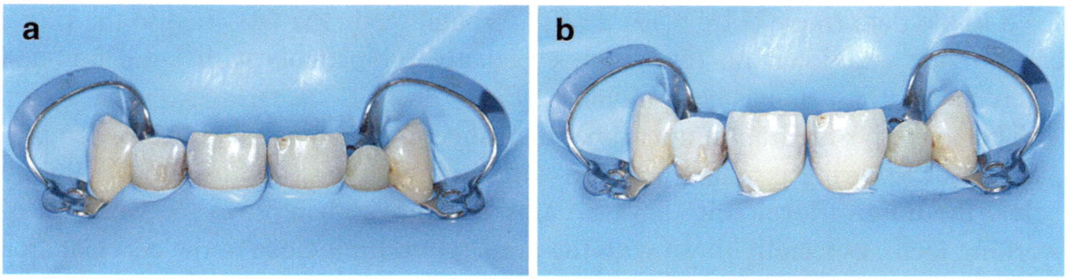

Fig. 3.32 Rubber dam sheet applied to the upper frontal group before and after inversion (**a**) and applying dental floss ligatures (**b**)

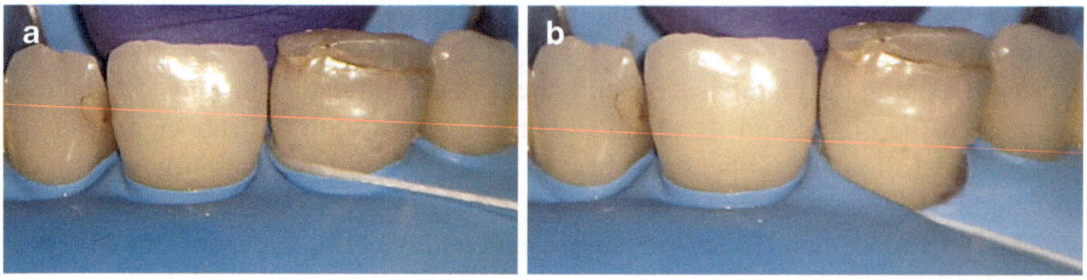

Fig. 3.33 Rubber dam sheet before (**a**) and after inversion using dental floss (**b**)

isolation. If the sheet is inverted in the sulcus, then an obtuse angle is formed between the tooth crown and the dam sheet's inner face, preventing saliva infiltration more effectively (Fig. 3.32b). The inversion of the sheet in the sulcus can be achieved with:

- Simple floss or knot dental floss (Fig. 3.33a, b)
- Air spray
- Spatula
- Teflon tape

• Check the circular sealing of the sheet around the crown.

3.3.1.5 Application of Additional Means of Fixation, Retention, and Sealing

Dental floss ligatures, Teflon tape, rubber liquid dam, elastic cords or rings, pieces cut out of the dam foil, additional clamps, and interdental wedges/PENE.

Dental Floss Ligatures

These can be used to achieve a better fixation of the sheet on the isolated mesial tooth and to position the rubber dam sheet apically in the sulcus on the tooth needing treatment. Ligatures can be single or double, consisting of two wires. The floss length required for a ligature can be approximated by positioning its end at the elbow level (Fig. 3.34). The ligatures can be made in several ways (Figs. 3.35 and 3.36). After their fixation on the tooth, the excess can be cut out or stretched and fixed to the dam frame (Fig. 3.37). For the frontal teeth, the floss tied to the frame can provide additional lip retraction, especially for patients with large lips and where an elastic sheet has been mounted (Fig. 3.38).

The apical positioning of the rubber dam sheet on the tooth is critical when preparing and restoring proximal cavities with a gingival margin close to or slightly below the gingiva level (Fig. 3.39). A floss ligature can improve the isolation of working teeth, especially those with the preparation limit close to the cervical area where salivary infiltration is more likely. Because of this, we recommend ligatures on all teeth with proximal cavities (Fig. 3.40).

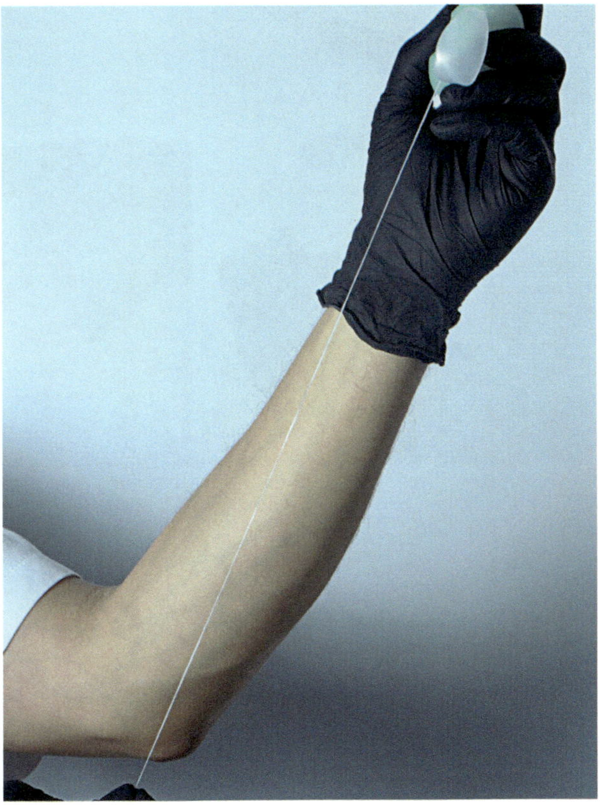

Fig. 3.34 Measuring the dental floss needed to make a ligature

Teflon Tape

The Teflon tape (Fig. 3.41) is frequently used to apically relocate the rubber dam sheet margins or to close the areas where the dam sheet did not fit tightly on the tooth (Fig. 3.42).

Rubber Liquid Dam

The liquid rubber dam can apply the clamp to the tooth in cases of atypical coronal anatomy and seal areas where the sheet does not fit perfectly on the tooth (Fig. 3.43).

Elastic Cords and Rings

The elastic cords and rings used to fix the rubber dam sheet can be for dental usage or general usage. Their usage is simple and effective, and many clinicians prefer them. In their absence, the clinician can make an elastic cord by cutting a narrow strip of rubber dam sheet from the margin of the sheet (Fig. 3.44).

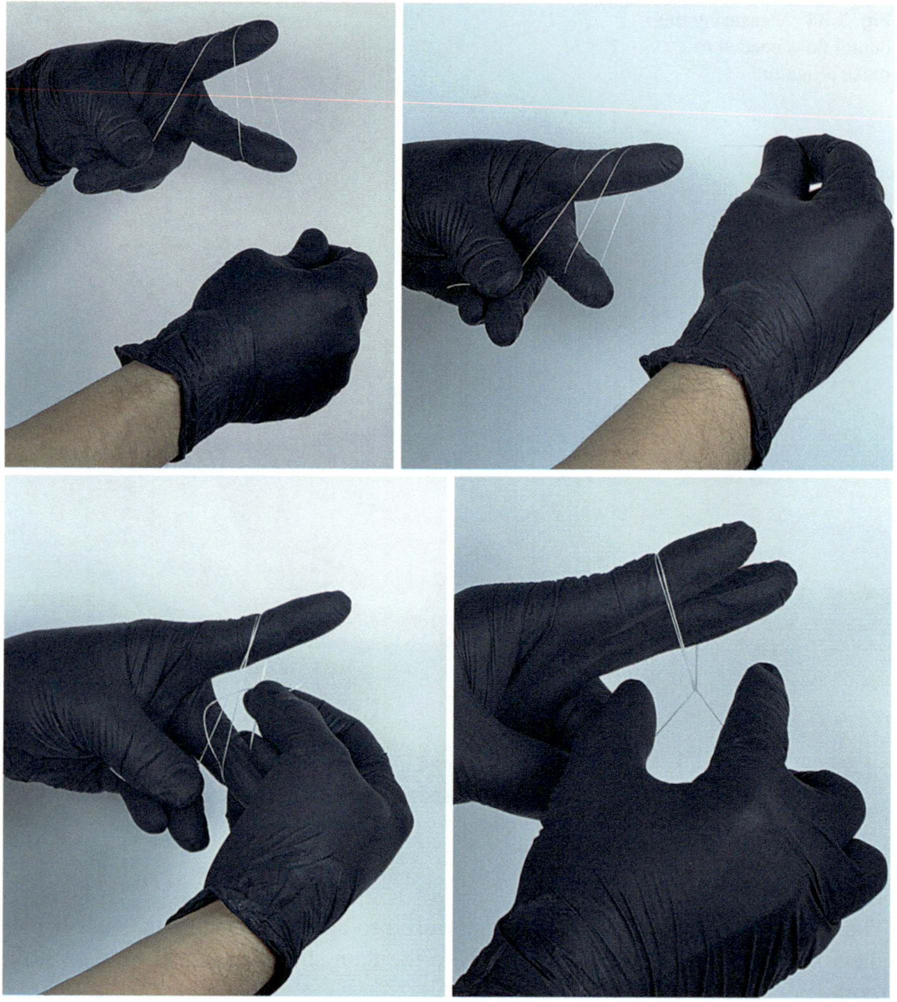

Fig. 3.35 Possible technique for a double floss ligature

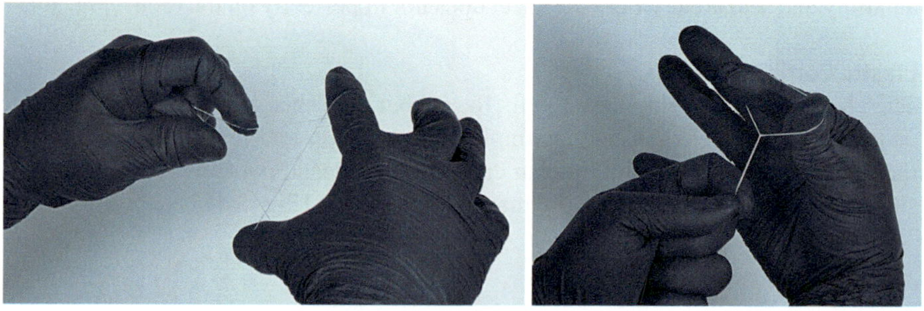

Fig. 3.36 Possible technique for a dental floss ligature

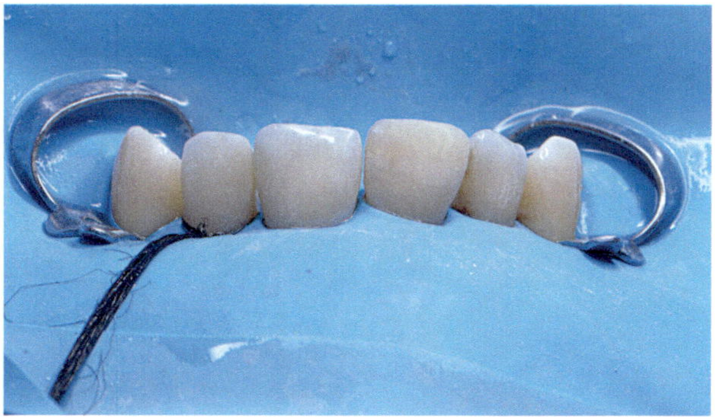

Fig. 3.37 Holding the excess floss of a ligature and securing it to the dam frame

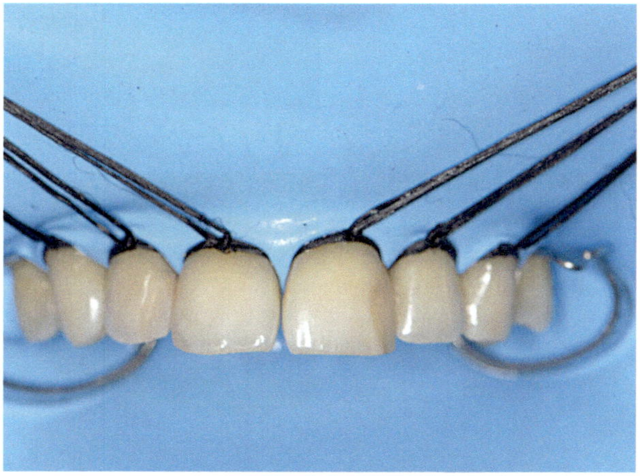

Fig. 3.38 Upper front group isolation with ligatures on each tooth and fixing the excess floss on the dam frame

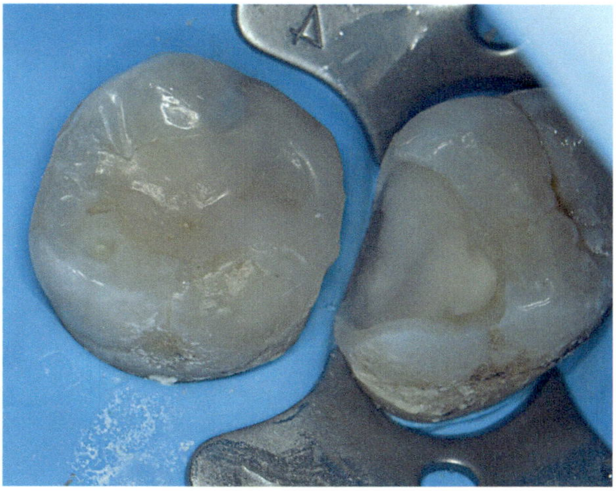

Fig. 3.39 Rubber dam isolation of a molar with a subgingival margin cavity

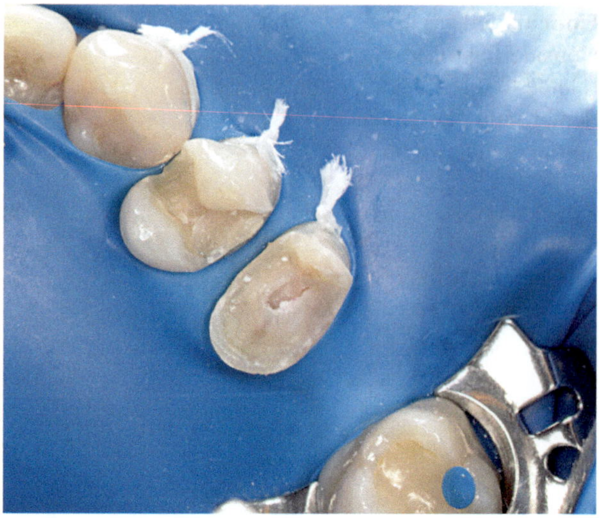

Fig. 3.40 Group isolation with ligatures on each tooth

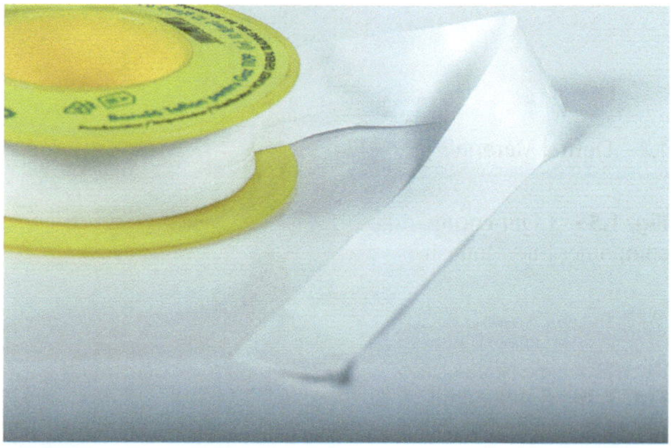

Fig. 3.41 Teflon (PTFE) tape roll

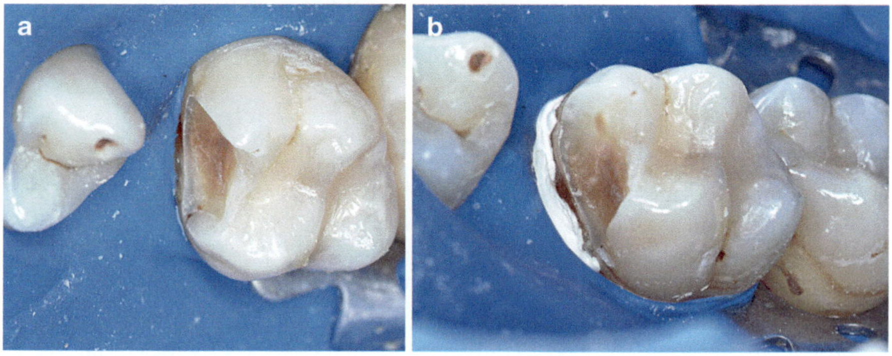

Fig. 3.42 Untight sealing in the gingival area (**a**) completed by applying a Teflon tape cord (**b**)

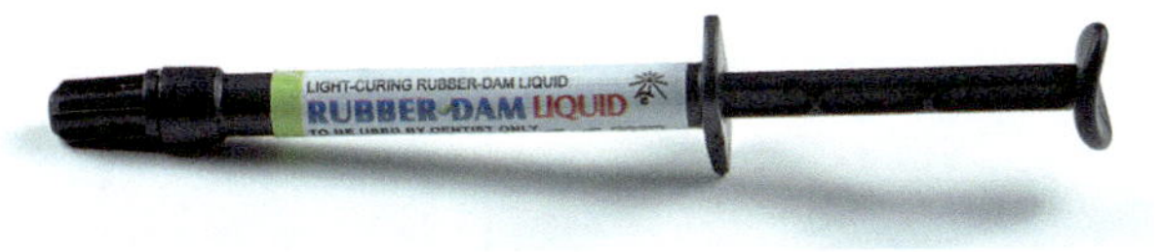

Fig. 3.43 Liquid rubber dam syringe

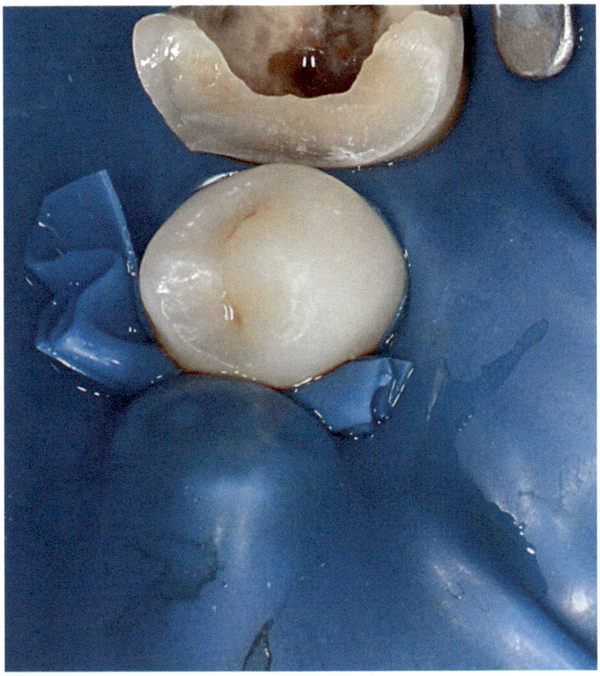

Fig. 3.44 Cord made by rubber dam sheet

Additional Clamps

The mesial fixation of the rubber dam sheet can also be achieved by applying additional clamps (Fig. 3.45a). Moreover, the apical positioning of the rubber dam sheet can be achieved by applying type B gingival tissue retractors (Fig. 3.45b).

Additional Customizations

The rubber dam isolation is not indicated for patients with permanent or temporary respiratory problems. If, however, the mouth-breathing patient agrees to the use of the dam, a perforation should be made in the upper part of the sheet (Fig. 3.46a).

The upper part of the rubber dam sheet should not cover the nostrils, limiting the patient breathing (Fig. 3.46b), but it should be stretched, folded, or cut to free the nostrils (Fig. 3.46c).

A disposable textile or paper protector can be placed under the dam sheet to protect the cheeks, absorb perspiration, or avoid direct contact between the skin and the rubber dam sheet material in case patients are allergic to these materials (Fig. 3.47a–c).

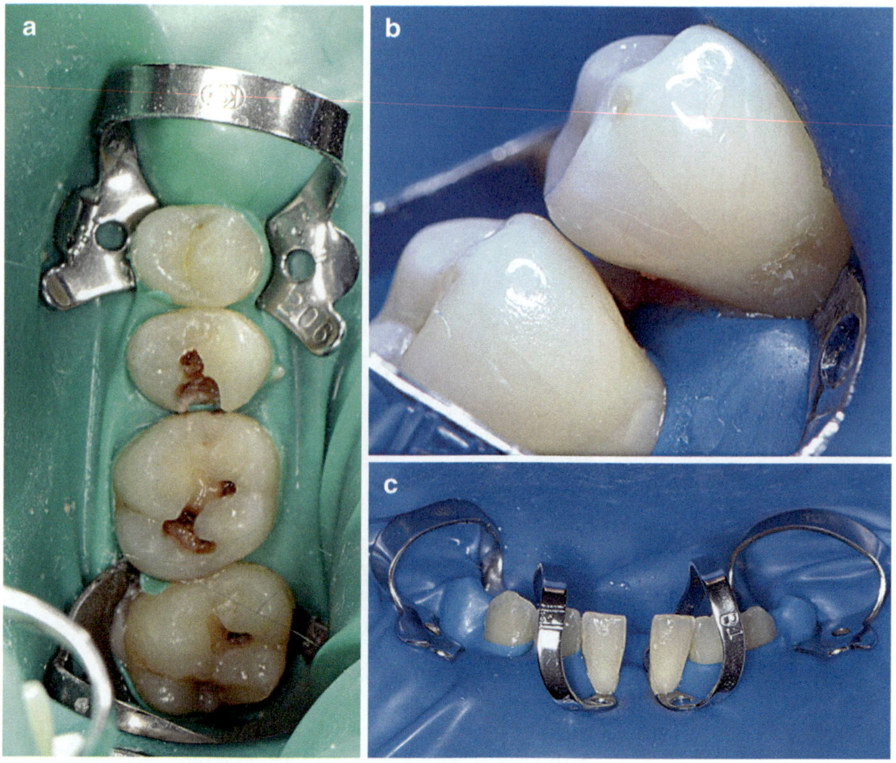

Fig. 3.45 Supplementary clamp applied on a premolar (**a**) and B4 gingival tissue retractor on premolar (**b**) and central incisors (**c**)

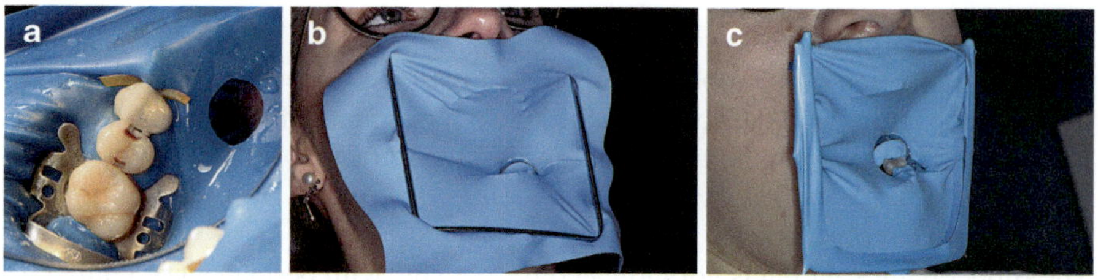

Fig. 3.46 Rubber dam sheet with a perforation for air access (**a**); improperly fitted sheet that partially covers the nostrils and prevents breathing (**b**); sheet folded at the base of the nose to prevent covering of nostrils (**c**)

The lower part of the dam sheet can be lifted on the frame and anchored to the top edge to form protective pockets where water or other liquids used during the treatment can be collected. This prevents them from spilling onto the patient's face or clothing (Fig. 3.48).

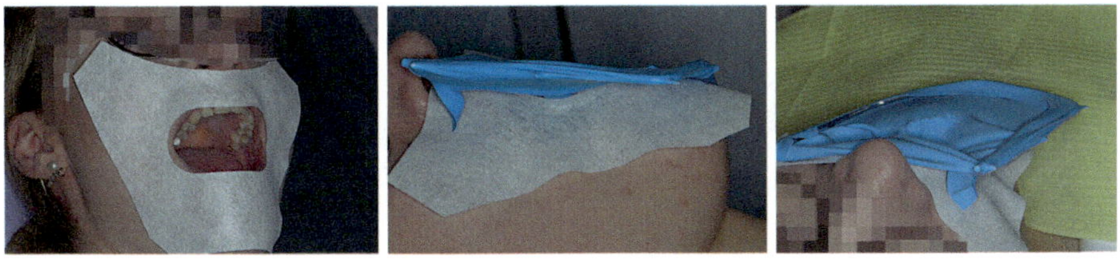

Fig. 3.47 Paper protection was placed over the patient's face under the rubber dam sheet

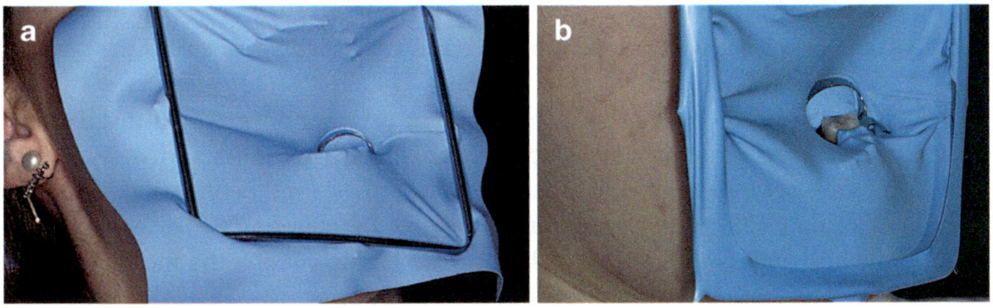

Fig. 3.48 Rubber dam sheet applied to the metal frame (**a**) with pockets at the bottom to prevent liquid leakage (**b**)

Fig. 3.49 Isolation of the upper arch with a split dam in quadrant 2

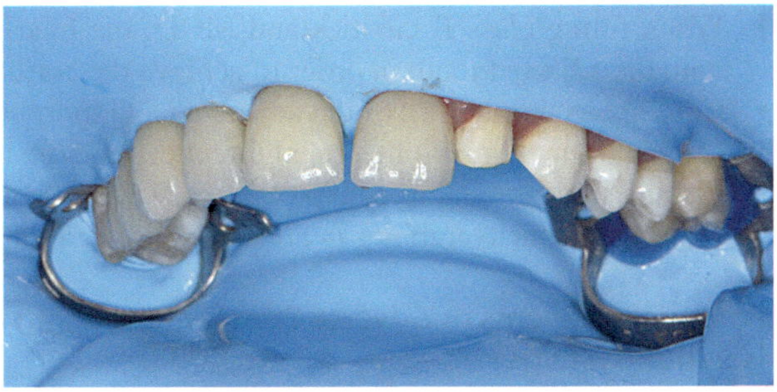

The split dam isolation technique is preferred for specific procedures (e.g., no prep veneer cementation, cementation of crowns on vertiprep abutments) where preparations are not clearly defined, and their limits identification is difficult. Thus, the rubber dam is cut with scissors to make the gingiva visible and to avoid the interference of prosthetic work with the clamps, rubber dam, or auxiliary means of isolation. The isolation, in this case, is not ideal, but some of the advantages of using the rubber dam system are present (e.g., soft tissue retraction, preventing touching the teeth with tongue or mouth closing) (Fig. 3.49).

Isolation Particularities for Direct Restoration

In restorative dentistry, group isolation of at least three teeth, one mesial and one distally positioned to the tooth being worked on (Fig. 3.50), is preferred to achieve

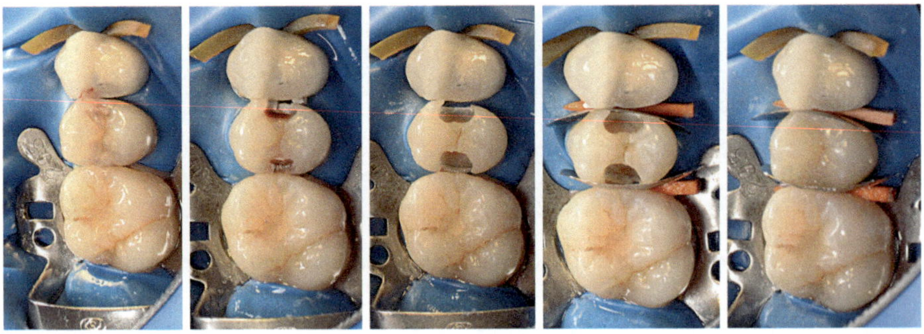

Fig. 3.50 Group isolation with a rubber dam and elastic cord to restore a premolar

better visibility and access [27]. Furthermore, in the case of proximal-distal cavity restorations, it is recommended to place the dam clamp on a tooth as distally as possible, preferably two teeth distally positioned, to provide sufficient space for matrix system placement [28]. When preparations open to neighboring teeth, the neighboring tooth whose cavity will be opened must also be included in the mesial or distal isolation. Group teeth isolation offers several advantages:

- When preparing class II cavities and MOD, the dentist has the opportunity to examine the proximal surfaces of neighboring teeth, which are often affected by caries.
- When filling class II cavities and MOD, the matrices must come into contact with the adjacent tooth in order to achieve the correct contact.
- Continuous monitoring of the adjacent teeth morphology to achieve an aesthetically and functionally integrated direct occlusal restoration.
- Placing the dam clamp next to the tooth being worked on gives more working space and maneuverability in all stages: preparation, matrix fitting, and filling.

Potential Accidents or Adverse Effects of Installing the Rubber Dam Isolation Systems

The clamps fitting must be done carefully because their sudden use can traumatize the marginal periodontium leading to consecutive gingival retraction [29]. Applying clamps on teeth with cervical demineralization may cause enamel loss at this level [30].

At the periodontal level, avulsion can occur accidentally. If clamps are placed on prosthetically restored teeth, the ceramic work may accidentally break off, which is why metal clamps should not be placed over prosthetic work. If necessary, plastic clamps can be used, which are less aggressive.

Difficulties that may occur	Potential solutions
The rubber dam is not entirely cut open when the perforator is pressed, and the cut piece is still trapped inside (Fig. 3.51)	Trying to pull it off easily can lead to pinching and may cause the dam to tear. Tightening the perforator may achieve a better cut, or it may be decided to change the perforator with a new one

Difficulties that may occur	Potential solutions
The clamp cannot be stabilized on the tooth because of the crown shape	Applying a liquid rubber dam or any composite resin to the tooth above the clamp tines prevents the clamp from coming off the tooth; use a clamp with subgingival tines
The papilla is not covered with a rubber dam (Fig. 3.51)	Try arranging the sheet with a spatula or with a less sharp explorer. If the interdental distance at the cervical level is larger, then replacing the sheet with a new one is recommended, where the perforations will be made at a larger distance than those on the template
The rubber dam does not fit onto the tooth in a circular motion for a tight seal because the perforations are too close together (Fig. 3.52)	Gently move the dam clamp for repositioning and allow the sheet to mold to the tooth or fill it with rubber liquid dam or Teflon tape.
The concave anatomy of the proximal surface of some teeth, especially upper molars, prevents the sheet from fitting to the tooth (Fig. 3.53)	Top up with liquid dam or Teflon tape

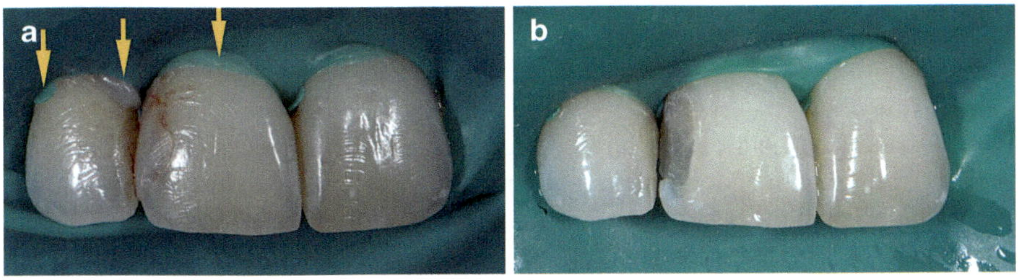

Fig. 3.51 Improper application of rubber dam sheet that has not been completely cut out and does not cover the papilla (**a**); image after deficiency correction (**b**)

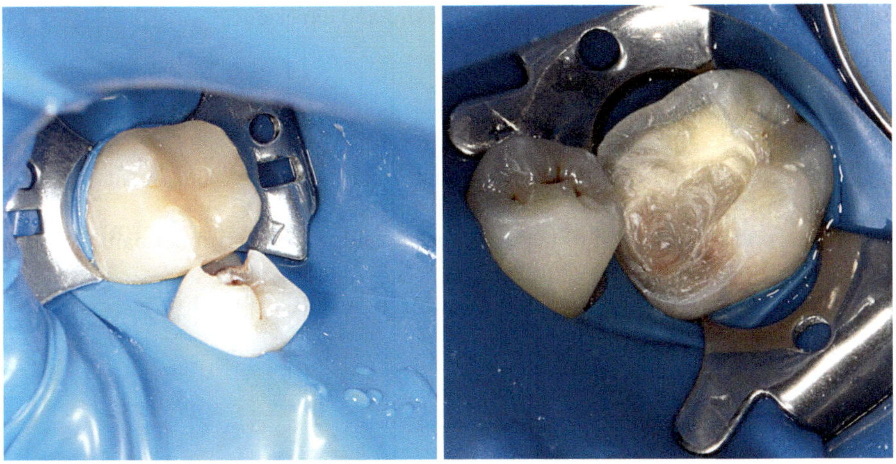

Fig. 3.52 Aspect of inadequate isolation due to increased interdental distance at the cervical level and perforations in the rubber dam made too close

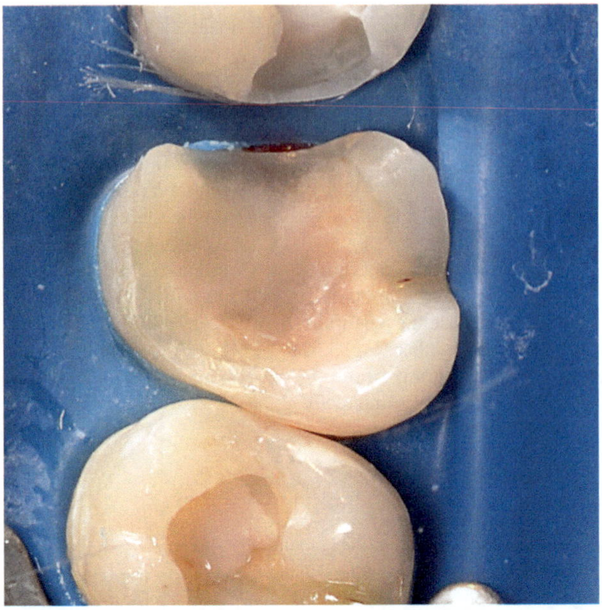

Fig. 3.53 Aspect of a rubber dam sheet isolation that does not fit tightly into the concave morphology of the molar proximal area

Conclusion

Direct restorations and cementation of ceramic prosthetic pieces (onlays, crowns, veneers), along with endodontic treatments, are the main procedures for which the rubber dam isolation is commonly used. Although old as a concept, rubber dam isolation remains the golden standard in isolating the operating field from the salivary and oral anatomical environment. In addition, the isolation provides optimal conditions for the dentist to focus on the treatment: visibility, access, and continuity of treatment because the patient is not tempted to close the mouth or stop the dentist from working. The cases in which the doctor cannot use dam isolation are extremely rare and are often solved by the dentist's desire and experience.

Review Questions

1. What are the main advantages of rubber dam isolation for direct and indirect restorations?
2. What are the main phases of rubber dam isolation, and what do they consist of?
3. What auxiliary means of fixation, retention, and sealing of rubber dam isolation are used, and how are they performed?
4. What are the advantages of isolating a group of teeth for restorative treatments?

3.4 Adjacent Teeth Protection Techniques (Pre-distancing and Wedging)

3.4.1 Wedging and Pre-distancing

Main idea: Pre-distancing is achieved by positioning a wooden or solid plastic interdental wedge during the preparation of proximal cavities.

The purpose of teeth pre-distancing during the preparation (Figs. 3.54 and 3.55) is to get more benefits:

- Doing a gradual pre-distancing during cavity preparation is necessary to position the sectional matrix and to obtain a tight contact point [31].
- Protection of the interdental papilla can be traumatized by the rotating burr sliding during the proximal cavity preparation. Injury to the interdental papilla causes bleeding, especially if it is swollen, which is extremely common with proximal caries.
- Maintaining a tight seal achieved with the rubber dam sheet by eliminating the possibility of piercing the sheet with the burr in the interdental area during proximal cavity preparation.
- Enlarging the interdental space so that the risk of touching the adjacent tooth with burrs decreases during preparation.
- Shaping a smooth gingival margin without accidentally creating pits by sliding the burr over the gingival margin (Fig. 3.55).

When the class II cavity preparation or mirror cavities are prepared, the wedge may be damaged, and it cannot be subsequently used for matrix fixation. It should be replaced with a new wedge (Fig. 3.56).

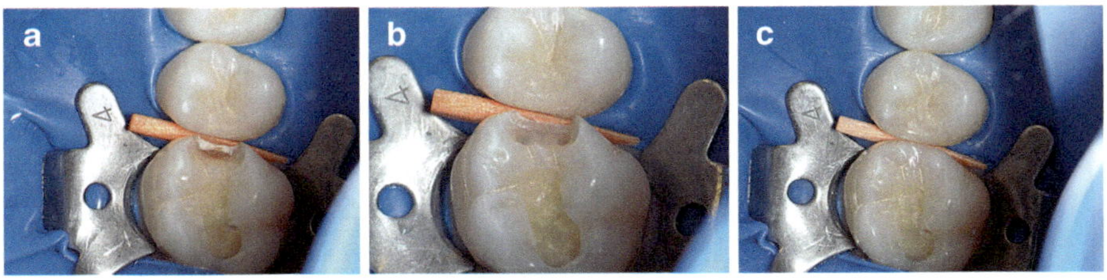

Fig. 3.54 Steps of proximal cavity preparation in the presence of interdental wedges: initial aspect (**a**), during preparation (**b**), final cavity prepared (**c**)

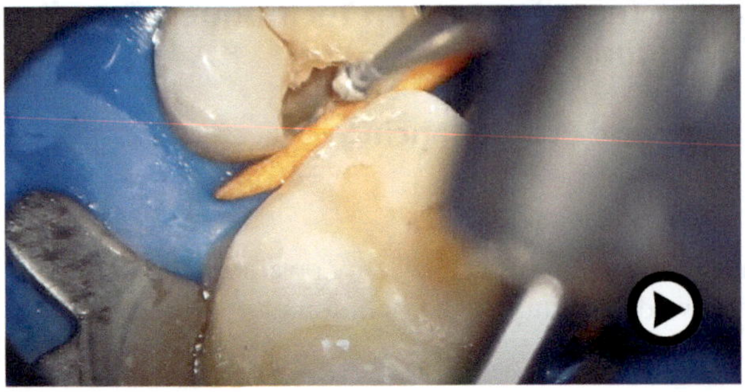

Fig. 3.55 Class II cavity preparation with wedges in place (▶ https://doi.org/10.1007/000-bqk)

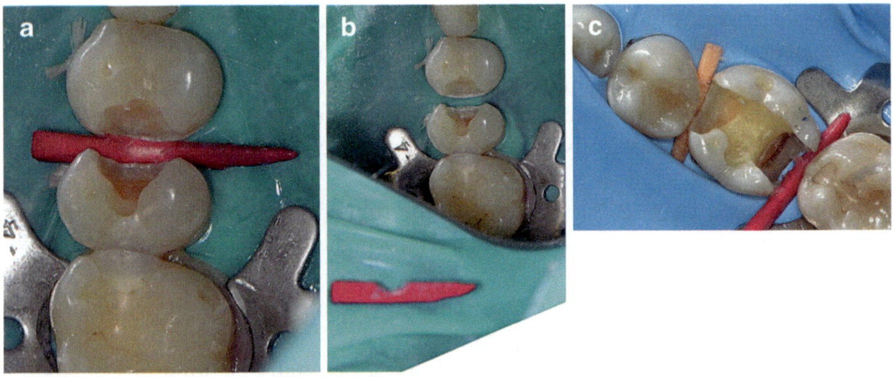

Fig. 3.56 Preparation of symmetrical proximal cavities: image during preparation (**a**); removal of the damaged wedge (**b**). Preparation of a MOD cavity in the presence of interdental wedges (**c**)

Difficulties that may appear	Potential solutions
Failure to install the wedge from the beginning and the rubber dam sheet perforates (Fig. 3.57)	A new rubber dam sheet can be applied, or the perforated sheet can be used, but an assumed inadequate isolation
Impossibility to insert the interdental wedge	Choosing another wedge or thinning the wedge with burs
The wedge comes out during preparation, and it is gradually pushed back	This happens when the tip of the wedge hooks into the rubber dam sheet, which is tensioned by it. The stretched rubber dam sheet will gradually pull the wedge out between the teeth. Correct wedge positioning

Conclusion

Using interdental wedges is a quick, inexpensive procedure that has only advantages for the operator and for the treatment, which is why we recommend it in all cases of proximal preparations.

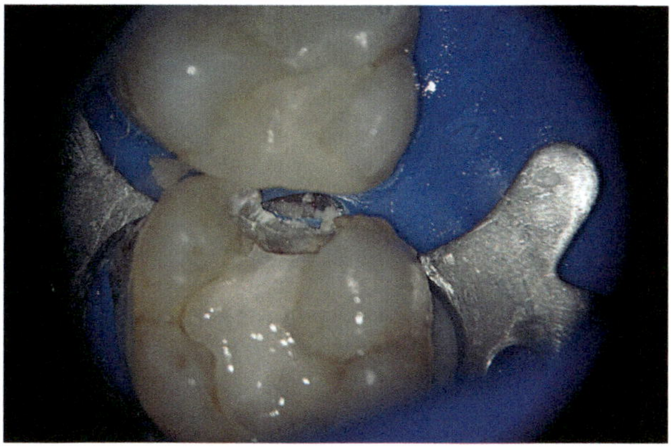

Fig. 3.57 Aspect of a rubber dam sheet interdentally perforated with burrs while preparing a proximal cavity

3.4.2 Wedge Guards

Main idea: Touching the adjacent tooth with the burr during the preparation of proximal cavities can be prevented by wedge guards with metal protection. These can be also made by combining a classic wedge with a flat metal strip (straight matrix tape).

When working with high-speed (turbine) burs for proximal cavity preparation, there is a risk of unintentionally touching the neighboring tooth with the burr. This is undesirable malpractice that often goes unnoticed. Published studies indicate a frequency of this malpractice is 74% in experienced dentists and 94% in students when the preparation is done without protecting the neighboring tooth [32]. The percentage drops below 50% if metal protection strips and wedges are used (Fig. 3.58).

Metal wedge guards can be prefabricated or made from a classic wedge with a straight piece of the metal strip (Fig. 3.59a).

In the case of Palodent V3 WedgeGuards, the metal bands can be removed after the cavity preparation has been completed. The wedge will remain available in position for the matrix mounting phase (Fig. 3.59b).

Difficulties that may occur	Potential solutions
Triggering the gingival bleeding when the wedge is being removed	Gingival bleeding subsides spontaneously, and the blood that covers the rubber dam sheet is washed away with the water spray
Repeated perforation of the metal strip	This signals that the neighboring tooth is in danger of being touched by the burr and that the operator must work more carefully—Possibly using magnification

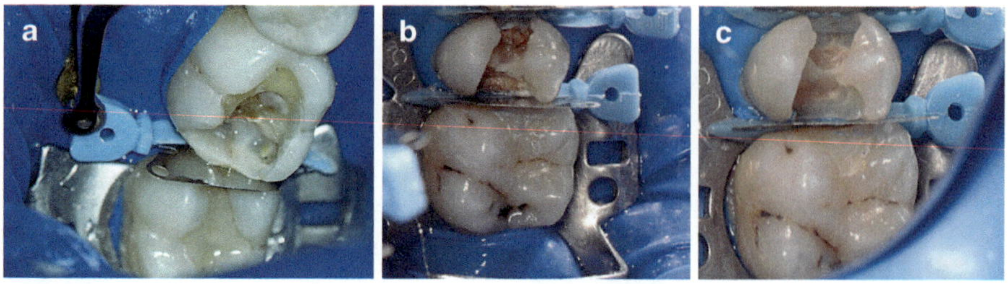

Fig. 3.58 Preparation of proximal cavities in the presence of wedge guards with metal protection (**a–c**)

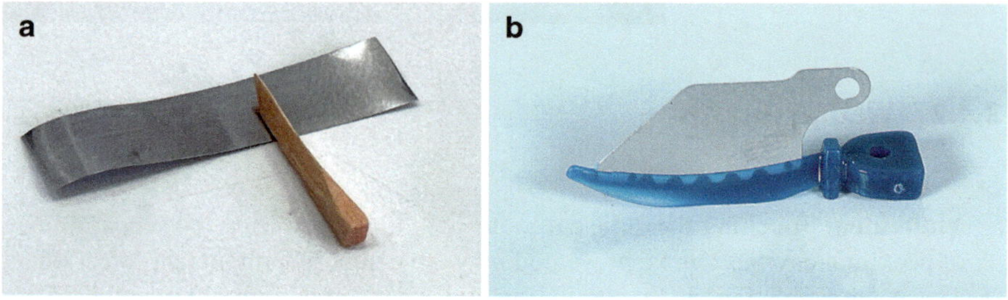

Fig. 3.59 Interdental wooden wedges and flat metal matrix tape (**a**); dedicated interdental wedge with removable metal protection (**b**)

Conclusion

Protecting the adjacent teeth when preparing the proximal cavities is recommended in all cases, and the lack of it is only desirable when using a method of magnification that provides better control.

3.5 Cavity Design and Preparation Techniques

Main idea: Cavity design for composite resin restorations are not currently determined by the material's physical properties. The main criteria for cavity design are removing carious tissue and the mechanical strength of the remaining structures. Therefore, there are no standard cavities for composite resin restorations.

According to Black's principles, cavity preparation follows specific universally recognized characteristics. Many names (Prime, Bronner, Markley, Rodda, Gilmore, and Modern) have developed the design and shape of cavities prepared on teeth. The first deviation from Black's concepts was in 1951, supported by Markley [33] and later by other authors [34, 35], who introduced multiple revisions. The cavities we prepare today no longer follow many of the recommendations made by these authors, well-established in the literature, and it is most often a "minimally invasive" preparation.

The cavities could have a minimum depth or even some small areas of enamel that are unsustained by the dentin at the cavo-superficial edge. Large areas of thin unsupported enamel must be removed. The cavity base does not require the placement of a material for its planning. Unsupported dentin enamel from the proximal gingival edge should not be removed because this may lead to interdental papilla bleeding and, more importantly, to enamel loss. Otherwise, the cavity may end up with dentin edges, providing inferior composite adhesion.

Furthermore, marginal ridges are part of a circumferential occlusal frame that is resistant to occlusal forces and, once interrupted, will weaken the dental crown. Any cavity shape that preserves the marginal ridges is much stronger than the one from which the ridges are missing, especially since, at least in the lower teeth, they come into direct contact with the cusps of the antagonists and take up the occlusal forces.

Cavity preparation is a procedure that consists of removing the demineralized enamel and infected dentin. Four main stages of this procedure can be identified (Fig. 3.60) that will precede the restoration (Figs. 3.61 and 3.62):

- Cavity opening or removal of an old, inadequate restoration
- Removal of infected dentine
- Providing strength and assessment of residual tooth tissue and removal of large enamel areas that are not supported by dentin or that are structurally compromised
- Finishing cavity edges

Due to the use of adhesive materials, making cavities according to Black's rules is no longer necessary. However, some of the principles and some of the preparation steps remain valid:

1. Opening the carious process—with rotary instruments.
2. Removal of altered dentin—with manual and rotary instruments.

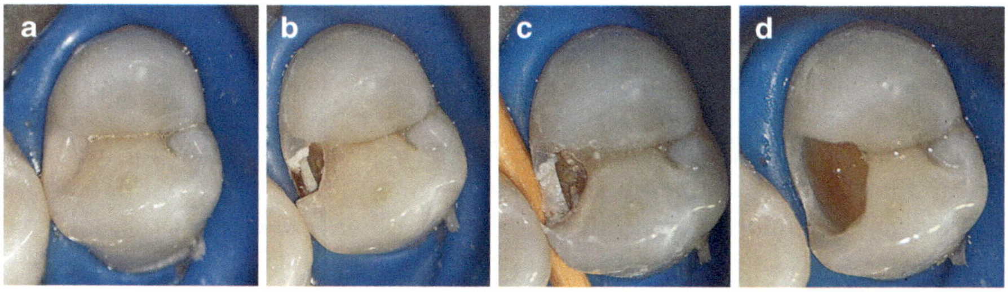

Fig. 3.60 Cavity preparation steps: opening the carious process (**a**); removing the infiltrated dentin (**b**); evaluating and optimizing the cavity (**c**); finishing the edges (**d**)

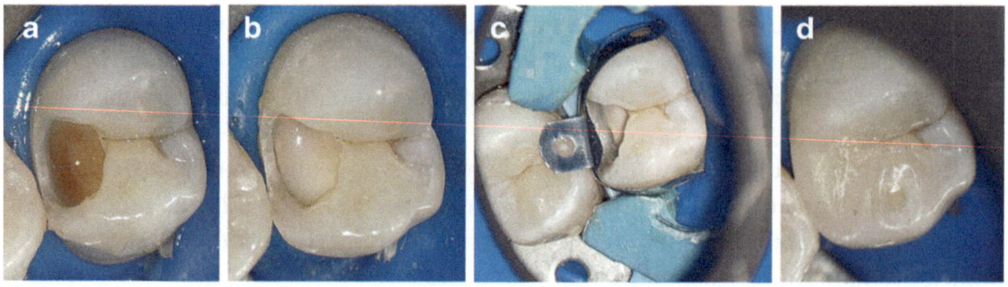

Fig. 3.61 Cavity restoration steps: disinfection (**a**); liner application (**b**); matrix in place (**c**); adhesive system and restorative material (**d**)

3. Performing preventive extension—when it does not contradict the minimally invasive principles. A cavity does not have to be extended by removing healthy tissue only to obtain edges in self-cleansing areas, even though the advantages of such a restoration are certain (visible and accessible margins allow the dentist to remove the excess material and a good finish and the patient to maintain the proper hygiene).
4. Ensuring retention—is less important and has no benefits for adhesive restorations. On the contrary, making a retentive shape undermines mechanical strength by the unjustified removal of dental tissue.
5. Ensuring strength—creating cavities that provide sufficient material thickness and eliminating large areas of thin enamel not supported by dentin.
6. Finishing cavity edges—to achieve smooth contours on which restorative materials achieve good marginal sealing.
7. Checking, cavity cleaning by water flushing/air spray, and disinfecting the cavity with CHX.

Cavities are generally prepared with high-speed (in enamel) and low-speed (in dentin) rotary instruments, but ultrasound tools, laser, chemical methods, and air abrasion are becoming increasingly common. The recommended instrument for infected dentin removal in deep cavities is a manual instrument like Black spoons or dental excavators, which provides better control and can prevent the accidental opening of the pulp chamber.

Regardless of the classification method or the prepared cavity naming, some mandatory characteristics of the prepared cavities must be taken into consideration even with conservative or minimally invasive preparations:

- They need to have a minimum occlusal depth of 1.5 mm to ensure the mechanical strength of the composite resin layer.
- Ensuring minimum enamel bridge widths of 1.5 mm when preparing multiple cavities on the same occlusal surface.
- The cavities' internal angles will be rounded so they do not create any tensions in the restorative materials.
- Cavity shapes should be as round as possible and not geometric/rectangular to reduce stress on the restorative materials.

- The remaining enamel layer should be sufficiently thick and supported by dentin to have the necessary strength.
- Cusps too thin to withstand occlusal forces should be removed, and direct or indirect cusp protection should be achieved.
- All cavity edges must be smooth, free of demineralized enamel areas (white spots), and free of cracks or fractures. These are finished by gentle rounding, but it is unnecessary to bevel them, except for aesthetic reasons on the frontal teeth (see Sect. 3.6.2) (Fig. 3.62).

In order to achieve a good marginal sealing of the restoration that prevents microleakage, and the emergence of marginal secondary caries, a circumferential area of a minimum 1 mm width of sound enamel (and hard dentin), free of irregularities, major unsupported areas, and demineralized white spots and cracks, on which a good adhesion can be achieved, is required (Fig. 3.63).

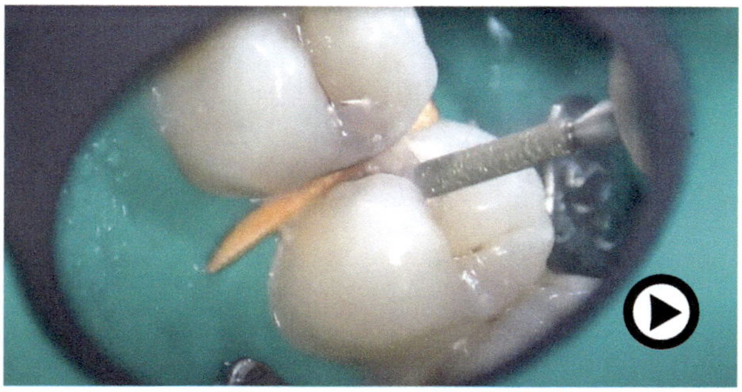

Fig. 3.62 Preparation of two mirror cavities, prewedging, converting into class I cavities, sculpting morphology, and pigment application (▶ https://doi.org/10.1007/000-bqj)

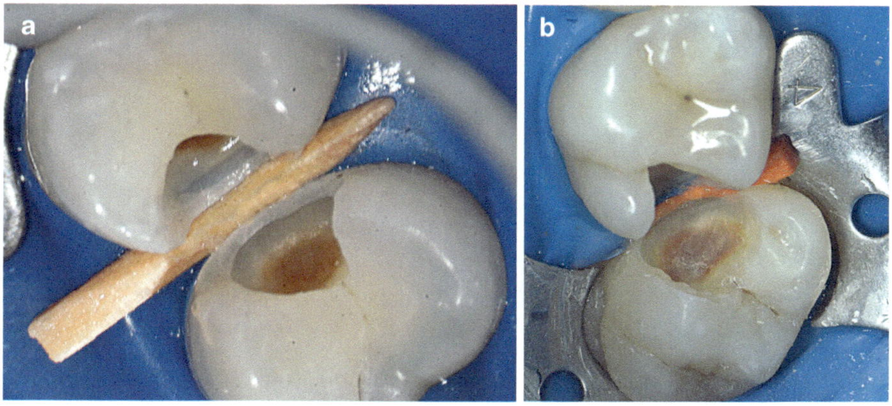

Fig. 3.63 Prepared proximal cavities for direct restoration: cavity enamel margins; the 1.5 mm wide circumferential dentin "band" of healthy hard tissue (**a, b**)

Difficulties that may occur	Potential solutions
White chalky spots of demineralized enamel (Fig. 3.64)	Given the low hardness of the demineralized enamel, these must be removed with turbine burs or even with low-speed burs
Enamel cracks (Fig. 3.65)	The area containing the crack should be included in the cavity preparation, removing the crack, because this is a future pathway for bacterial infiltration that will affect the success of the long-term restoration
Thin edges (Fig. 3.66) or cracked edges (Fig. 3.67) that can easily fracture and where the composite is challenging to adapt, not having a regular contour	These areas result from the proximal contour preparation of the cavity with round or cylinder burrs (Fig. 3.68a). The edges can be straightened using flame burrs with low risk of touching adjacent tooth walls (Fig. 3.68b)

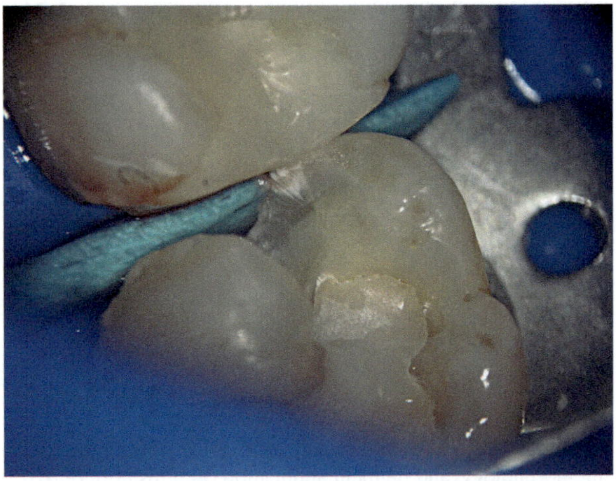

Fig. 3.64 Demineralized white spot enamel area

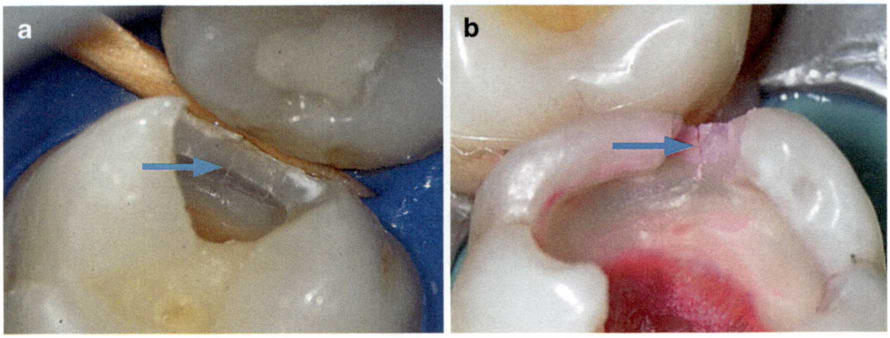

Fig. 3.65 Cracks in the enamel of the proximal gingival margin (**a**); crack identification by infiltrating the caries detector (**b**)

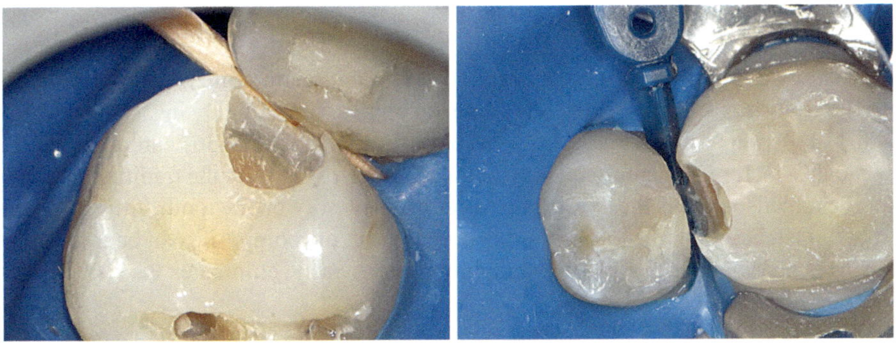

Fig. 3.66 Improperly prepared proximal cavities, with thin edges of the enamel walls and multiple cracks through the entire enamel thickness at the gingival margin level

Fig. 3.67 Improperly prepared proximal cavity with cracked enamel edges, thin, and without mechanical strength

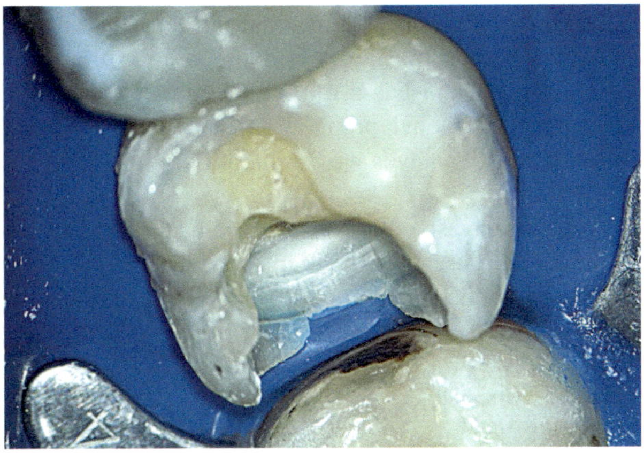

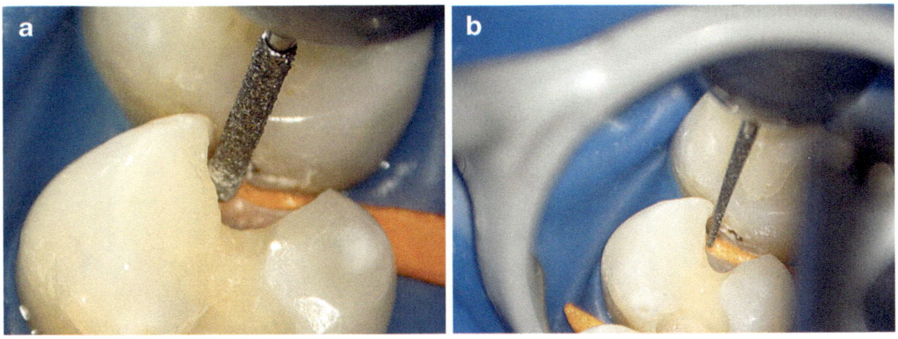

Fig. 3.68 Preparing the proximal box with cylinder diamond burr (**a**) and finishing the enamel edges with a fine flame diamond burr (**b**)

3.5.1 Disk Preparation

The cavity configuration plays a vital role in restoration durability. Class II cavities' traditional "box" shape creates sharp interior angles. A minimally invasive proximal "disklike" preparation (Fig. 3.69) proposed by David Clark [36] can alleviate the typical C-factor problems because it avoids the sharp angles of the traditional preparation and also allows the composite to act in a new way on the tooth, sitting "on the tooth" instead of "in the tooth." In this preparation, the composite can be injected in a single phase, which saves time and, more importantly, eliminates the risk of gaps between layers (see Sect. 4.10).

3.5.2 Tunnel Preparation

Another alternative to the classic "box" preparation is the "tunnel" preparation between the occlusal and proximal surfaces, passing under the marginal edge, which remains intact (Fig. 3.70). This preparation is recommended when the marginal edge is intact and has a minimum thickness and height of 1.5 mm, ensuring its strength. The tunnel preparation has many advantages and disadvantages [37]. Among the advantages we can mention:

- It is less invasive, leaving the occlusal mechanical strength contour of the tooth intact by preserving the marginal edge.
- Preserves the dental contact point intact in many cases.

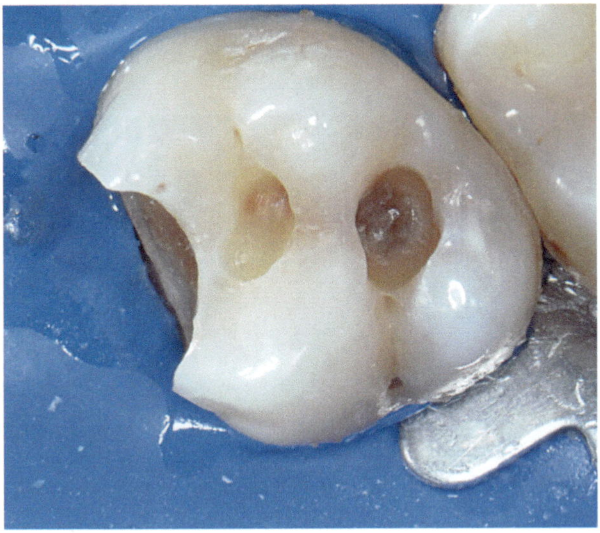

Fig. 3.69 Minimally invasive proximal "disklike" preparation to avoid preparing a "box," which sacrifices more dental tissue

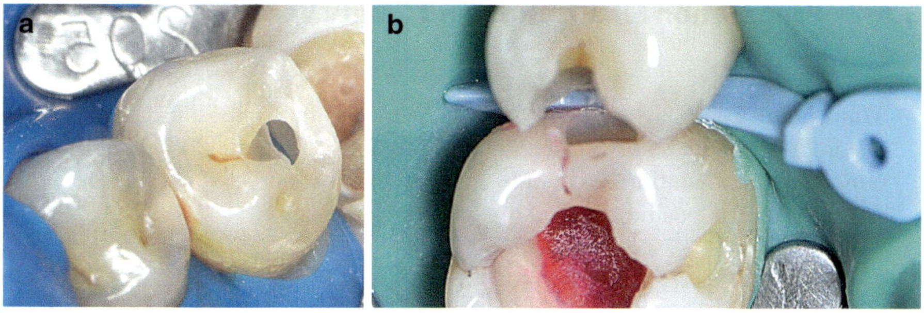

Fig. 3.70 Proximal tunnel-like preparations with preservation of the marginal edge (**a**) and (**b**)

The disadvantages associated with this type of preparation are:

- Limiting the access and visibility
- Decreased control of the obtained proximal morphology
- Marginal edge fracture risk

As a relatively complex preparation, studies have shown that the clinician's experience plays a decisive role in the success of restorations using this type of cavity [38]. It is a paradox that although this type of preparation is less invasive, preserving the marginal edge, the restoration failure rate in these cavities is higher than in other posterior restorations [39, 40]. The most common causes of failure include fracture of the remaining marginal edge and secondary caries. The most likely explanation is the lack of proper assessment of the remaining marginal edge strength. In addition, the atypical shape makes it challenging to evaluate the obtained cavity and, subsequently, the filling. These restorations should be avoided rather than recommended, the *cassette/box type* preparation being more predictable [41].

Conclusion

There are no standard ways of making preparations that are going to be directly restored with composite resins. The cavities' shape is dictated by minimally invasive and conservative principles, by cleaning the carious areas and preservation of hard, healthy dental tissues resistant to occlusal mechanical forces. Therefore, the tooth's degree of damage and the doctor's individual decision for each case will largely dictate the long-term prognosis of future restorations.

Review Questions

1. What might be some of the important general characteristics of cavity preparation?
2. What are the features and advantages of proximal "disklike" shape preparation?
3. What are the advantages and disadvantages of proximal tunnel preparation?

3.6 Preparation Finalization and Cavity Verification

Main idea: The final stage of cavity preparation for composite resin direct restoration involves several simple procedures, including checking for removal of caries-infiltrated dentin, enamel beveling, and creating interdental space for matrix positioning and thickness compensation.

3.6.1 Verification of Cavities with Caries Indicators

Checking the Cavity Preparation Stage with Caries Indicators (Figs. 3.71 and 3.72).

Since the 1970s, a technique was developed that exploited the infiltrating and staining properties of fuchsin, which was then introduced into the clinical practice in order to differentiate the two layers of dentin: the heavily infected outer carious dentin, which must be removed, and the uninfected, demineralized, damaged dentin, which can be preserved [42, 43]. Because of its carcinogenic potential, fuchsin-based staining was replaced by another stain that could dye only the bacterially infected tissue. It has been shown that the absence of staining does not mean the absence of bacteria [44, 45], so these caries indicator solutions do not bind in bacteria-infected dentin but in the dentin organic matrix that is less mineralized

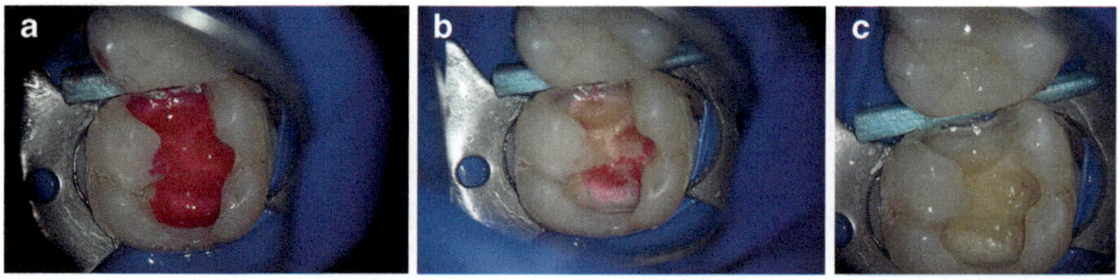

Fig. 3.71 Evaluation of infiltrated dentin removal with caries indicator: application in the cavity (**a**); aspect after immediate indicator rinsing (**b**); final image of the cavity (**c**)

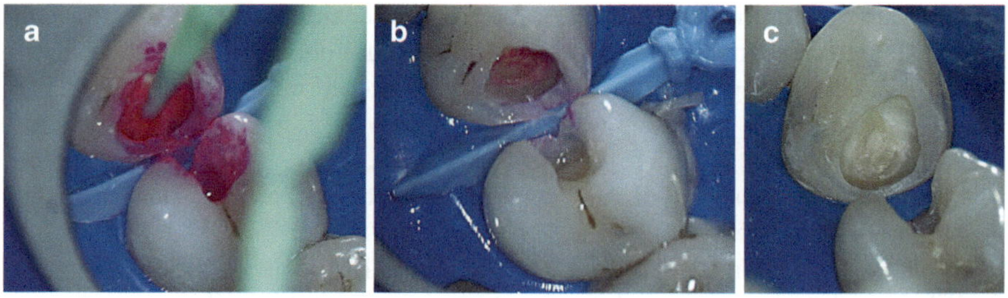

Fig. 3.72 Caries detector application with a microbrush (**a**); lightly stained aspect of the cavity base after washing out the caries detector (**b**); final image of the cavity (**c**)

[46]. Thus, the indicator will stain the healthy hard dentin in the dentinoenamel junction area and the circumpulpar dentin of caries-free, freshly extracted teeth. This is due to the abundant presence of an organic matrix that retains the stain. Therefore, these caries detectors must be used with great care, knowing their limitations. Otherwise, there is a risk of excessive and unjustified removal of dental hard tissue.

However, according to other investigations, caries detectors may be beneficial in detecting caries, and when they are not used during cavity preparation, carious tissues may remain undiagnosed by the clinician [47, 48]. Whenever it is possible to use caries indicators, this should be done in parallel with the use of an explorer to identify more effectively the dentinal areas that need to be removed. The staining produced by the caries indicator should be assessed in terms of color intensity and the high contrast areas indicating the carious dentin. It has been investigated whether the caries indicator can influence the subsequent adhesion of restorative materials, thereby increasing microleakage. The published results excluded the decrease of adhesion on both enamel and dentin [49], although some studies have found decreases when using certain composite resins [50].

The caries detector is most easily applied with a microbrush by brushing over the entire internal surface of the cavity, and then the surface is quickly washed off with a strong jet of water. The areas where the stain has remained firmly fixed after washing are assessed, and then a decision is made on which of these areas the additional dentin should be removed. In making this decision, the clinician should bear in mind the avoidance of opening the pulp chamber and the principle that complete bacterial removal is not always necessary—as it has limited clinical relevance [51]. Thus, removing only the areas of a more intense color, where the indicator has bonded more firmly into the degraded collagen, can lead to the best results.

Difficulties that may occur	Potential solutions
Confusion between the color of the caries indicator fixed in certain areas and the opening of the pulp chamber when using a red color indicator	Change the indicator that has a different color
Accidental opening of the pulp chamber when the stained dentin is excessively removed from all areas where the caries indicator has set	If the pulp chamber has been opened, direct capping is recommended when the opening complies with the indications for this procedure (recent, uncontaminated, small diameter, healthy pulp)

Conclusion

A combination of visual examination and conventional explorer use is the most effective method of assessing the dentin to be removed during cavity preparation. Subsequent use of the caries detector may result in the unnecessary removal of healthy dental tissue. The clinician should perform this procedure with great clinical judgment to preserve the lightly stained areas and remove the dentin from heavily stained areas.

3.6.2 Cavity Beveling

The cavity edge shape prepared for restoration with composite resins is the subject of much discussion among clinicians and researchers. The edges of the opening of the cavity can be kept straight with an angle of about 90°, or they can be beveled. Beveling is described as obliquely sectioning enamel prisms without interrupting the dentinoenamel junction, using diamond burs that can have different shapes (Fig. 3.73). For specific bevel shapes (e.g., straight), different angles are recommended by the literature (e.g., 45–60°) in correlation with different lengths of extension on the occlusal or buccal surface. The burr shape used will also give the shape of the bevel. The beveling can be limited to a part of the enamel layer or extended to its total thickness by operating the burr deep into the cavity. There are now a wide variety of recommendations for what bevel types should be used to achieve the best possible aesthetics in the anterior area.

Beveling is a mandatory step for preparing the cavities in the frontal teeth for aesthetic reasons. Among the possible bevel types commonly used for directly restored cavities, we can mention:

- Straight, at 45° [52]
- "Infinite" beveling [53]
- Concave
- Irregular

The straight bevels can be made with cylinder burs and tapered or flared burs, and the concave ones with round or oval burs.

However, the beveling of the edges can also be considered a less conservative approach that may harm the tooth-material interface quality [54]. However, most studies and authors stipulate that the beveling improves adhesion and prevents microleakage and the development of secondary caries because beveling removes

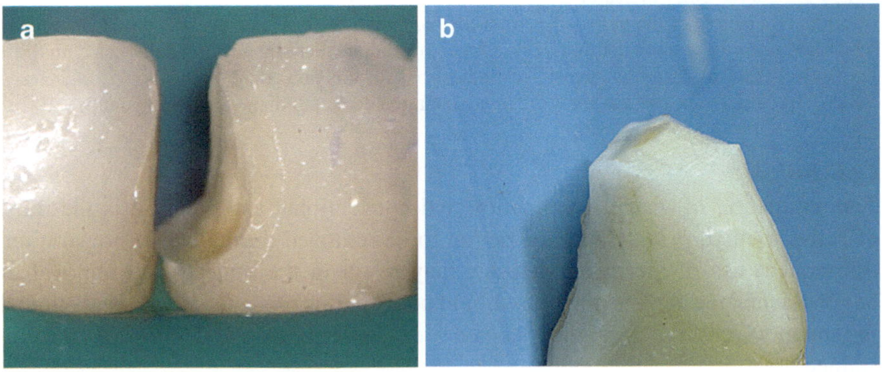

Fig. 3.73 Class IV cavity on upper central incisor (**a**) and lower central incisor (**b**) with concave beveled enamel edges, done with a round and olive diamond burr

the aprismatic enamel layer [55]. Beveling will enlarge the available enamel area for adhesion and improve the integration of the restoration shade with the tooth [56]. This is especially important in the anterior aesthetic area.

As for the posterior teeth beveling, information is conflicting. The existence of a bevel conforms to a progressively thinned edge of the composite resin in the occlusal surface layer, which does not affect the strength of the material under occlusal pressure forces [57]. However, the edges of the occlusal cavities that will be restored with composite resins do not require beveling [58].

The importance of increasing the enamel surface area available for adhesion has not been so strictly necessary, as adhesives have improved over the years—beveling is no longer so necessary from this point of view. Therefore, beveling of cavity occlusal edges is not recommended by some authors [59, 60] because of the minimally invasive reasons (unnecessary removal of the hard dental tissue) but also because of workflow, making it challenging to identify the cavity margin. Moreover, the aesthetic problem of the posterior teeth differs from the anterior teeth because of their positioning and different anatomy.

We believe that beveling is generally not necessary, and we do not recommend it on the cavity's occlusal margins of posterior teeth because:

- It increases the further loss of healthy dental tissue
- It increases the surface area of final restorations, increasing susceptibility to wear
- This can lead to the formation of a thin layer of composite resin at the edge of the restoration that may be vulnerable to fracture
- After beveling, a poorer defined peripheral contour is obtained, and it is harder for the clinician to notice, which may not be suitable for obtaining good obturation and finishing

Difficulties that may occur	Potential solutions
Difficult access with burs in the gingival margin area	Use of longer burs or abandoning beveling
Obtaining thin enamel edges that have no resistance	Removing enamel edges that are too thin

Conclusion

Beveling in the frontal teeth is necessary for aesthetic reasons. There is a wide range of bevel types and shapes that clinicians use depending on the clinical case, the recommendations of composite resin manufacturers, previous personal experience, and individual documentation from the literature. Beveling increases the enamel area available for adhesion, and it can be performed where it is deemed necessary. The decision to perform the beveling should consider the absolute need to extend the available area for adhesion and preserve healthy tooth structures. The enamel edges of the obtained preparation and composite resin restoration must be thick enough to be mechanically resistant. Each clinical case must be evaluated individually according to the composite resin used for the restoration, taking into account the specific indications of the manufacturers.

3.6.3 Separation of Teeth

Separation of teeth before the cavity filling stage (which also involves proximal surfaces) can improve working conditions for the operator and the clinical results obtained. These are directly related to the patient's periodontal health at the interdental papilla level.

The reasons why separation of teeth can be helpful at all stages of a direct restoration are as follows:

- At the examination stage for clinical or radiological diagnosis in order to remove radiographic overlaps.
- At the cavity preparation stage, slight changes in the position of a tooth that has migrated over time into the proximal carious cavity of the neighboring tooth. Cases of severe positional changes should also be carefully evaluated from a periodontal, orthodontic, and occlusal point of view.
- At the direct restoration stage, in order to create a space for the matrix insertion and to obtain a tight contact.
- In the final stage, it allows the finishing of the restorations or removes some material debris that may be stuck in the interdental space.

The separation can be achieved slowly, predominantly through orthodontic techniques that are less demanding, painless, and nonaggressive for the periodontium and the patient: elastic rubber orthodontic bands, interdentally placed pieces of rubber dam sheet, wire ligatures, gutta-percha, overcontoured crowns, or excess fillings.

The rapid separation is achieved in the same session when the tooth is restored. The most popular method of rapid tooth separation is by using dental wedges (Fig. 3.74) or matrix rings that separate by the pressure they exert on the teeth (Fig. 3.75), but there are also special instruments that are less used by clinicians: the Elliot separator (Fig. 3.76), the Ferrier separator, the Ivory separator, etc.

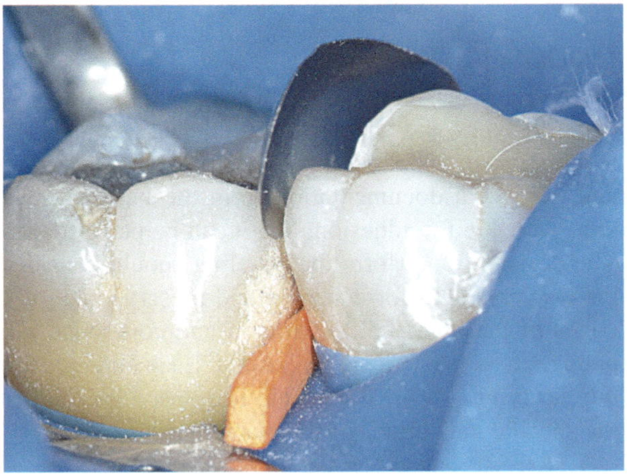

Fig. 3.74 Teeth pre-distancing by inserting a wooden interdental wedge

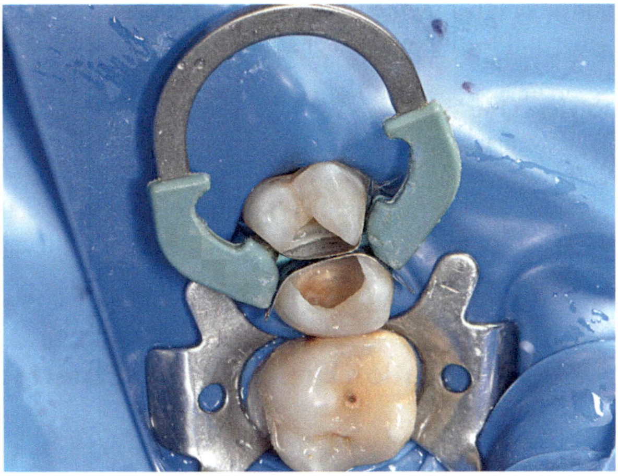

Fig. 3.75 Teeth pre-distancing by fitting a Palodent matrix ring that rests on the two teeth

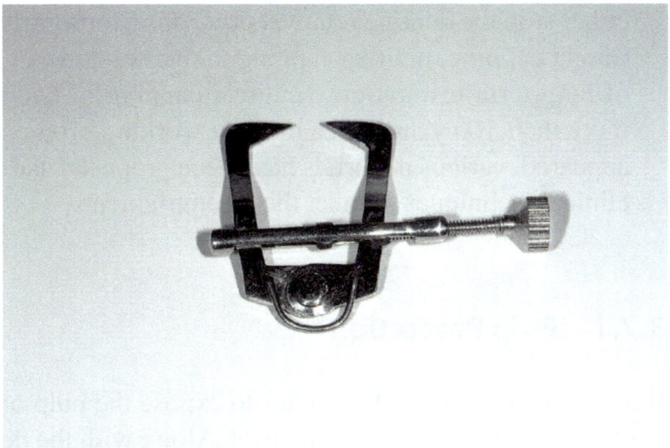

Fig. 3.76 Elliot separator used for teeth spacing

In the case of modern matrix systems, the rings that have glass-fiber-reinforced plastic, rubber, or silicone tines can also achieve tooth separation by the pressure they apply to the teeth they come into contact with.

Difficulties that may occur	Potential solutions
The wedge does not have enough space for interdental insertion	The wedge can be changed to a smaller size, or it can be thinned with a burr
The matrix ring cannot be stabilized and slips due to the coronary anatomy	The ring can be stabilized by adding a rubber liquid dam or any composite resin that adheres to the tooth and ring

Conclusion

Teeth should be separated in all cases of class II and MOD cavity restorations to achieve a good contact of the future restoration. This is paramount in creating space to compensate for the thickness of the matrices used for direct restorations that involve proximal surfaces. Separation of teeth by any of the methods indicated above, or other methods recommended and practiced by clinicians, may be easier to achieve if teeth pre-distancing has been done at the time of cavity preparation.

Review Questions

1. How are cavities checked with caries indicators?
2. How is cavity beveling of front teeth done?
3. What are the reasons why beveling of posterior teeth is not recommended?
4. What are the reasons why the separation of teeth can be helpful at all stages of a direct restoration?

3.7 Preparation Limitation and Expectation Techniques

Main idea: The principles of minimally invasive dentistry and the desire to preserve pulp vitality forces the dentist, in certain cases of deep caries, to either stop the dentine removal procedure, thus limiting the cavity preparation (direct capping, indirect capping in one session), or postponing the execution of long-term restorations (indirect capping in two or more sessions). In the more than 100 years since the first working protocols in restorative dentistry appeared, various materials have been proposed and used according to various clinical techniques to meet these requirements.

3.7.1 Pulp Protection

Black's theory stated: "It is better to expose the pulp of a tooth than to leave it covered only with softened dentin" [61]. Along with the development of the concept of minimally invasive dentistry and dental materials, the clinical approach has become much more conservative [62].

Moreover, dental tissues are limited, and their volume cannot be increased or expanded, which is why their preservation is essential. The treatment of deep caries often involves massive enamel and dentin removal. The sacrifice is even more pronounced when there are complications with these caries, irreversible pulpal pathology, or gangrene/necrosis. Therefore, the attention of clinicians and researchers has been and is mainly focused on avoiding pulp damage to maintain dental vitality [63].

The amount of dentin that needs to be removed when cleaning a carious process and preparing a cavity has always been a topic of research and debate in dentistry [64, 65]. It is not yet apparent how much carious/unhealthy dentin can be left at the base of the cavity in order to allow pulp healing [66] or to prevent irreversible pulp inflammation induced by this remaining unhealthy dentin.

We will use the generic term "carious/unhealthy dentin" to refer to demineralized dentin from a carious lesion, which includes both "affected" dentin (collagen structure preserved, absence of bacteria) and "infected" dentin (collagen structure irreparably degraded, presence of bacteria).

Ideally, cleaning a carious lesion involves completely removing the affected and bacteria-infected dentin. Clinically, however, the difference between the two types of dentin is sometimes difficult or even impossible. In practice, this removal can be achieved by several methods, including:

- Mechanically, rotary with low-speed burs (contra-angle handpiece)
- With ultrasonic loops/tips
- Abrasion with blasting particles
- Manually, with excavators or Black spoons
- Chemical application of various gel-like substances
- By laser

All cleaning techniques remove the dentin with different degrees of effectiveness, but it is not yet known how these techniques could differentiate between areas of infiltrated, infected, or necrotic dentin and areas of healthy dentin that can be preserved [67]. Only the chemical gels out of these methods (e.g., Carisolv, RLS Global, Sweden) remove the smear layer, leaving the dentinal tubules opened for adhesion. However, conventional manual mechanical cleaning with excavators offers the best combination of cleaning efficiency, control, and minimal invasiveness in deep cavities [67].

The evolution of cavity cleaning and preparation techniques has fallen far behind the development of dental materials and adhesive restorative techniques.

3.7.1.1 The Thickness of the Remaining Dentin Layer

The need for dental pulp protection during restorative treatments is directly correlated, anatomically speaking, with the thickness of the remaining dentin layer at the base of the prepared cavities [68].

If following a cavity preparation, the thickness of the remaining dentin layer between the cavity base and the pulp is less than 1 mm, then the pulp vitality may be impaired [69], and if the remaining dentin falls below 0.5 mm, then the pulp of young teeth may be irreversibly affected [70, 71].

The degree of pulp damage increases directly proportional to the decrease in thickness of the remaining dentin layer. Therefore, to maintain tooth vitality and achieve stable long-term results, it is crucial to maintain a dentin layer as thick as possible at the cavity base and a highly controlled reduction of enamel areas to comply with the principles of minimally invasive preparation [72].

The isolation of a carious process from the salivary environment by a tight coronal restoration will prevent bacterial nutrient sources [73]. Healthy pulp has an excellent ability to defend itself against acids and bacterial toxins through neodentinogenesis, significantly when aided by its coating with a bioactive material. Therefore, the complete removal of the damaged dentin is not always necessary for long-term success [74] if there is a good seal against the salivary environment provided by a durable crown restoration [75].

Total removal of carious dentin from the base of a deep cavity can lead to pulp exposure, an incident that should be regarded as iatrogenesis [76].

In order to see if there is the possibility of direct or indirect capping, the following conditions must be met [77, 78]:

- Healthy vital pulp without previous spontaneous pain.
- Pain caused by hot or cold stimuli must disappear when the stimulus is removed.
- There are no periapical lesions of endodontic origin.
- Complete isolation of the operating field from the salivary environment.

If certain conditions are being met, indirect capping is always preferable to direct capping for several reasons:

- The risk of opening the pulp chamber and exposing the pulp decreases by 98%.
- There is no evidence that the partial removal of carious dentin can influence the restoration longevity and pulp symptomatology.
- There is sufficient evidence that the complete removal of carious dentin is not necessary for long-term success if the crown restoration seals tightly [79].
- There is less chance of bacteria from the carious dentin reaching the pulp [80].
- The risk of pulp bleeding disappears. For direct pulp capping, this can lead to the poor long-term success [81].
- It has a better chance of long-term success than direct capping.

Conclusion
The procedure of capping the pulp with various recommended materials placed either directly over the pulp ("direct capping") or over a thin layer of dentin ("indirect capping") is performed in order to maintain the pulp vitality, preventing an endodontic treatment when the pulp is healthy and asymptomatic.

Review Questions
1. What are the reasons why pulp protection is needed for deep cavities?
2. What are the reasons why the indirect capping technique is preferable to direct capping?

3.7.2 Indirect Capping

Main idea: Indirect capping is a procedure that involves permanently covering a thin layer of dentin that is kept close to the pulp (affected or possibly infected). It is possible to perform the permanent restoration in the same session or to postpone it for another session (at a pre-determined time interval), in which additional dentin removal may be done or not.

Indirect capping, first proposed by Pierre Fauchard more than 200 years ago [82], was defined as the application of a sealant (varnish or adhesive) or liner (cement or resins in a maximum layer of 0.5 mm) over preserved demineralized dentin in order to avoid pulp exposure [83]. The concept has come back to the fore in the era of minimally invasive dentistry, especially since multiple studies have shown that the partial removal of carious dentin versus total removal does not influence the long-term success of restorations [84, 85].

The treatment called “indirect caping” or “indirect pulp capping” has been defined in German literature as the treatment of a thin layer of remaining caries-free dentin in the vicinity of the pulp chamber [86] in deep cavities.

The English literature defines *indirect capping* as a permanent covering of a thin layer of dentin kept close to the pulp (affected or possibly infected), a procedure performed in one or two sessions. In the second session, the complete excavation can be performed or omitted [87, 88].

Given that there is a thin layer of dentin whose health status may be uncertain, there is a risk of irreversible pulp inflammation. Microorganisms can cause this, either the bacteria left in the dentin layer or those newly infiltrated after the first session (between appointments). Another possible cause may be the cytotoxicity of the used materials.

Several techniques for performing indirect capping are commonly used, either in one or two steps [89]:

3.7.2.1 Indirect Capping in One Session [90]

Cleaning the Cavity

This technique is based on removing infected dentin (demineralized, with denatured collagen structure, infiltrated with bacteria, irreversibly destroyed) and preserving the affected dentin layer (which is also demineralized, but with the collagen structure still intact, without bacteria, with potential for remineralization). The theory makes sense, but in clinical practice, it is not easy to differentiate between the two types of dentin.

A way to differentiate the two types of dentin could be using caries indicator substances, which mainly infiltrate into the dentin that has a denatured collagen structure and is bacteria-infected. Although their fidelity may be questionable, there are currently no better quantitative techniques that can be applied clinically, easily, and quickly, even during the treatment.

Another option may be to differentiate according to the operator’s clinical sense to remove the wet dentin with the amorphous structure and keep it dry and fibrous, which has some moderate resistance to excavator scraping (Fig. 3.77). Although it is highly subjective and dependent on the operator and his experience, this is perhaps the most widely used method by clinicians.

Disinfection

Indirect capping is done under fair rubber dam insolation conditions. The clinical crown of the tooth and the carious lesion can be disinfected prior to the start of the procedure with low-concentration sodium hypochlorite (NaOCl 1–5%) or chlorhexidine (CHX 2%) to avoid cross-contamination. The same substances can disinfect

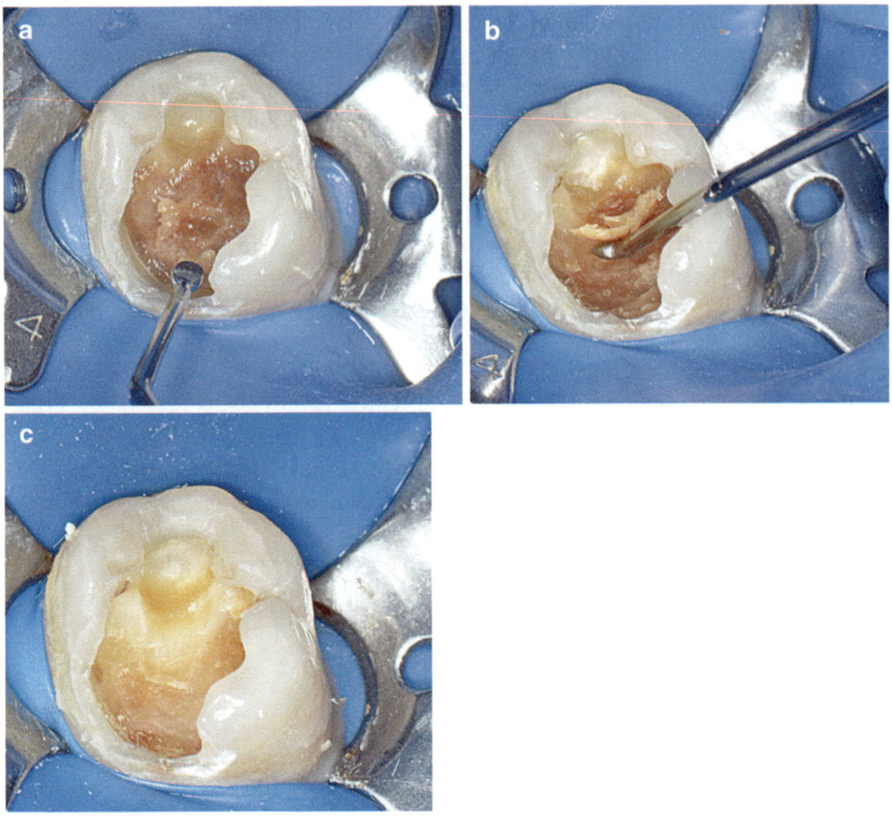

Fig. 3.77 Cleaning the floor of the cavity with a Black spoon (**a**) by scraping the infiltrated dentin (**b**); final cavity after manual cleaning (**c**)

the prepared cavity after using the water/air spray [91, 92]. There should be no concern about pulp damage if sodium hypochlorite in concentrations less than 5% is used for disinfecting the cavity[93].

The Dentine sealing and Filling

The sealing material used in indirect capping is intended to disinfect the remaining dentin layer from the pulp vicinity and to stimulate the formation of tertiary dentin [94]. If the pulp is in a stage of reversible pulpitis, indirect capping treatment is expected to create favorable conditions for pulp healing and inflammation remission.

Traditionally, calcium hydroxide has been recommended for indirect capping since the 1930s [95]. Due to the disadvantages of soluble calcium hydroxide suspensions, calcium disilicate types of cement (MTA, Biodentine) may be a better alternative for indirect pulp coating [96].

The damaged dentin is covered with a bioactive liner expecting to be remineralized and transformed into hard dentin. If this liner is the self-curing calcium hydroxide or classic MTA (Fig. 3.78), it must be fixed by coating with a GIc that extends

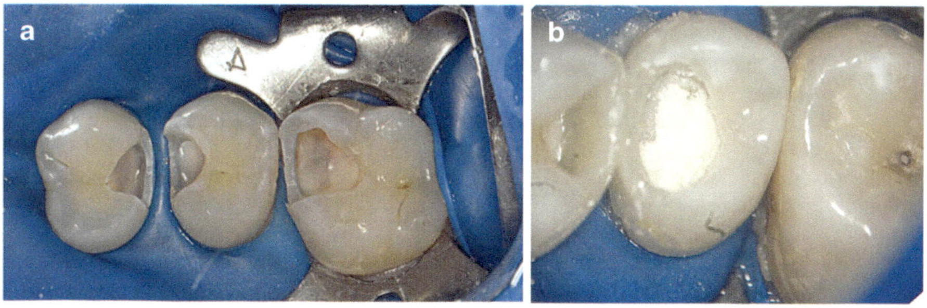

Fig. 3.78 Deep cavities where a liner was applied on the cavity floor: calcium hydroxide (**a**) and MTA (**b**)

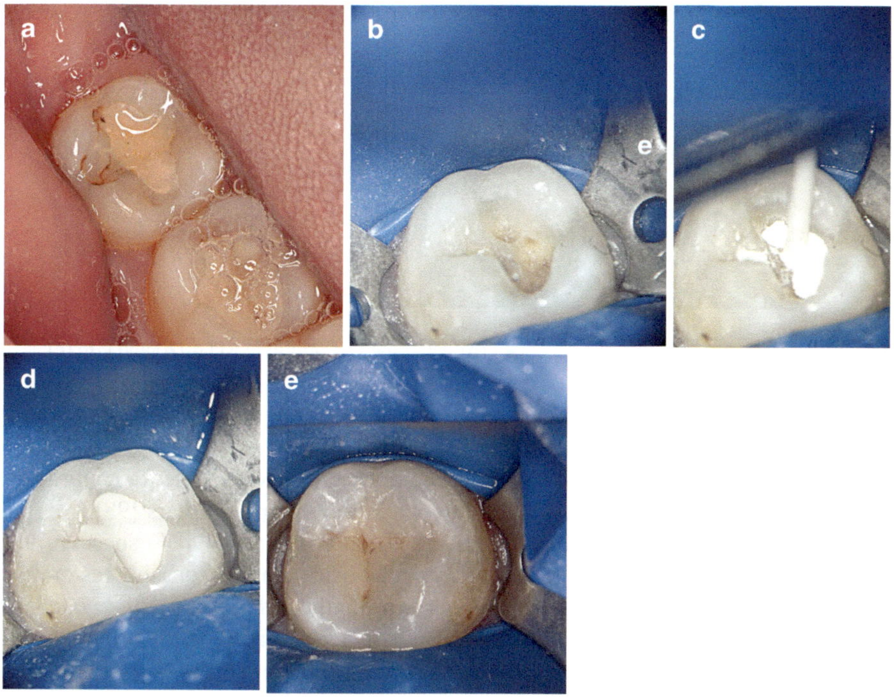

Fig. 3.79 Replacement of an old composite resin occlusal restoration on a lower molar: initial old restoration (**a**); prepared cavity (**b**); self-curing liner (**c**); GIc base (**d**); composite resin restoration (**e**)

into the area of healthy peripheral dentin—to be able to fix well through adhesion. The liner, the GIc base, and the composite resin (Fig. 3.79) will be used in this case. The final restoration will be done in the same session by applying an adhesive composite resin restoration over the GIc [97].

If indirect coronal restoration is planned, it is recommended to be postponed for 4–8 months from the date of indirect capping to monitor the treatment progress.

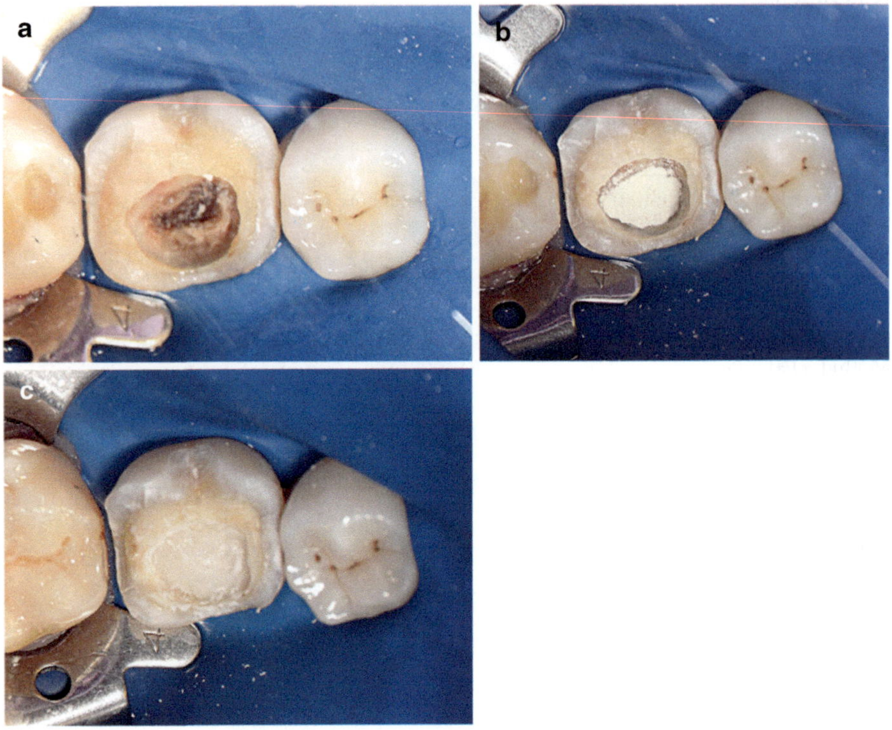

Fig. 3.80 Indirect capping in a deep cavity (**a**) performed by applying MTA (**b**) and GIc (**c**)

During this period, the tooth may receive a durable composite resin or GIc restoration (Fig. 3.80).

Although some studies indicate a significantly higher success rate for using MTA as a liner in indirect capping compared to calcium hydroxide, others [98] (Marina Agathi Petrou et al. in 2015) indicate identical (approximately 90%) success rates for calcium hydroxide and MTA. It is recommend using a nonabsorbable restorative material (MTA or Portland cement) and performing the indirect capping in one session by coronal sealing with durable restorative material, based on the principle that each reintervention may be an additional source of contamination.

Calcium hydroxide has been shown to remove the bacteria from the dentin it covers and to stimulate neodentinogenesis. At the same time, the GIc, used without the underlying calcium hydroxide layer (Fig. 3.81), is effective in providing favorable clinical and microbiological results when used as a liner in indirect capping [99]. For long-term success, the type of liner is less important than achieving an excellent circumferential cavity seal with a durable restoration that does not allow infiltration [100]. This evidence allows clinicians to achieve indirect capping in a single session with a simplified technique (light-curing GIc and composite resins).

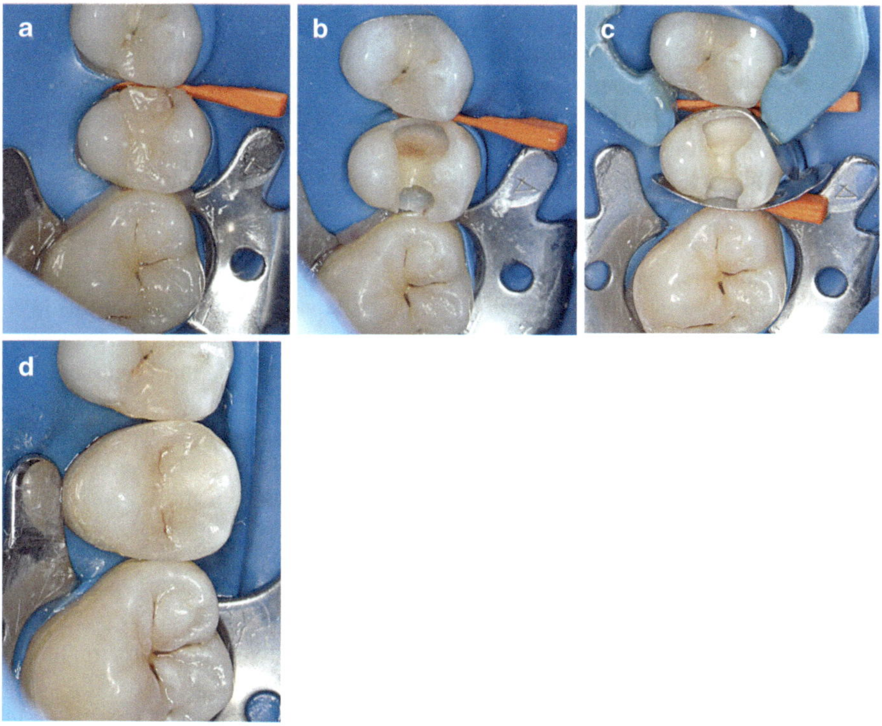

Fig. 3.81 Replacing an old, inadequate mesio-occlusal composite resin restoration on tooth 25 that also has caries on the distal surface: initial old restoration (**a**); cavity preparation (**b**); liner and matrices in place (**c**); final composite resin restoration (**d**)

Difficulties that may occur	Potential solutions
Performing an indirect capping technique in two sessions can compromise the treatment by the patient not attending the second session	Educating the patient or adopting a technique in one session
Retention of an amount of damaged and infiltrated dentin, combined with the coronal microleakage, can lead to pulp inflammation	Endodontic treatment.

Conclusion

In the case of a deep cavity, the clinician may clean the cavity thoroughly and perform a direct adhesive composite resin restoration with liner application or indirect capping in a single session. This involves the differential removal of dentin and the liner application.

3.7.2.2 Indirect Capping in Two Sessions [73]

Mount and Hume, authors of the "SiSta (Site & Stage)" classification of cavities, recommend the treatment of deep cavities by indirect capping in two stages:

1. In the first session, the infected dentin with the wet and amorphous aspect is removed from the cavity base, and a good circumferential cleaning of the walls down to the healthy hard dentin is done to allow a good adhesion that is necessary to stop salivary infiltration. The affected dentine is preserved in the expectation of remineralization, which will occur if its degree of mineralization exceeds 10%. Although it is impossible to clinically assess the exact degree of mineralization of the remaining dentin, dentin mineralized by at least 10% can be clinically perceived with an explorer or during excavation as a firm material that resists some degree of scraping. A temporary filling of bioactive material (e.g., calcium hydroxide or GIc) with good adhesive capacity is applied over this layer to achieve sound isolation from the salivary environment. This will be kept for at least 3 weeks but not more than 6 months.
2. In the second session, the pulp status is assessed, and if the pulp is asymptomatic and vital, the temporary filling is partially removed, and the permanent restoration is performed. This is a classic indirect capping option, but some authors indicates that the pulp assessment should be performed in the second session even earlier, after 7–10 days [101].

If the clinician deems it necessary (knowing the case details), they can remove the filling and decide to clean the dentin further. This indirect capping technique is recommended not only by the European Society of Endodontics (ESE) [88] but also by the American Association of Endodontists (AAE) [102], which assimilates the treatment of "indirect capping" with that of "stepwise excavation." Both associations recommend that indirect capping should be performed in two sessions at a maximum interval of 6 months (ESE) or 6–8 months (AAE) for the total removal of the first filling (fist appointments) and additional dental cleaning from the cavity base *(European Society of Endodontology: Quality guidelines for endodontic treatment: consensus report of the European Society of Endodontology. Int Endod J 2006; 39:921–930).*

Beyond the principles of minimally invasive dentistry and the primary dental concern of preserving vital teeth, indirect capping can have socioeconomic importance in maintaining the oral health status of the population. The economic impact is easier to quantify, especially in countries where the cost of treatment is state-subsidized and the cost of endodontic treatment is significantly higher than the cost of indirect capping. It is, therefore, more than not only a medical issue but also a financial pragmatism and social responsibility.

Difficulties that may occur	Potential solutions
Accidental opening of the pulp chamber	Direct capping or endodontic treatment
Accidental displacement of the liner	Repeat the procedure
The emergence of irreversible pulp symptoms	Endodontic treatment

Conclusion

The key difference between one-session and two-session capping is the waiting period until the final adhesive restoration is achieved, which is necessary to confirm the pulp's health. The recommended waiting period may vary from one author to another, each technique having its advantages and disadvantages. The restoration between sessions is preferably done with a long-lasting restorative material, most commonly GIc, as achieving excellent coronal sealing is essential.

The two-session technique is considered more conservative from a clinical point of view but more time-consuming and possibly more expensive for the patient, requiring two visits to the dentist. However, if pulp symptoms appear (irreversible pulpitis), regardless of whether the capping was done in one or two sessions and the duration between the two sessions, endodontic treatment is imminent.

Review Questions

1. What are the advantages, disadvantages, and steps to achieve indirect capping in one session?
2. What are the advantages, disadvantages, and steps to achieve indirect capping in two sessions?

3.7.3 Direct Capping

Main idea: Dental pulp exposed due to dental trauma, carious processes, or iatrogenic mechanical causes can be covered with bioactive materials placed directly over the pulp to maintain tooth vitality and avoid endodontic treatment.

According to the definition given by the American Association of Endodontists, mechanical exposure refers to an "accidental exposure of the pulp by maneuvers performed with rotary or manual instruments in the absence of penetrating caries."

Indications of direct capping [102]:

1. Permanent teeth that require restoration.
2. Recent accidental or traumatic mechanical exposure of dental pulp (vital and asymptomatic) (<1 mm; <24 h) (Fig. 3.82).
3. The exposure site allows the direct capping material to contact the exposed pulp directly.

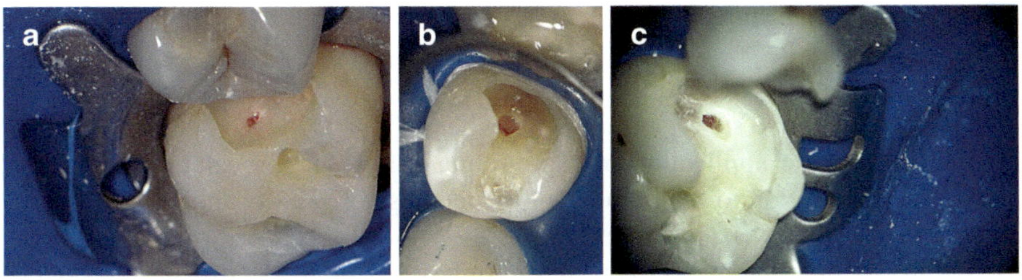

Fig. 3.82 Accidental pulp chamber openings during deep cavity preparation (**a–c**)

4. Slight bleeding, but controllable or absent, at the exposure site.
5. Mechanical exposure of pulp occurs under rubber dam isolation conditions.
6. A tooth can benefit from appropriate coronal restoration with good sealing.
7. The patient has been informed and he or she has accepted the possibility of pulp aggravation that could lead to endodontic treatment.

3.7.3.1 Bleeding Control

Most commonly, dental pulp exposures are also associated with bleeding that needs to be controlled and where hemostasis must be performed [103]. Heavy bleeding may be an indication of pulp inflammation and could make the direct capping procedure impossible to be done. Bleeding control is done by applying sterile pads and using solutions:

- The saline solution is most commonly used, being the least invasive for the pulp [104], but with poor hemostatic and disinfecting properties.
- Sodium hypochlorite (1–5%) is more invasive/aggressive to the pulp but with good hemostatic and disinfectant properties.
- Chlorhexidine has weak hemostatic proprieties but good antibacterial properties.

3.7.3.2 Materials

Materials that can be applied in direct capping over the exposed dental pulp facilitate the formation of repair dentin and maintain the dental pulp vitality. These can be:

- Self-curing calcium hydroxide
- Calcium disilicate or bioceramic types of cement: MTA (mineral trioxide aggregate) or Biodentine

As for the light-curing materials proposed for direct capping by various authors over time (adhesives, light-curing GIc), studies show that the remaining unpolymerized monomers have a cytotoxic effect on fibroblasts [105]. When near the pulp, they may diffuse directly to the pulp in the pulp exposure area or diffuse through the dentinal tubules, generating some degree of pulp inflammation [106]. Therefore, vital pulp therapy using light-curing adhesive resins is not indicated [107].

3.7.3.3 Direct Capping Protocol

If the criteria for performing the treatment are met (assuming the tooth is already anesthetized and it is isolated using a rubber dam), the protocol for performing direct capping that we recommend is:

1. Irrigation with saline solution.
2. Hemostasis with a sterile cotton wool pellet.
3. Preparation and application of capping material (MTA or calcium hydroxide) and its application to the pulp chamber opening. If MTA is applied, it is gently compressed with a paper cone).
4. Fixing the material by applying self-curing or light-curing GIc. Self-curing GIc should be applied without pressure so that it does not push the liner (direct capping material) into the pulp chamber.

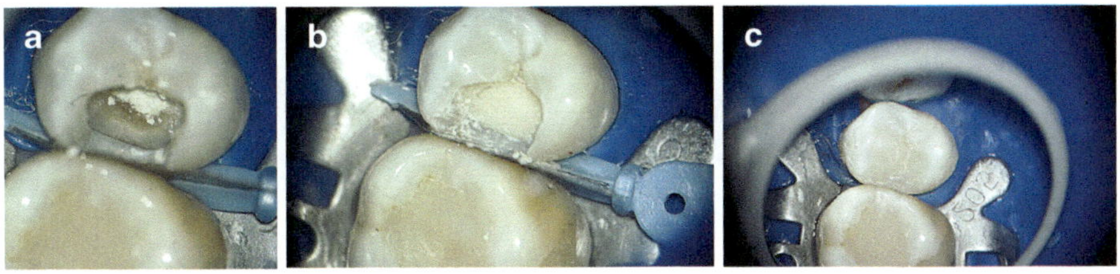

Fig. 3.83 Direct pulp capping of a premolar: MTA (**a**); GIc (**b**); composite resin restoration (**c**)

5. Placement of long-term adhesive restoration.

When fixing the MTA with self-curing GIc, the focus should be on the compaction pressure of the material so that the MTA is not pushed into the pulp chamber opening and pressing the pulp (Fig. 3.83).

When fixing the MTA with RMGIc, the focus will be on the temperature drop likely to be transmitted to the pulp. This can be done by blowing air gently after the first few seconds from the light-curing start or by choosing a low-power, short-session polymerization scheme [108, 109] (Fig. 3.84a–d). Recent studies that measure the temperature rise using this protocol (MTA + RMGIc) have shown that it remains below the threshold of pulp damage, which is 42.5 °C (i.e., an increase of 5.5° above body temperature [110]).

The treatment is identical even if only one pulp horn is accidentally opened and if there are two communications (Fig. 3.85).

3.7.3.4 Treatment Success

The chance of a successful treatment is higher when the exposure is due to mechanical causes, carried out accidentally during treatments than when the exposure is caused by caries [77, 111]. This is most likely explained by the fact that accidental mechanical exposures produce less bacterial contamination than carious processes, which may also be associated with pulp inflammation [70]. Patient age has frequently been associated with treatment success in favor of younger individuals, but the literature does not provide a consensus on this observation. Multiple studies have found no association between direct pulp capping success and age (Matsuo et al.).

Performing a long-lasting restoration with good sealing in the same session with direct capping is imperative, with success rates ranging from 47.3% for placement of a temporary restoration to 80.8% for long-term restoration, immediately after capping [112–114].

Difficulties that may occur	Potential solutions
Heavy bleeding impossible to stop	Abandoning direct capping and performing a pulpectomy. Most likely, the pulp is already suffering from irreversible inflammation
Pushing the MTA or self-curing CIS into the pulp chamber during compaction	It is most likely that bleeding will occur at this point, and the procedure should be stopped and resumed after the hemostasis has been performed. Otherwise, the tooth may develop irreversible endodontic symptomatology

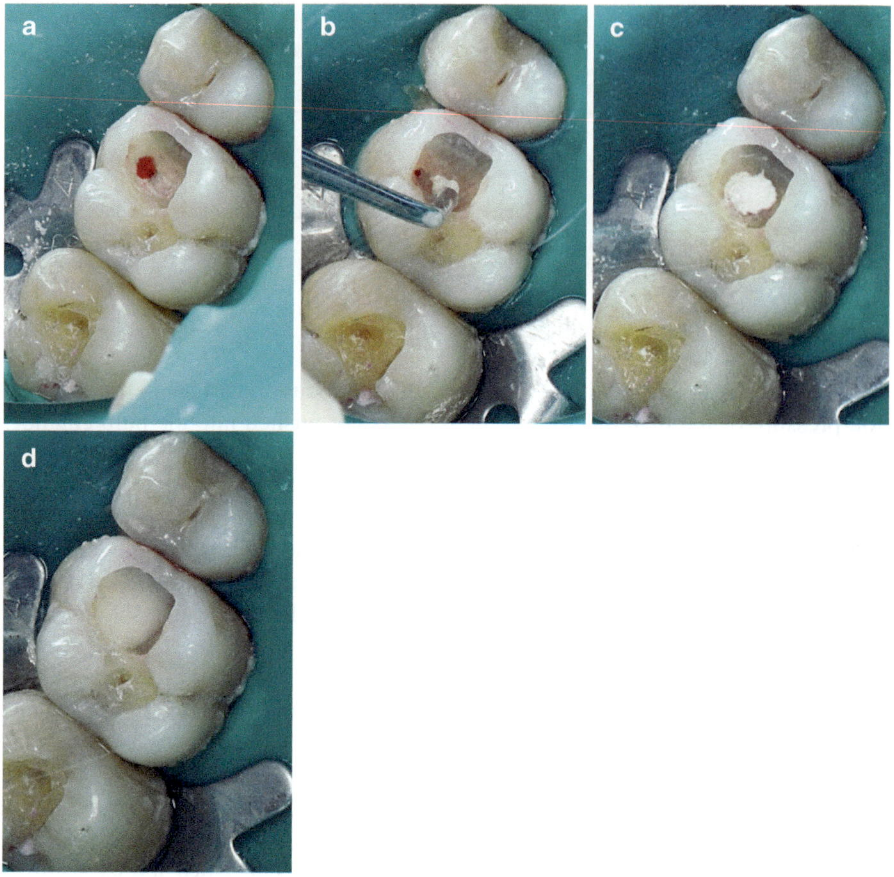

Fig. 3.84 Direct capping of a molar: immediate aspect after opening the pulp chamber (**a**); applying MTA with an obturator (**b**); aspect after applying MTA (**c**); applying GIc (**d**)

Conclusion

The literature on direct capping offers the following suggestions [115]:

1. Avoid pulp exposure. The chances of maintaining tooth vitality are excellent if the tooth is asymptomatic and sealed tightly with an adhesive restoration, even if we retain carious tooth tissue at the cavity base.
2. Control bleeding with distilled water, saline, CHX, or sodium hypochlorite. Water and saline are gentlest on the pulp, while sodium hypochlorite is more effective as a hemostatic and disinfectant.
3. MTA shows comparable results to calcium hydroxide in short-term studies.
4. Calcium hydroxide remains the gold standard for direct capping, with published longer-term studies that show a good cost-effectiveness ratio.
5. Making a restoration that provides a good seal against the salivary environment immediately after the direct capping in the same session prevents bacterial microleakage.

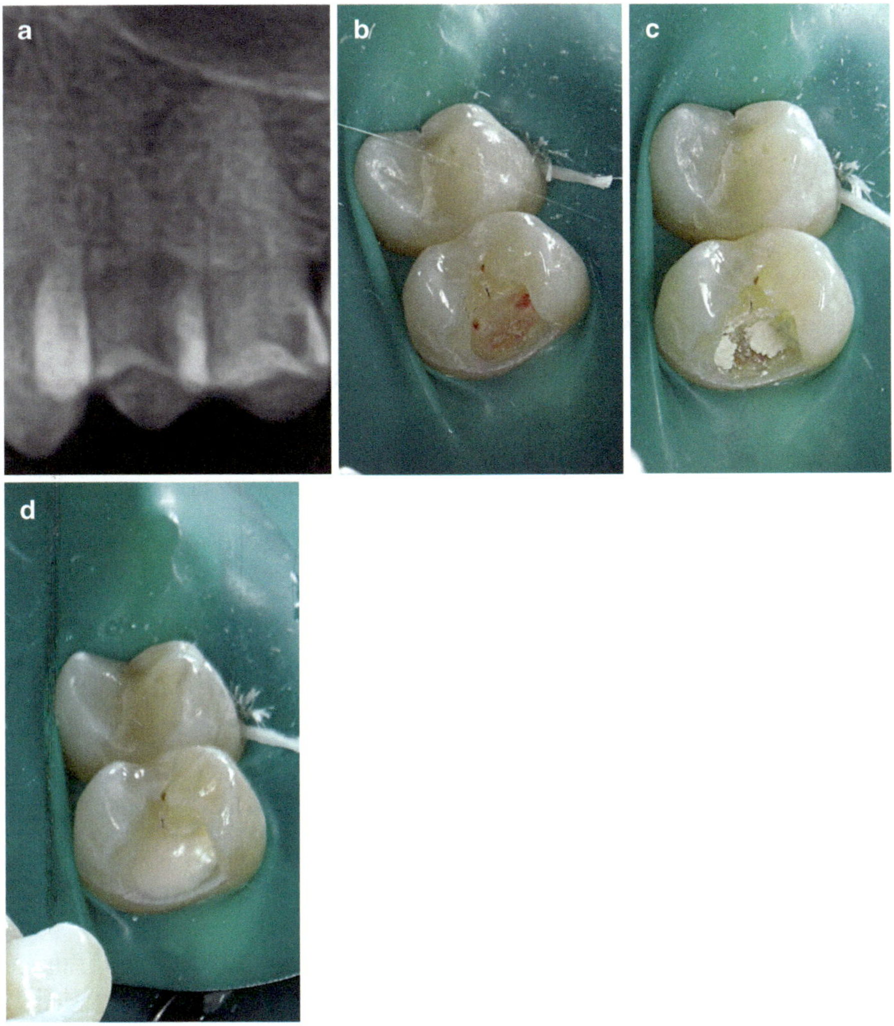

Fig. 3.85 Direct capping of a premolar: radiological aspect (**a**); aspect after the two-site opening of the pulp chamber (**b**); aspect after MTA application (**c**); GIc in place (**d**)

6. Fixing MTA with light-curing materials is a safe method for keeping the pulp temperature below the critical risk threshold of 42.5 °C (5.5 °C increase during light-curing).

Review Questions
1. What are the indications for direct capping?
2. How is bleeding control carried out in case of accidental opening of the pulp chamber?
3. What is the protocol for direct capping, and what materials are used?

References

1. Vanini L, Mangani F, Klimovskaia O. Conservative restoration of anterior teeth. ACME. 2007;
2. Manauta J. Custom rings updated. Styleitaliano. October 20, 2013. Accesat în data de 10 martie 2022 la. https://www.styleitaliano.org/jordi-manauta-custom-rings-updated/.
3. Bader J, Shugars D, Bonito A. Systematic reviews of selected dental caries diagnostic and management methods. J Dental Educ. 2001;65:960–8.
4. Schwendicke F, Tzschoppe M, Paris S. Radiographic caries detection: a systematic review and meta-analysis. J Dent. 2015;43(8):924–33.
5. Kois JC. The restorative-periodontal interface: biological parameters. Periodontol. 2000;1996(11):29–38.
6. Schätzle M, Land NP, Anerud A, Boysen H, Bürgin W, Löe H. The influence of margins of restorations of the periodontal tissues over 26 years. J Clin Periodontol. 2001;28(1):57–64.
7. Jorgic-Srdjak K, Plancak D, Maricevic T, Dragoo MR, Bosnjak A. Periodontal and prosthetic aspect of biological width part I: Violation of biologic width. Acta Stomatol Croat. 2000;34:195–7.
8. Magne P, Spreafico RC. Deep margin elevation: a paradigm shift. J Esthet Restor Dent. 2012;
9. Matthews DC, Tabesh M. Detection of localized tooth-related factors that predispose to periodontal infections. Periodontol. 2000;2004(34):136–50.
10. Schmidt JC, Sahrmann P, Weiger R, Schmidlin PR, Walter C. Biologic width dimensions – a systematic review. J Clin Periodontol. 2013;40:493–504.
11. Dragoo MR. Resin-ionomer and hybrid-ionomer cements: part II, human clinical and histologic wound healing responses in specific periodontal lesions. Int J Periodontics Restorative Dent. 1997;17:75–87.
12. Stetler KJ, Bissada NF. Signifcance of the width of keratinized gingiva on the periodontal status of teeth with submarginal restorations. J Periodontol. 1987;58:696–700.
13. Tao J, Wu Y, Chen J, Su J. A follow-up study of up to 5 years of metal-ceramic crowns in maxillary central incisors for different gingival biotypes. Int J Periodontics Restorative Dent. 2014;34:e85–92.
14. Herrero F, Scott JB, Maropis PS, Yukna RA. Clinical comparison of desired versus actual amount of surgical crown lengthening. J Periodontol. 1995;66:568–71.
15. Nugala B, Kumar BS, Sahitya S, Krishna PM. Biologic width and its importance in periodontal and restorative dentistry. J Conserv Dent. 2012;15(1):12–7.
16. Yiğit Özer S, İbrahim U, Bahşi E. Surgical extrusion of a complete crown fractured tooth: a case report. Int Dent Res. 2011;1(2):70–4.
17. Becker BD. Intentional replantation techniques: a critical review. J Endod. 2018;44(1):14–21.
18. Elkhadem A, Mickan S, Richards D. Adverse events of surgical extrusion in treatment for crown-root and cervical root fractures: a systematic review of case series/reports. Dent Traumatol. 2014;30:1–14.
19. Das B, Muthu MS. Surgical extrusion as a treatment option for crown-root fracture in permanent anterior teeth: a systematic review. Dent Traumatol. 2013;29(6):423–31.
20. Kindelan SA, Day PF, Kindelan JD, Spencer JR, Duggal MS. Dental trauma: an overview of its influence on the management of orthodontic treatment. Part 1. J Orthod. 2008;35(2):68–78.
21. Faria LP, Almeida MM, Amaral MF, Pellizzer EP, Okamoto R, Mendonca MR. Orthodontic extrusion as treatment option for crown-root fracture: literature review with systematic criteria. J Contemp Dent Pract. 2015;16:758–62.
22. Bach N, Baylard JF, Voyer R. Orthodontic extrusion: periodontal considerations and applications. J Can Dent Assoc. 2004;70(11):775–80.
23. González-Martín O, Solano-Hernandez B, Torres A, González-Martín S, Avila-Ortiz G. Orthodontic extrusion: guidelines for contemporary clinical practice. Int J Periodontics Restor Dent. 2020;40:667–76.
24. Stevens BH, Levine RA. Forced eruption: a multidisciplinary approach for form, function, and biologic predictability. Compend Contin Educ Dent. 1998;19(10)

25. Carvalho CV, Bauer FP, Romito GA, Pannuti CM, De Micheli G. Orthodontic extrusion with or without circumferential supracrestal fiberotomy and root planing. Int J Periodontics Restorative Dent. 2006;26(1):87–93.
26. Heintze SD, Rousson V. Clinical effectiveness of direct class II restorations – a meta–analysis. J Adhes Dent. 2012;14(5):407–31.
27. Boushell LW, Walter R, Wilder AD Jr. Preliminary considerations for operative dentistry. In: Heyman HO, Swift Jr EJ, Ritter AV, editors. Sturdevant's art & science of operative dentistry. 6th ed. Missouri: Elsevier; 2012. p. 186–215.
28. de la Peña VA, García RP, García RP. Sectional matrix: step-by-step directions for their clinical use. Br Dent J. 2016;220(1):11–4.
29. Sirajuddin S, Narasappa KM, Gundapaneni V, Chungkham S, Walikar AS. Iatrogenic damage to periodontium by restorative treatment procedures: an overview. Open Dent J. 2015;9:217–22.
30. ACB M, Restrepo M, Azevedo ER, RCL C, Santos-Pinto L, ACC Z. Effect of Rubber Dam Clamps on Demineralized Cervical Enamel of Permanent Teeth. J Dent Child (Chic). 2018;85(1):3–7.
31. Loomans BA, Opdam NJ, Roeters FJ, Bronkhorst EM, Burgersdijk RC, Dörfer CE. A randomized clinical trial on proximal contacts of posterior composites. J Dent. 2006;34(4):292–7.
32. Milic T, George R, Walsh LJ. Evaluation and prevention of enamel surface damage during dental restorative procedures. Aust Dent J. 2015;60(3):301–8. quiz 421
33. Markley MR. Restorations of silver amalgam. J Am Dent Assoc. 1951;43(2):133–46.
34. Almquist TC, Cowan RD, Lambert RL. Conservative amalgam restorations. J Prosthet Dent. 1973;29:524–8.
35. Osadetz CJ. Conservative amalgam instrumentation. Ontario. Dent. 1997;55(11):18–21.
36. Clark D. The injection-molded technique for strong, esthetic class II restorations. Inside Dent. 2010;6(1)
37. Wiegand A, Attin T. Treatment of proximal caries lesions by tunnel restorations. Dent Mater. 2007;23:1461–7.
38. Pilebro CE, van Dijken JW. Analysis of factors affecting failure of glass cement tunnel restorations in a multi-center study. Clin Oral Investig. 2001;5(2):96–101.
39. Pilebro CE, van Dijken JW, Stenberg R. Durability of tunnel restorations in general practice: a three-year multicenter study. Acta Odontol Scand. 1999;57(1):35–9.
40. Hasselrot L. Tunnel restorations in permanent teeth. A 7 year follow up study. Swed Dent J. 1998;22(1–2):1–7.
41. Summitt's Fundamentals of Operative Dentistry. In: Hilton TJ, Ferracane JL, Broome JC, editors. Jr. Dos Santos Summitt's fundamentals of operative dentistry: a contemporary approach. fourth ed. Quintessence Pub Co; 2013.
42. Fusayama T. Two layers of carious dentin: diagnosis and treatment. Oper Dent. 1979;4:63–70.
43. Ansari G, Beeley JA, Reid JS, Foye RH. Caries detector dyes – an in vitro assessment of some new compounds. J Oral Rehabil. 1999;26(6):453–8.
44. Anderson MH, Loesche WJ, Charbeneau GT. Bacteriologic study of a basic fuchsin caries-disclosing dye. J Prosthet Dent. 1985;54(1):51–5.
45. Zacharia MA, Munshi AK. Microbiological assessment of dentin stained with a caries detector dye. J Clin Pediatr Dent. 1995;19:111–5.
46. Boston DW, Graver HT. Histologicial study of an acid red caries disclosing dye. Oper Dent. 1989;14:186–92.
47. Boston DW, Liao J. Staining of non-carious human coronal dentin by caries dyes. Oper Dent. 2004;29(3):280–6.
48. Franco SJ, Kelsey WP. Caries removal with and without a disclosing solution of basic fuchsin. Oper Dent. 1981;6(2):46–8.
49. Piva E, Meinhardt L, Demarco FF, Powers JM. Dyes for caries detection: influence on composite and compomer microleakage. Clin Oral Investig. 2002;6(4):244–8.
50. Demarco FF, Matos AB, Matson E, Powers JM. Dyes for caries detection influence sound dentin bond strength. Oper Dent. 1998;23(6):294–8.

51. Lennon AM, Buchalla W, Rassner B, Becker K, Attin T. Efficiency of 4 caries excavation methods compared. Oper Dent. 2006;31(5):551–5.
52. Vargas M. Conservative aesthetic enhancement of the anterior dentition using a predictable direct resin protocol. Pract Proced Aesthet Dent. 2006;18(8):501–7.
53. Fahl N Jr. Achieving ultimate anterior esthetics with a new microhybrid composite. Compend Contin Educ Dent Suppl. 2000;(26):4–26.
54. Soliman S, Preidl R, Karl S, Hofmann N, Krastl G, Klaiber B. Influence of cavity margin design and restorative material on marginal quality and seal of extended class II resin composite restorations in vitro. J Adhes Dent. 2016;18(1):7–16.
55. Coelho-De-Souza FH, Camargo JC, Beskow T, Balestrin MD, Klein-Júnior CA, Demarco FF. A randomized double-blind clinical trial of posterior composite restorations with or without bevel: 1-year follow-up. J Appl Oral Sci. 2012;20(2):174–9.
56. Meurer JC, Rizzante FA, Maenossono RM, FMG F, JFS B, Ishikiriama SK. Effect of cavosurface angle beveling on the exposure angle of enamel prisms in different cavity sizes. Microsc Res Tech. 2020;83:304–9.
57. Apel Z, Vafaeian B, Apel BD, Hussain A. Occlusal stresses in beveled versus non-beveled tooth preparation. Biomed Eng Adv. 2021:2.
58. Lang LA, Burgess JO, Lang BR, Wang R-F. Wear of composite resin restorations in beveled and nonbeveled preparations. J Dent Res. 1995;74:165.
59. Lynch CD, Opdam NJ, Hickel R, et al. Guidance on posterior resin composites: Academy of Operative Dentistry – European Section. J Dent. 2014;42(4):377–83.
60. Lynch CD, Shortall AC, Stewardson D, Tomson PL, Burke FJ. Teaching posterior composite resin restorations in the United Kingdom and Ireland: consensus views of teachers. Br Dent J. 2007;203(4):183–7.
61. Black GV. Operative dentistry. Chicago: The technical procedures in filling teeth; 1908.
62. Ricketts D, Lamont T, Innes NP, Kidd E, Clarkson JE. Operative caries management in adults and children. Cochrane Database Syst Rev. 2013;(3):CD003808.
63. Gilboe DB, Teteruck WR. Fundamentals of extracoronal tooth preparation. Part I. Retention and resistance form. J Prosthet Dent. 1974;32(6):651–6.
64. Mertz-Fairhurst EJ, Curtis JW Jr, Ergle JW, Rueggeberg FA, Adair SM. Ultraconservative and cariostatic sealed restorations: results at year 10. J Am Dent Assoc. 1998;129(1):55–66.
65. Banerjee A. Applications of scanning microscopy in the assessment of dentine caries and methods for its removal. PhD Thesis. University of London; 1999.
66. Buchalla W, Frankenberger R, Galler KM, et al. Aktuelle Empfehlungen zur Kariesexkavation. Wissenschaftliche Mitteilung der Deutschen Gesellschaft für Zahn-erhaltung (DGZ). Deutsche Zahnärztliche Zeitschrift. 2017;72:484–94.
67. Banerjee A, Kidd EA, Watson TF. Scanning electron microscopic observations of human dentine after mechanical caries excavation. J Dent. 2000;28(3):179–86.
68. Romeo G, Bresciano M. Diagnostic and technical approach to esthetic rehabilitations. J Esthet Restor Dent. 2003;15(4):204–16.
69. Cox CF, Bergenholtz G, Heys DR, Syed SA, Fitzgerald M, Heys RJ. Pulp capping of dental pulp mechanically exposed to oral microflora: a 1-2 year observation of wound healing in the monkey. J Oral Pathol. 1985;14(2):156–68.
70. Murray PE, Windsor LJ, Smyth TW, Hafez AA, Cox CF. Analysis of pulpal reactions to restorative procedures, materials, pulp capping, and future therapies. Crit Rev Oral Biol Med. 2002;13(6):509–20.
71. Wisithphrom K, Murray PE, About I, Windsor LJ. Interactions between cavity preparation and restoration events and their effects on pulp vitality. Int. J. Periodontics Restor. Dent. 2006;26:596–605.
72. Oztürk E, Bolay S. Survival of porcelain laminate veneers with different degrees of dentin exposure: 2-year clinical results. J Adhes Dent. 2014;16(5):481–9.
73. Mount JG, Hume WR, Wolff SM, Hien CN. Preservation and restoration of tooth structure. Wiley Blackwell; 2016. p. 200.

74. Schwendicke F, Dorfer CE, Paris S. Incomplete caries removal: a systematic review and meta-analysis. J Dent Res. 2013;92(4):306–14.
75. Sawicki L, Pameijer CH, Emerich K, Adamowicz-Klepalska B. Histological evaluation of mineral trioxide aggregate and calcium hydroxide in direct pulp capping of human immature permanent teeth. Am J Dent. 2008;21(4):262–6.
76. Hilton TJ, Summitt JB. Pulpal considerations. In: Hilton TJ, Ferracane JL, Broome JC, editors. Summitt's fundamentals of operative dentistry, A Contemporary Approach. Fourth ed. Quintessence; 2013. p. 131–53.
77. Baume LJ, Holz J. Long term clinical assessment of direct pulp capping. Int Dent J. 1998;31:251–60.
78. Hilton TJ. Keys to clinical succes with pulp capping: A literature review. Oper Dent. 2009;34:615–25.
79. Ricketts DN, Kidd EA, Innes N, Clarkson J. Complete or ultraconservative removal of decayed tissue in unfilled teeth. Cochrane Database Syst Rev. 2006;(3):CD003808. Update in: Cochrane Database Syst Rev. 2013;3:CD003808.
80. Horsted-Bindslev P, Lovschall H. Treatment outcome of vital pulp treatment. Endod Top. 2002;2(1):24–34.
81. Swift EJ, Trope M, Ritter A. Vital pulp therapy for the mature tooth – Can it work? Endod Topic. 2003;5:49–56.
82. Bogen G, Chandler N, Kuttler S. Vital pulp therapy. In: Ingle's endodontics. 6th ed. Ontario: BC Decker; 2008. p. 1310–29.
83. American Academy of Pediatric Dentistry. Manual 2005-2006. Guideline to pulp therapy for primary and young teeth. Pediatr Dent. 2005;7(suppl.7):130–4.
84. Foley J, Evans D, Blackwell A. Partial caries removal and cariostatic materials in carious primary molar teeth. A randomised controlled clinical trial. Br Dent J. 2004;197:697–701.
85. Ribeiro CC, Baratieri LN, Perdigão J, Baratieri NM, Ritter AV. A clinical, radiographic, and scanning electron microscopic evaluation of adhesive restorations on carious dentin in primary teeth. Quintessence Int. 1999;30(9):591–9.
86. Schäfer E, Hickel R, Geurtsen W, et al. Offizielles Endodontologisches Lexikon – mit einem Anhang für Materialien und Instrumente. Der Deutschen Gesellschaft für Zahnerhaltung Endodontie. 2000;9:129–60.
87. Babbush CA, Fehrenbach MJ, Emmons M, editors. Mosby's dental dictionary. 2nd ed. St. Louis: Mosby Elsevier Publishing; 2008.
88. European Society of Endodontology. Quality guidelines for endodontic treatment: consensus report of the European Society of Endodontology. Int Endod J. 2006;39:921–30.
89. Thompson V, Rg C, Fa C, et al. Treatment of deep carious lesions by complete excavation or partial removal. J Am Dent Assoc. 2008;139(6):705–12.
90. Summitt's Fundamentals of Operative Dentistry. In: Hilton TJ, Ferracane JL, Broome JC, editors. Jr. Dos Santos Summitt's fundamentals of operative dentistry: a contemporary approach. Quintessence Pub Co; 2016.
91. Bogen B, Chandler N. Vital pulp therapy. In: Ingle J, Bakand L, Baumgartner J, editors. Ingle's endodontics. Hamilton: BC Decker Publishing; 2008. p. 1310–29.
92. Cao Y, Bogen G, Lim J, Shon WJ, Kang MK. Bioceramic materials and the changing concepts in vital pulp therapy. J Calif Dent Assoc. 2016;44:278–90.
93. Rosenfeld EF, James GA, Burch BS. Vital pulp tissue response to sodium hypochlorite. J Endod. 1978;4:140–6.
94. Ricucci D, Loghin S, Lin LM, Spangberg LS, Tay FR. Is hard tissue formation in the dental pulp after the death of the primary odontoblasts a regenerative or a reparative process? J Dent. 2014;42:1156–70.
95. Hermann B. Ein weiterer Beitrag zur Frage der Pulpenbehandlung. Zahnärztl Rundsch. 1928;37:1327–76.
96. Akhlaghi N, Khademi A. Outcomes of vital pulp therapy in permanent teeth with different medicaments based on review of the literature. Dent Res J (Isfahan). 2015;12:406–17.

97. Dammaschke T, Galler K, Krastl G. Current recommendations for vital pulp treatment. Dtsch Zahnärztl Z Int. 2019;1:43–52.
98. Petrou MA, Alhamoui FA, Welk A, Altarabulsi MB, Alkilzy M, Splieth CH. A randomized clinical trial on the use of medical Portland cement, MTA and calcium hydroxide in indirect pulp treatment. Clin Oral Investig. 2014;18(5):1383–9.
99. Duque C, Negrini TC, Sacono NT, Spolidorio DM, de Souza Costa CA, Hebling J. Clinical and microbiological performance of resin-modified glass-ionomer liners after incomplete dentine caries removal. Clin Oral Investig. 2009;13(4):465–71.
100. Pinto AS, de Araújo FB, Franzon R, et al. Clinical and microbiological effect of calcium hydroxide protection in indirect pulp capping in primary teeth. Am J Dent. 2006;19(6):382–6.
101. Iliescu A, Gafar M. Cariologie şi Odontoterapie restauratoare. Editura Medicală. 2006;
102. American Association of Endodontists. Guide to clinical endodontics. Fifth ed; 2013.
103. Matsuo T, Nakanishi T, Shimizu H, Ebisu S. A clinical study of direct pulp capping applied to carious-exposed pulps. J Endod. 1996;22(10):551–6.
104. Costa CA, Edwards CA, Hanks CT. Cytotoxic effects of cleansing solutions recommended for chemical lavage of pulp exposures. Am J Dent. 2001;14(1):25–30.
105. Modena KC, Casas-Apayco LC, Atta MT, et al. Cytotoxicity and biocompatibility of direct and indirect pulp capping materials. J Appl Oral Sci. 2009;17(6):544–54.
106. Pashley DH. Consideration of dentine permeability in cytotoxicity testing. Int Endod J. 1988;21(2):143–54.
107. Costa CA, Hebling J, Hanks CT. Current status of pulp capping with dentin adhesive systems: a review. Dent Mater. 2000;16(3):188–97.
108. Millen C, Ormond M, Richardson G, Santini A, Miletic V, Kew P. A study of temperature rise in the pulp chamber during composite polymerization with different light–curing units. J Contemp Dent Pract. 2007;8(7):29–37.
109. Malčić AI, Pavičić I, Trošić I, Simeon P, Katanec D, Krmek SJ. The effects of bluephase LED light on fibroblasts. Eur J Dent. 2012;6(3):311–7.
110. Petrovic V, Stasic NJ, Komlenic V, Savic-Stankovic T, Latkovic M, Miletic V. Temperature changes in the pulp chamber induced by polymerization of resin-based dental restoratives following simulated direct pulp capping. Chem Industry. 2019;73(4):239–48.
111. Al Hiyasat A, Barrieshi-Nusair K, Al-Mari M. The radiographic outcome of direct pulp capping procedures performed by dental students. J Am Dent Assoc. 2006;137:1699–705.
112. Besic F. The fate of bacteria sealed in dental cavities. J Dent Res. 1943;22:349–54.
113. Baume LJ, Holz J. Long term clinical assessment of direct pulp capping. J Int Dent J. 1981;31(4):251–60.
114. Pinto AS, de Araújo FB, Franzon R, Figueiredo MC, Henz S, García-Godoy F, Maltz M. Clinical and microbiological effect of calcium hydroxide protection in indirect pulp capping in primary teeth. Am J Dent. 2006;19(6):382–6.
115. Hilton TJ. Keys to clinical success with pulp capping: a review of the literature. Oper Dent. 2009;34(5):615–25.

Part II

Direct Restorations

The Interdental Contacts: Direct Restoration Techniques of the Proximal Walls by the Centripetal Method

4

Proximal contact, or interdental contact area, has been defined as the tooth surface where a proximal face of a tooth comes into contact with the adjacent tooth [1]. As a terminology, the term "contact point" is widely used, a term perhaps even more popular than "contact surface"; in reality, it is the area or surface of interdental contact. This chapter will focus on the main aspects that must be taken into account to obtain good interdental contacts: techniques for anterior and posterior teeth related to the types of materials, layering strategies, and type of matrix used.

This chapter starts from the premise of applying the centripetal technique [2] for all types of restorations made in cavities that also involve the proximal areas and marginal ridges: class I (Fig. 4.1), MOD (Fig. 4.2), or mirror cavities (Figs. 4.3 and

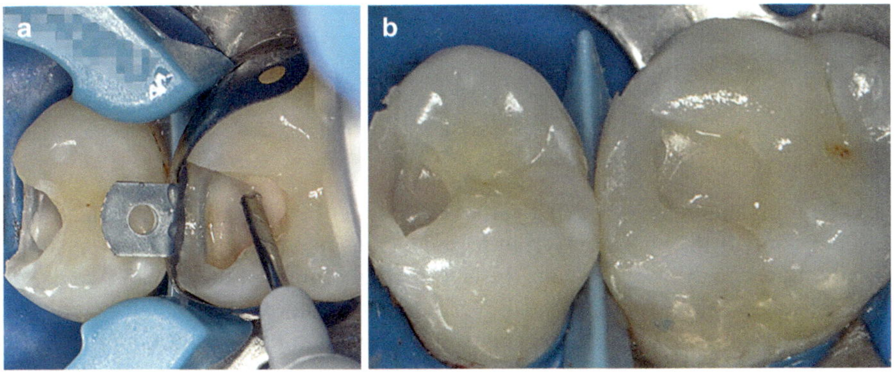

Fig. 4.1 Class II mesio-occlusal cavities on premolar and molar (**a**) transformed into class I cavities by the centripetal technique, initial restoration of the proximal walls (**b**)

Supplementary Information The online version contains supplementary material available at https://doi.org/10.1007/978-3-031-55899-3_4. The videos can be accessed individually by clicking the DOI link in the accompanying figure caption or by scanning this link with the SN More Media App.

© The Author(s), under exclusive license to Springer Nature Switzerland AG 2024

M. Bud, *Direct Restorations*, https://doi.org/10.1007/978-3-031-55899-3_4

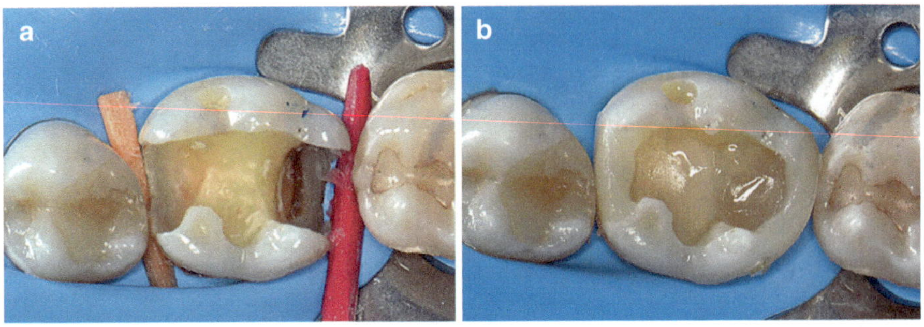

Fig. 4.2 MOD cavity on lower first molar (**a**) transformed into a class I cavity (**b**)

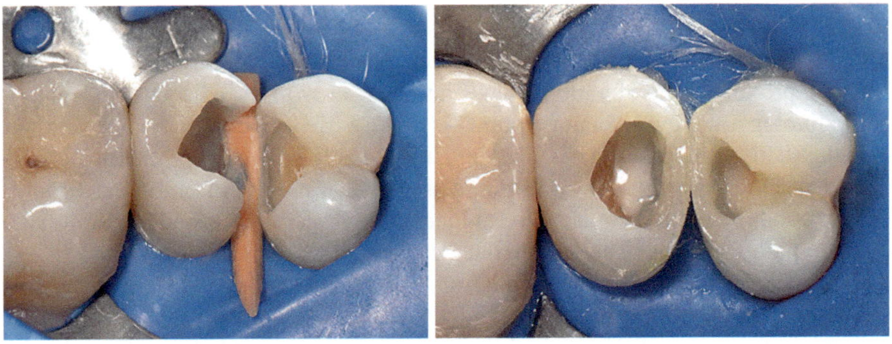

Fig. 4.3 Proximo-occlusal mirror cavities on premolars

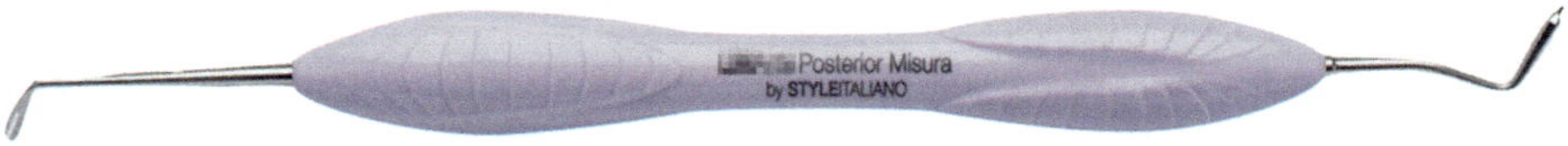

Fig. 4.4 Restoration of the proximal walls

4.4). This technique requires, firstly, the restoration of the proximal walls in a single stage by one of the chosen layering techniques using appropriate matrix systems. Then follows, in the second stage, the layering/bulk filling of the obtained cavity. In the last stage, the morphology of the last applied composite layer will be created. Even when using bulk packable composites, we recommend performing the occlusal morphology as a separate step in order to be able to pay the necessary attention to modeling the appropriate anatomical relief.

4.1 General information

4.1.1 Proximal Wall Morphology

The morphology of a composite restored proximal wall will be determined by the shape and conformation of the matrices on the tooth. Thus, it is preferable to use matrices that are as anatomical as possible and as well-adapted to the dental surfaces as possible. Even under these conditions, there is the possibility of a concave deformation of the matrices in the contact area, more common in circular ones than in sectional ones [3]. This most likely occurs due to insufficient space created by pre-distancing for matrix placement.

4.1.2 Height of Proximal Walls/Marginal Ridge

The level (height) at which the marginal ridge should be placed differs from case to case. This information should be obtained before cavity preparation if the original marginal ridge is partially or fully preserved. If its level is identical to the level of the adjacent tooth, special instruments can be used to help place the two marginal ridges at the same level. One such tool available on the market is the "Posterior Misura" from the LM-Arte modeling kit, which allows horizontal and vertical measurements of the proximal wall to be restored from the composite, depending on the marginal ridge of the adjacent tooth. This tool has one of the spatula-like tips sectioned down the middle allowing it to sit on the matrix. Sliding will establish the level of the composite applied for wall reconstruction at the level of the marginal ridge of the adjacent tooth [4]. The opposite tip of the instrument allows the measurement of the depth of 1.5 mm, required for the last occlusal layer of the composite.

4.1.3 Layering of Materials for the Restoration of Proximal Walls

The specialized literature has always paid particular attention to the method of layering and the materials used in the centripetal technique for restoring the proximal walls, with particular attention to the gingival edge of class II cavity preparations.

The gingival margin area of the proximal cavities is one of strategic importance, considering that 80–90% of secondary caries are located at the gingival margin of the second- and fifth-class cavities [5]. The causes can be multiple, and the gingival margin area of class I cavities can present specific characteristics, among which we can mention:

- Multiple cracks in the enamel (if not removed, then they can be infiltration paths).
- Areas without enamel so that the adhesion of the restoration is achieved only on the dentin, therefore, in weaker conditions, and in some cases even on the sclerotic or root dentin that provides even more unfavorable support for the adhesion.
- The distance between this area and the tip of the light guide of the polymerization lamp is more significant than in the case of any other point, which is why deficiencies in the polymerization of the composite may occur.
- Areas inaccessible to curing light when using metal matrices that can prevent the light from adequately curing the composite.
- Sharp or irregular angles where packable composites are difficult to adapt to seal the cavity margins well.

- Frequent salivary microinfiltrations occurring during adhesion, sometimes undetectable without magnification, sometimes favored by the juxtagingival or even subgingival position of the gingival margin. In these areas, adhesion is compromised right from the start, usually being the starting point of future marginal caries.
- Difficulties in adapting matrices that lead to fillings with excess material, sometimes impossible to observe clinically in the absence of radiological examinations. This excess can create food retention and the aspect of marginal secondary caries or caries on the adjacent tooth.
- Difficulties in handling the materials in this area due to the sometimes tiny dimensions of the proximal cavities, which make access of the instruments difficult. Thus, packable composites can be difficult to be placed and compact in this area.
- Difficult visual control of materials placed on the gingival margin in the absence of magnification. In the presence of magnification, it can be checked whether the material has sealed the area and whether the material has inclusions or air voids.

The general disadvantages associated with packable composites, such as polymerization shrinkage, are added to the location and unique characteristics of the gingival margin region disadvantages.

Thus, to partially or totally solve the inconveniences mentioned above, multiple restoration techniques have been proposed over time which vary either in the method of stratification/application of the packable composite, the type of materials, or both.

Classically, the centripetal technique describes restoring the proximal wall with packable composite resin. Analyzing different evaluation criteria (marginal integrity, infiltration, resistance, etc.) in vivo and in vitro studies has demonstrated promising results, even superior to the classic centripetal technique by modifying it with other materials placed on the gingival margin: conventional flowable composite, bulk flowable composite, conventional GIc, RMGIc, giomers, etc. Thus, we can currently describe a classic centripetal technique and a wide range of "modified" centripetal techniques, widely used, among which we mention:

- Centripetal technique with oblique or split layering of the conventional packable composite (see Sect. 4.4) and bulk technique with packable composite (Fig. 4.5a).
- Centripetal technique with flowable composite on the gingival margin polymerized prior to adding the first layer of the packable composite (Fig. 4.5b).
- The centripetal technique with flowable composite on the gingival margin polymerized simultaneously with the packable composite (snowplow) (Fig. 4.5c).
- Centripetal technique with flowable/packable bulk and packable conventional composite: marginal ridge technique (Fig. 4.5d).
- Open sandwich centripetal technique with GIc/RMGIc/giomers and packable composite (Fig. 4.5e).

In this chapter, we will present these techniques in detail.

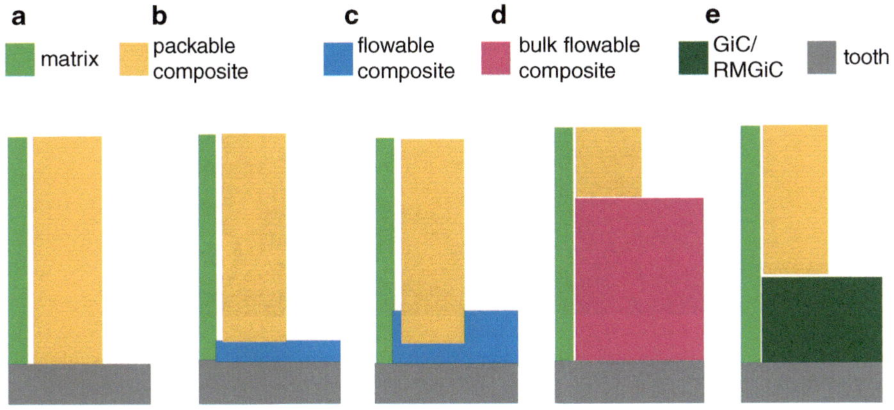

Fig. 4.5 Schematic representation of some possible methods to restore the proximal wall: bulk packable composite or oblique layering of conventional packable composite (**a**); addition of a flowable composite layer on the base of the cavity or only in the gingival margin area (**b**); the "snowplow" technique with flowable composite polymerized simultaneously with the packable one (**c**); reducing the depth of the cavity by applying flowable or packable bulk and subsequent restoration of the marginal ridge (**d**); reduction of cavity depth by application of GIc/variants of GIc "open sandwich" and subsequent restoration of the proximal wall (**e**)

4.2 Techniques for Posterior Teeth Where Material and Layering Technique Vary

4.2.1 Centripetal Technique with Classic Oblique and Split-Layered Packable Composite

Main idea: In the case of class II or MOD cavities, restoring a proximal wall with packable composite is achieved by successive additions using the oblique (zigzag) technique.

Regardless of the type of layering chosen for the restoration of the proximal wall, the matrix must be well-adapted along the entire contour of the cavity. Additional means can be used (e.g., Teflon tape) (Fig. 4.6).

The oblique technique involves multiple layers of packable composite placed in an oblique pattern to restore large walls and avoid to link two opposite walls. To fully restore with packable composite, the linking of opposite walls should be avoided to decrease the C-factor. In most cases, three oblique layers [6] are sufficient: the first "triangle" between the gingival margin and one of the vertical walls, the second triangle is formed between the other vertical wall and the composite already placed and polymerized, and the third will be the marginal ridge itself. All these three layers also come into contact with the matrix.

Another possible incremental technique to restore the proximal wall by conventional packable composite is the vertical stratification starting from the two vertical walls of the proximal cavity (oral and buccal), known as "split" [7].

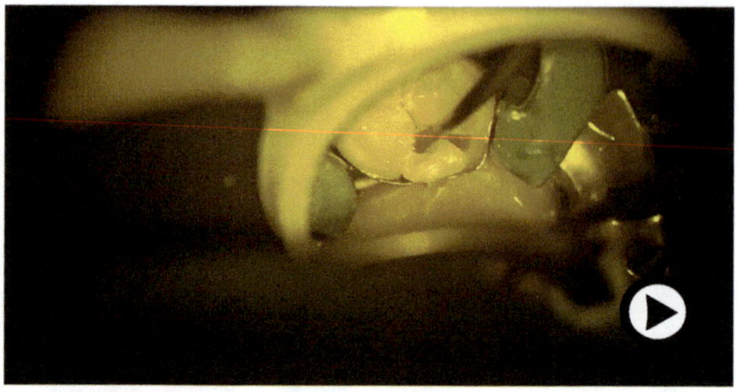

Fig. 4.6 Centripetal technique with oblique-layered packable composite (▶ https://doi.org/10.1007/000-bqp)

4.2.1.1 Working Technique

In the case of a class II cavity (Fig. 4.7), the first composite layer will be placed on the gingival margin, obliquely, going up toward one of the vertical walls (buccal or oral) (Fig. 4.7a). The composite can be applied with a spatula or obturator and condensed with a microbrush to avoid leaving voids, after which it will be completely polymerized. The second layer will be placed immediately above it, in a similar manner, but toward the opposite wall (Fig. 4.8b). The last applied layer will define the occlusal part of the wall, which will be the marginal ridge (Fig. 4.8c). The thickness of the layers usually does not exceed 1.5 mm, according to the manufacturer's instructions. In most cases, three increments are sufficient if the wall destruction is not very extensive [6].

In the case of mirror cavities, both matrices are applied for proper space distribution, and after the restoration of the first tooth wall, the corresponding matrix is removed. Thus, during the restoration of the wall of the second tooth, only one matrix will be present to achieve a close contact point.

Difficulties that may arise	Possible solutions
The level of the initial marginal ridge was not recorded before cavity preparation	In this situation, the level is dictated by the morphology of the rest of the occlusal surface or is identical to that of the adjacent tooth. The final level will be given at the time of the occlusion adjustments
The teeth have changes in position, or the marginal ridge was absent, and the initial level of the marginal ridge could not be known	In this situation, a symmetrical unitary morphology of the tooth is observed, placing the crest level symmetrically with the opposite or adjacent one. The occlusal adjustment stage will establish the correct position of the marginal ridge
The small size of the proximal box of the cavity makes an oblique or "split" stratification impossible	A simplified horizontal layering of the proximal wall can be used, or the centripetal technique can be abandoned, applying the material throughout the cavity

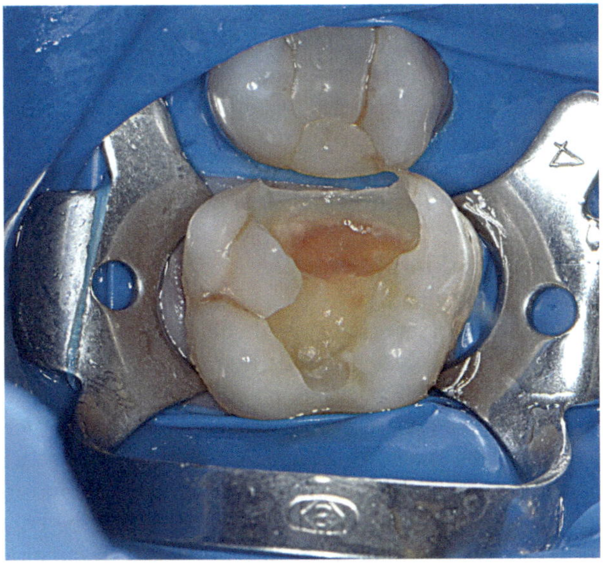

Fig. 4.7 Initial aspect of a mesio-occlusal cavity prepared on a molar

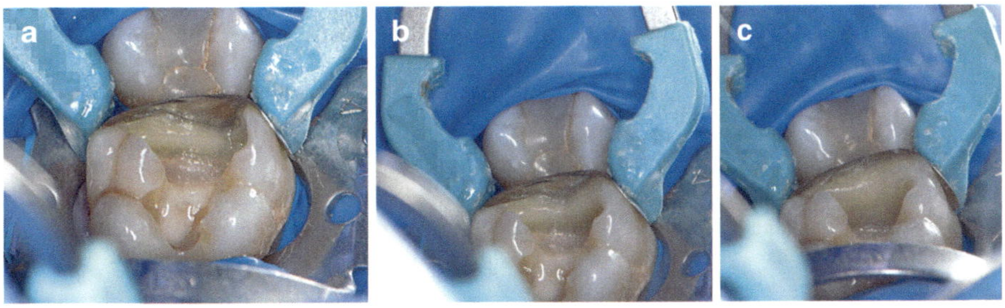

Fig. 4.8 Application of the first layer of composite following the oblique centripetal technique of the proximal wall (**a**); followed by the second layer (**b**) and the last increment in the marginal ridge area (**c**)

4.2.2 Flowable Composite on Gingival Margin Technique with Separate Polymerization

Main idea: Applying a layer of flowable composite to the gingival margin in the area of the angle formed with the matrix can improve marginal sealing and decrease microinfiltration. This technique diminishes the voids at the enamel-composite interface and compensates for the polymerization shrinkage of the packable composite.

Microinfiltration is one of the most common problems in restorative dentistry [8], being among the major causes of marginal secondary caries and postoperative sensitivity [9]. Polymerization shrinkage and voids induced at the composite-enamel interface may be among the causative factors of microinfiltration [10]. Various ways of decreasing the polymerization shrinkage of composites have been proposed to reduce the C-factor, including using flowable composites with higher elasticity (low elastic modulus) [11, 12].

4.2.2.1 Working Technique

In the case of class II cavities, after cavity preparation, disinfection, and pulp protection, if necessary (Fig. 4.9), then the mounting of the matrices and the application of the adhesive system are carried out. The flowable composite is applied to the gingival margin (Fig. 4.10), positioning the applicator tip against the base of the cavity and then gently lifting as the material is injected. Magnification can be beneficial at this stage. By adjusting the microscope to an intermediate magnification level, the delicate application of the flowable composite layer can be achieved, and the tightness sealing of the cavity angles may be controlled. Using loupes or the microscope for a magnified image, the clinician can easily eliminate possible air bubbles created during application. After application, the flowable composite is cured according to the manufacturer's instructions. Continue with oblique layering to restore the entire proximal wall, followed by restoration of the class I cavity obtained (Fig. 4.11).

Difficulties that may arise	Possible solutions
Application of too much flowable composite and its leakage toward the occlusal before its polymerization	The excess is removed using a microbrush, as the flowable composite should not reach the occlusal surface to absorb the occlusal forces due to the low filling
The aspect of air bubbles generated by the injection of the flowable composite	A sharp instrument (explorer or Fissura-like tool from the composite modeling kit) can be used to spread the flowable composite and remove air bubbles, and then continue application keeping the tip close to the base of the cavity

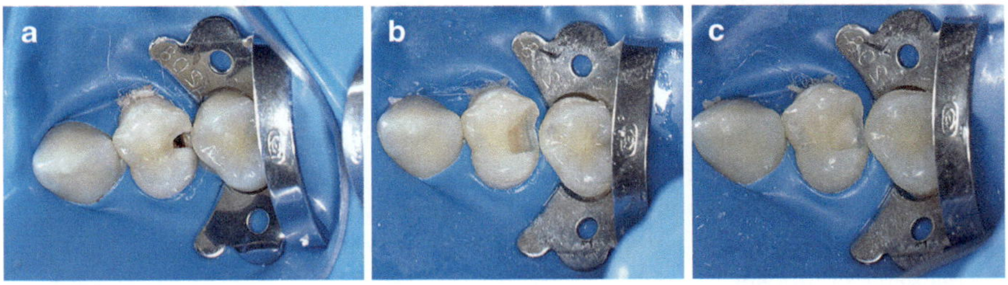

Fig. 4.9 Initial image of a distal carious lesion on tooth 24 (**a**); occluso-distal cavity prepared (**b**); liner applied (**c**)

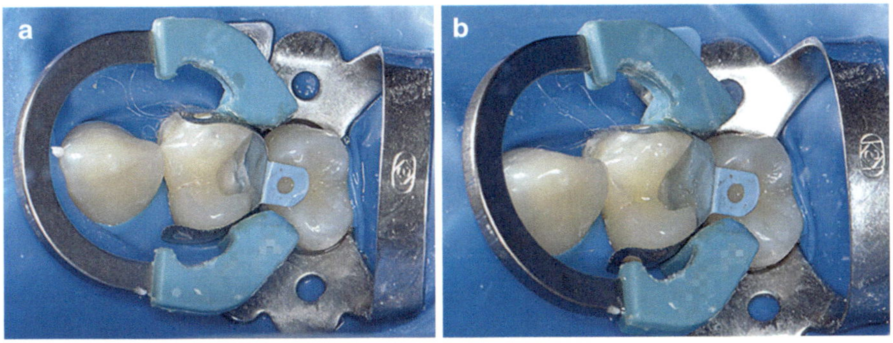

Fig. 4.10 Sectional matrix fixed with ring and interdental wedge (Palodent Plus) (**a**); flowable composite layer on the gingival margin (**b**)

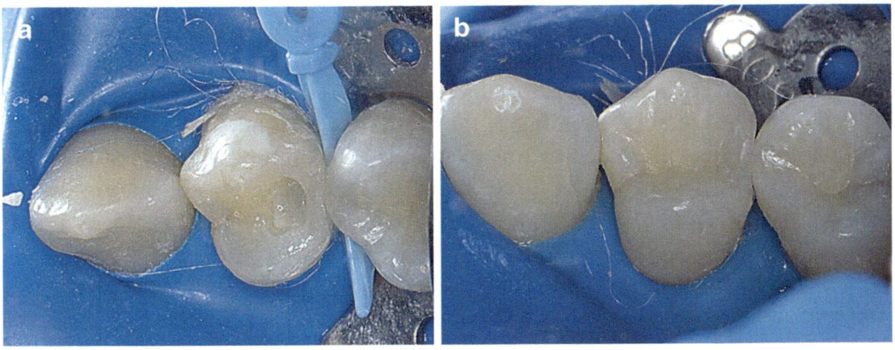

Fig. 4.11 Class I cavity obtained after restoration of the proximal wall (**a**) and final aspect of the restoration (**b**)

4.2.3 Technique with Flowable Composite on the Gingival Margin Simultaneously Polymerized with the First Layer of Packable Composite Applied (Snowplow)

Main idea: This technique involves the application of a layer of flowable composite on the gingival margin and its polymerization simultaneously with that of the packable composite layered over it (over the flowable composite).

The snowplow technique consists of the simultaneous polymerization of the flowable composite (Fig. 4.12a, b) and the packable one applied over it (Fig. 4.12c). This technique has proven superior results compared to the technique in which the flowable composite applied to the gingival margin is polymerized separately [13, 14], leading to the elimination of voids in this area [15]. On the contrary, some studies demonstrate the opposite, obtaining better results by separately polymerizing the

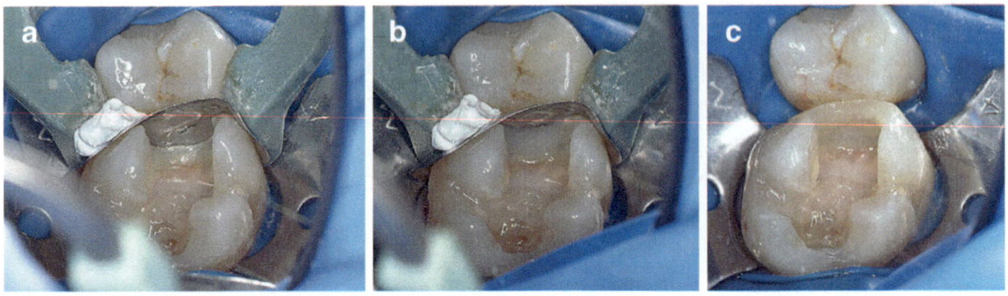

Fig. 4.12 Ocluso-mesial cavity prepared on tooth 26 (**a**); flowable composite applied on the gingival margin (**b**); proximal wall (**c**)

flowable composite applied to the gingival margin [16]. These results can be explained by the contraction forces of the packable composite during polymerization that can affect the adhesion of the underlying uncured flowable composite by traction. Another explanation could be that, in general, packable composites (being relatively sticky) can remain attached and pulled back with the modeling instrument which they were applied if not adequately compacted.

In the absence of a tight sealing of the matrix on the tooth at the gingival level, the hydraulic effect produced by this technique can result in a surplus of flowable composite. The frequency of excess material at the gingival margin varies between 16.5% and 75%, being one of the frequent problems of posterior restorations [17].

Nevertheless, there are few studies published about using uncured mixture of flowable and packable composites with conflicting opinion [18, 19].

4.2.3.1 Working Technique

Applying a packable composite over an uncured flowable composite can push the latter due to hydraulic pressure, helping to better marginal sealing of the restoration [20]. Thus, a thin layer of flowable composite is applied in the proximal box of the gingival margin (Fig. 4.13a) spreading it to seal the gingival margin to the matrix. Then the first increment of the packable composite is applied, from which the first layer of the proximal wall will be restored by the oblique technique, pressing the flowable composite (Fig. 4.13b). It will be pushed into the angles of the cavity and ensures a tight sealing of the future restoration. There is a possibility that part of the flowable composite flows back toward the occlusal (Fig. 4.13c). It must be cleaned before polymerization because it is not recommended to take occlusal forces (Fig. 4.14a). The following layers are applied (Fig. 4.14b, c) until the proximal wall is fully restored (Fig. 4.15).

Difficulties that may arise	Possible solutions
Extrusion of the flowable composite due to the pressure exerted by applying the packable composite	Careful check with magnification of the matrix's tight fit on the cavity's contour and the gingival margin
Reflow of flowable composite throughout the cavity when pressed with packable composite	Too much flowable composite may have been placed—Remove some of it with a microbrush

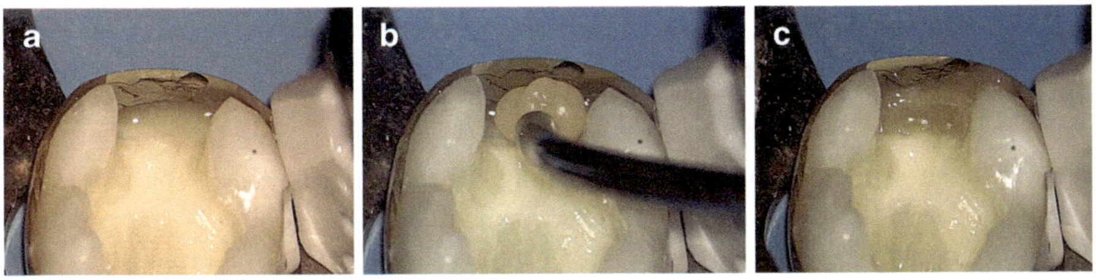

Fig. 4.13 Class II cavity in which a layer of flowable composite was applied to the gingival margin (**a**); applying an increment of conventional packable composite which will have a hydraulic effect on the uncured flowable composite (**b**); reflow of flowable composite toward the occlusal (**c**)

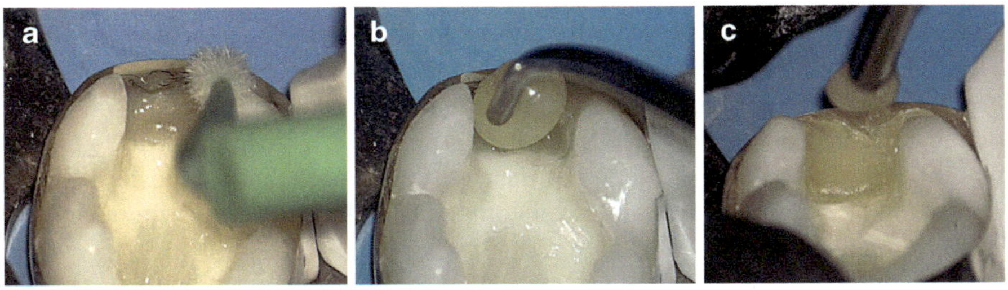

Fig. 4.14 Removal of excess flowable composite reflowed toward the occlusal (**a**); applying a new increment of packable composite to restore the proximal wall (centripetal technique) (**b**); applying the last increment of packable composite (**c**)

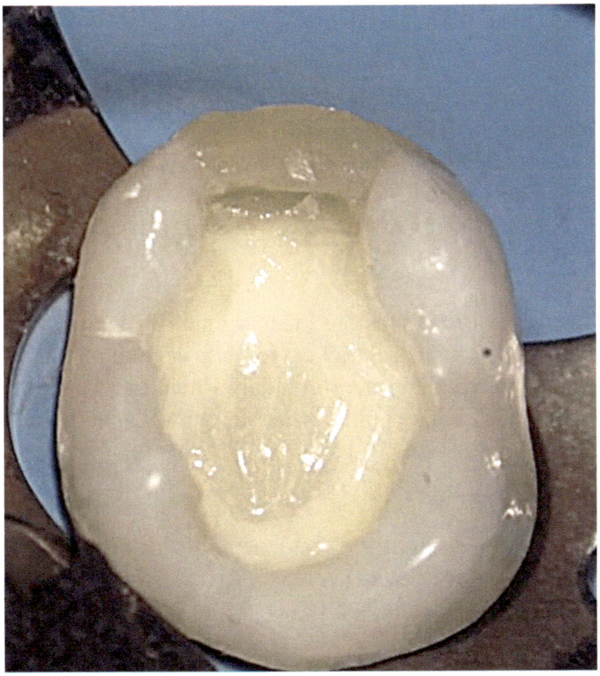

Fig. 4.15 Proximo-occlusal cavity after the complete restoration of the proximal wall by the "snowplow" technique

4.2.4 Flowable Bulk and Packable Conventional Composite Technique: Marginal Ridge Technique

Main idea: This technique involves filling the class II cavity with bulk composite (flowable or packable) up to 1.5 mm from the occlusal surface, and after its polymerization, the marginal ridge is restored. Thus, a class I cavity with a depth of 1.5 mm will be obtained and restored.

Bulk composites may be light-cured in layers of 4–5 mm, and they are increasingly used due to multiple clinical (good shrinkage and polymerization stress) and ergonomic (quick and easy to apply) advantages. Flowable bulk composites (e.g., SDR, Dentsply Sirona) combine these advantages with those of flowable composites, reducing polymerization shrinkage by up to 60–70% compared to a conventional flowable composite [21]. Thus, the use of SDR as a liner on the gingival margin, followed by the restoration of the cavity with packable composite, reduces infiltration at the gingival margin level compared to the classic layering technique of conventional packable composite [22].

A study by Czasch et al. (2013) showed that for flowable bulk composites (SDR, Surefill, Dentsply Sirona), polymerization shrinkage was reduced by up to 20% and polymerization stress by up to 80% compared to conventional packable composite resins [23].

4.2.4.1 Working Technique

Stage 1

In the case of a class II cavity, the sectional matrix fixed with a ring and interdental wedge is applied; pulp protection is performed, if necessary; and then the adhesive system is applied. The cavity is subsequently filled with bulk composite (flowable or packable) up to 1.5 mm from the occlusal surface and is polymerized according to the manufacturer's instructions (Fig. 4.16a).

Stage 2

The next step is to restore the marginal ridge with a conventional packable composite resin to obtain a class I cavity with a depth of 1.5 mm that will be easy to restore. If the matrices are more contoured than the standard sectional ones, they help to restore the contact points when neighboring teeth are spaced (increased interproximal distances) (Fig. 4.16b).

Stage 3

The continuation of the restoration of this cavity represents the application of the last layer of composite necessary to restore the occlusal morphology using an occlusal modeling technique.

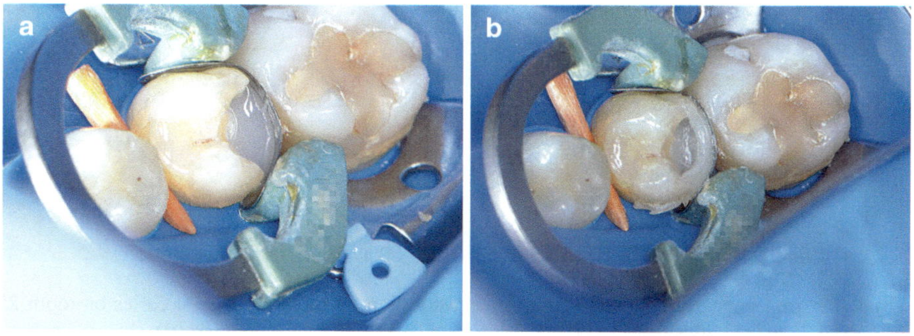

Fig. 4.16 Class I cavity filled with bulk flowable composite (SDR) up to 1.5 mm from the occlusal surface (**a**); image after restoration of the marginal ridge with conventional packable composite (**b**)

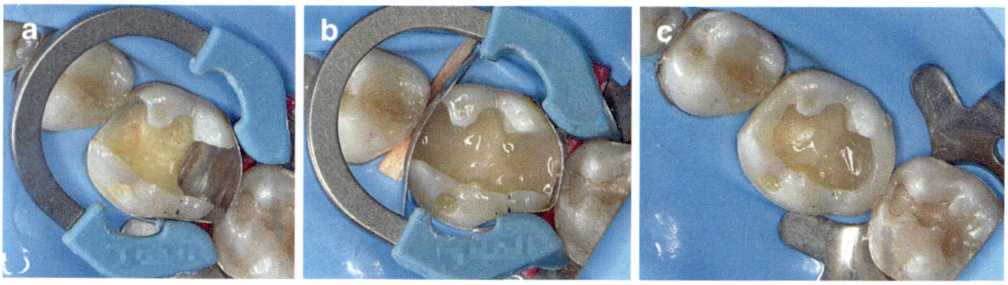

Fig. 4.17 MOD cavity prepared on a lower molar (**a**); the image after filling the cavity with a bulk flowable composite (SDR) up to 1.5 mm from the occlusal surface (**b**); restoration of the marginal ridges, mesial and distal, by packable composite (**c**)

In the case of MOD cavities, the technique is similar, the two marginal ridges being individually restored to obtain a class I cavity with a depth of 1.5 mm (Fig. 4.17). Applying the matrix and ring to restore one wall and only the matrix without the ring in the opposite cavity is preferable. Then the first contact area is restored, and the used ring is removed and reapplied in the opposite area. Placing two rings simultaneously, both mesially and distally, results in a separation effect in opposite directions and diminishes the effect in the applied contact area.

In the case of mirror cavities (Fig. 4.18), obtained either by removing carious processes or by removing old inadequate fillings, the restoration is carried out similarly. Thus, after the preparation of the cavity, the installation of the sectional matrices, the disinfection, and pulp protection (Fig. 4.19a–c), the bulk composite is applied, and the marginal ridge is successively restored, gradually removing the matrices (Fig. 4.20a–c). In this way, class I cavities are obtained in which the last layer of composite will be applied to restore the occlusal morphology through one of the occlusal modeling techniques (e.g., the technique of successive cusps, the technique of essential lines, etc.).

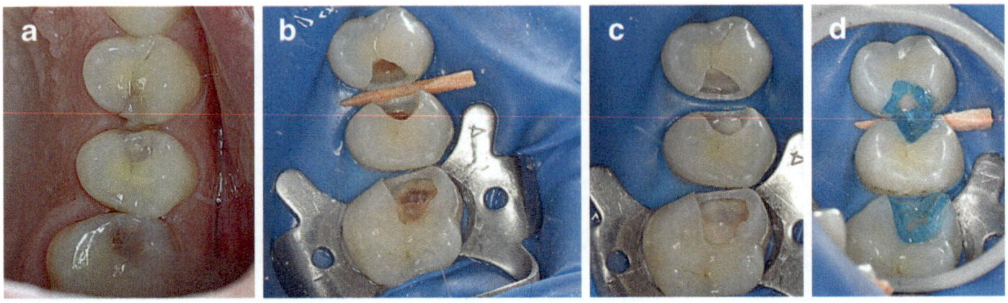

Fig. 4.18 Improper occluso-distal composite restoration on tooth 24; mesial caries on tooth 25 and tooth 26 (**a**); cavities prepared (**b**) and liner applied (**c**); selective etching (**d**)

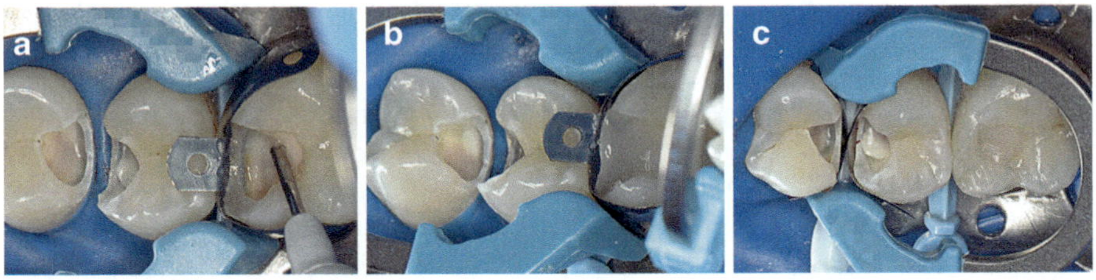

Fig. 4.19 Sectional matrix fixed with ring and interdental wedge on tooth 26 (**a**); bulk flowable composite (SDR) up to 1.5 mm away from the occlusal surface (**b**); restoration of the marginal ridge on tooth 26 by packable composite and application of matrices on the premolars (**c**)

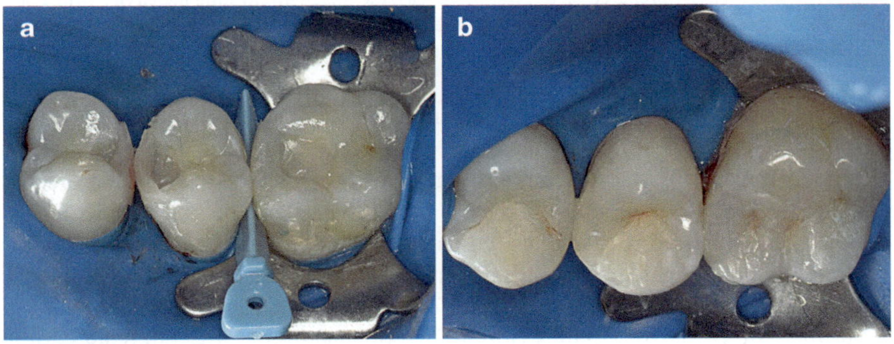

Fig. 4.20 Class II cavities transformed in class I (**a**); final restorations on teeth 24, 25, and 26 (**b**)

Difficulties that may arise	Possible solutions
Arbitrary positioning of the matrices to mirror cavities	Arranging the matrices so that the space is evenly distributed
The impossibility of determining the level of the marginal ridges if initially they were not preserved without a landmark	The level will be set according to the present ridges, and the final adjustment will be made during the occlusal adjustments stage

Difficulties that may arise	Possible solutions
The cavity obtained after bulk applications has less than 1.5 mm deepness for applying the packable composite	Removing it before polymerization with a microbrush or redistributing it in the cavity with a suitable tool (explorer, obturator, spatula)

4.2.5 Open Sandwich Technique (with GIc/Giomers/Flowable Composites)

Main idea: The open sandwich technique consists of placing in the subgingivally extended proximal cavity, a layer of glass ionomer cement that comes in contact with the matrix and subsequently in contact with the external environment of the tooth. The rest of the cavity is filled with composite resins.

The "open sandwich" technique initially described by Suzuki and Jordan [24] involves placing a layer of glass ionomer cement in the class I cavity that comes in contact with the matrix and then the composite material. The GIc material will be in contact with the external environment of the tooth. By contrary, the technique is called a "closed sandwich" if the GIc is completely embedded in the composite material (so the GIc does not come into contact with the matrix).

This technique has been proposed as the most suitable solution for restoring proximal cavities extended up to the level of the cementoenamel junction or below it [25], where there is no possibility of adhesion to the enamel. Although the open sandwich technique has been proven to provide the lowest microinfiltration of all restorative techniques currently available [26], the results are not stable over time [27]. The junction area between the GIc and composite resin should not be placed at the level of the contact point but below this level [28] (Fig. 4.21). GIc modified with resins

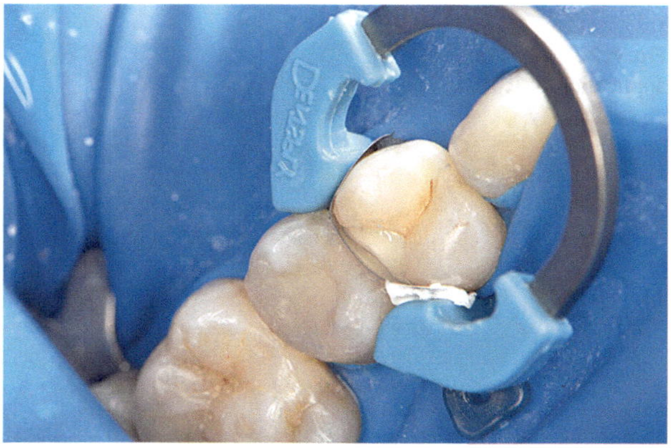

Fig. 4.21 Schematic representation of the thickness of the material layers in the case of the "open sandwich" technique relative to the interdental contact

have better mechanical and dentin adhesion properties than the conventional self-curing GIc described in the original technique [29] and can be used with greater success in the open sandwich technique [20]. In addition to superior mechanical and adhesion properties to self-curing variants, RMGIc presents several significant advantages for the open sandwich technique:

- They are easy to apply, being premixed, and packed in syringes.
- They set fast by photopolymerization.
- They are resistant to moisture in the long term.

Conditioning with orthophosphoric acid on the surface layer of RMGIc does not improve the adhesion of the composite that will be applied over it [30, 31]. In contrast, applying an adhesive between the RMGIc and the composite material significantly improves their adhesion [32, 33]. The technique is also known as "composite-laminated GIc" or "sandwich." This technique is recommended in patients at high risk of caries because it improves marginal sealing and releases fluoride [34].

4.2.5.1 Work Technique

The cleaning and disinfection of the cavity are performed. After placing the GIc or RMGIc material in the cavity, its uniform distribution, the absence of air bubbles, and excess material are monitored—after which it is polymerized (Fig. 4.22). The maximum filling level with this material must be below the level of the future contact point. In practice, this point is located at the matrix's maximum convexity level. Then, the chosen adhesive system is applied, and later the composite material restores the proximal wall and the marginal ridge using the centripetal technique. A class I cavity is obtained in this way. This will be filled with composite resin, and the occlusal morphology will be achieved.

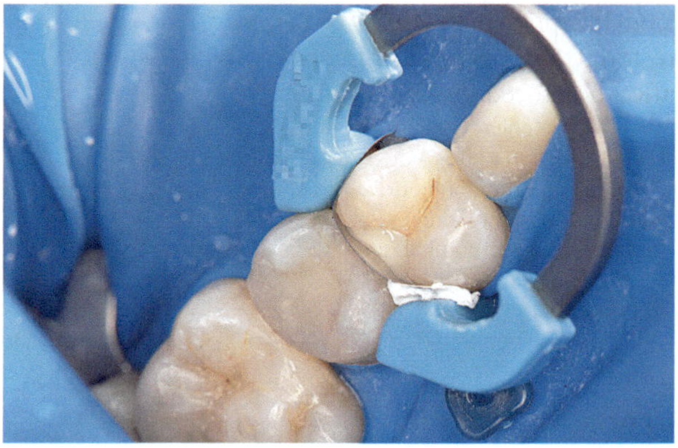

Fig. 4.22 Image after application of RMGIc in a class II cavity

Difficulties that may arise	Possible solutions
Increased waiting time for setting a self-curing GIc	Replacement with a light-curing GIc
Undesirable sticking of some GIc to the axial walls of the cavity when it is placed in the cavity	An explorer or bur can be used to remove the material

4.2.6 Bulk-Fill Technique

Main idea: Filling a cavity can be achieved by applying a bulk material from a single filling or two fillings, thus avoiding the layering technique required for conventional packable composites.

Using bulk composites (Fig. 4.23) allows the operator to decrease the working time by decreasing the number of increments required to fill cavities without introducing additional polymerization stress. Moreover, the marginal integrity of the restorations is not affected [35], and at the same time, the temperature transmitted to the pulp is maintained below the alarm threshold of 42.5 °C in the presence of a dentine layer of at least 0.5 mm [36] based on the cavity. This bulk application technique is possible due to the characteristics of bulk composite materials (see Sect. 1.2.2).

Flowable bulk composites are successfully used for fast and efficient cavity filling techniques, having good flow properties, elasticity, and adaptation to any cavity shape. Flowable bulk composites with reduced filler loading are generally not

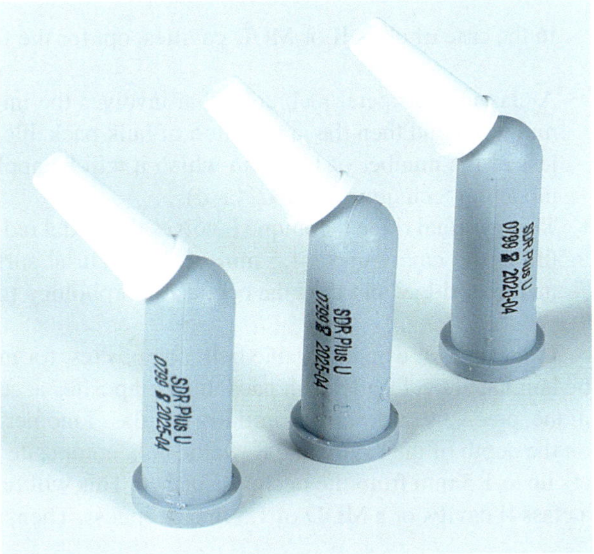

Fig. 4.23 Flowable bulk composite in compules

recommended for the occlusal surface subjected to forces. There are also exceptions, certain materials being indicated by the manufacturers, according to the instructions, for use also on certain areas subjected to forces (G-aenial flow, GC; SDR plus, Dentsply Sirona).

Although bulk materials can be applied and polymerized in layers of 4–5 mm, it is recommended that the first layer applied in the cavity is thin to avoid the increase in temperature transmitted to the pulp during polymerization [37]. Later, the cavity can be filled with a second layer up to the occlusal surface in the case of a packable bulk or up to 1.5 mm of the occlusal surface in the case of a flowable bulk (read the instructions of each material separately).

4.2.6.1 Working Technique

For packable bulk composites, the material can be applied to the cavity in one or more layers, depending on the depth of the cavity and the choice of a particular occlusal modeling technique. Thus, it is possible to apply a packable bulk composite:

- In a single layer, especially in superficial and medium cavities.
- In two layers: a first layer is applied to the base of the cavity and polymerized, followed by the second layer on which the occlusal morphology will also be achieved through the simultaneous cusp technique. The major disadvantage of this technique is brought by the fact that it requires the simultaneous modeling of the cusps according to the conventional method (the one used for amalgam) or the "essential lines" technique.
- In several layers: a first layer is applied to the base of the cavity and polymerized, followed by the second layer up to 1.5 mm from the occlusal surface and polymerized. Thus, it is possible to achieve cusp-by-cusp occlusal morphology, a technique that provides good control and aesthetic and functional results.

In the case of class II or MOD cavities, opt for the following:

- A classic centripetal technique that involves the initial restoration of the proximal walls and then the application of bulk packable composite material, regardless of the number of layers in which it will be applied and the chosen occlusal modeling technique (Fig. 4.24a–d).
- The marginal ridge technique involves the initial reduction of the cavity depth by filling the cavity up to 1.5 mm of the occlusal surface, then restoration of the marginal ridge, and then the occlusal morphology (see Sect. 4.7).

In the case of using flowable bulk composites, for most of the brands, they must be laminated occlusally with packable composites according to a "sandwich" technique, precisely as described initially for glass ionomer types of cement. Depending on the depth of the cavity, the flowable bulk composite is applied in one or two layers up to 1.5 mm from the occlusal surface. This will result in either a class I cavity, a class II cavity, or a MOD of 1.5 mm deepness. Then, the direct restoration will be

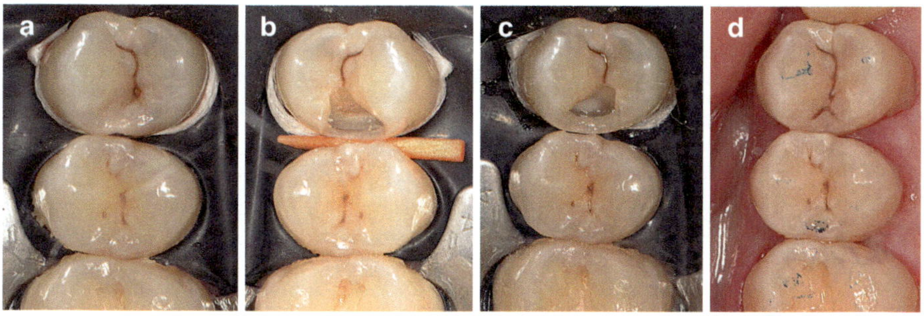

Fig. 4.24 Initial image of a distal carious lesion on tooth 14 (**a**); ocluso-distal cavity prepared (**b**); later transformed into a class I cavity by restoration of the distal wall (**c**); final image of the direct restoration on tooth 14 with application of brown pigment (**d**)

made from a packable composite by one of the techniques described (centripetal, simultaneous, successive, essential lines, etc.).

4.2.7 Injection Technique

Main idea: Filling a prepared cavity can be achieved by injecting a flowable composite with a packable heated composite using a transparent conformer (matrix or a clear stent).

Using the injection technique makes it possible to make direct restorations quickly and minimally invasively, with a predictable aesthetic result. The technique follows a straightforward procedure, with maximum control over each step.

The technique can be performed for class II cavities using transparent matrices (Fig. 4.25), but for more extensive frontal or lateral restorations, it is necessary to create a transparent stent (Fig. 4.26) based on a conventional or digital wax-up. A flowable composite is injected into this mold and light-cured (see Chap. 8).

The injection technique involves several peculiarities of proximal cavity preparation, the most important being the elimination of the concept of cavity preparation in occlusal and proximal slots/cassettes. If occlusal involvement occurs, the authors recommend that this cavity be prepared and filled separately, just like a class I cavity. Afterward, the proximal disk-shaped cavity will be prepared, flattened, and slightly deep so that the composite is applied “on the tooth” rather than “in the tooth.” In this way, the C-factor is significantly reduced or even eliminated.

The injection of the composite imposes certain particularities, such as:

- Less geometric preparation of a proximal cavity.
- Use of a transparent anatomically shaped matrix.
- Thin applicator tips for flowable composite (G20).

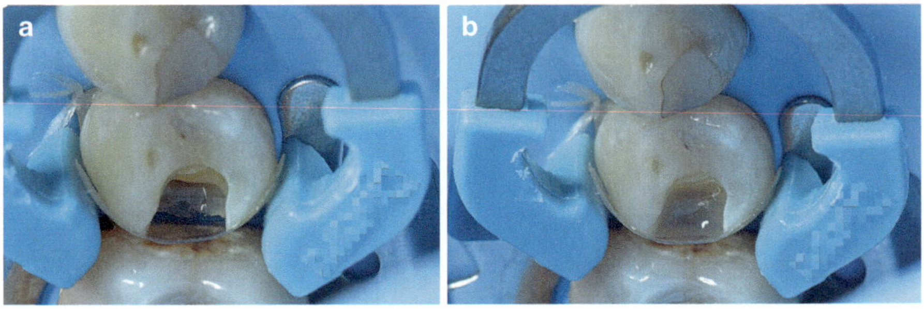

Fig. 4.25 Image of a class II cavity with clear celluloid sectional matrix fixed with ring and interdental wedge (**a**); injection of flowable composite (**b**)

Fig. 4.26 The transparent silicone stent made using a wax-up

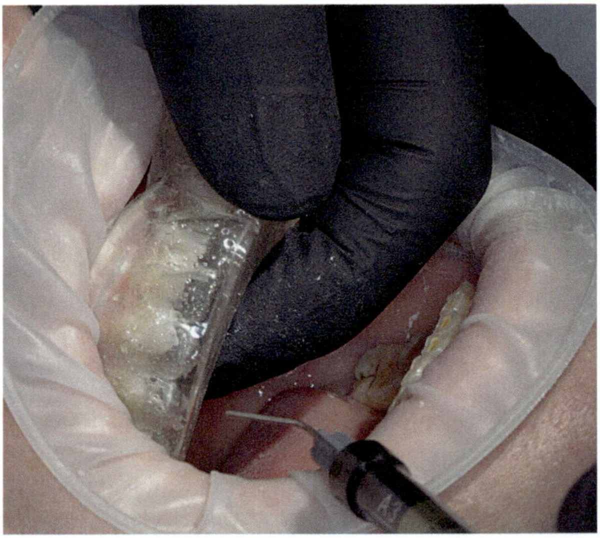

- Heating the packable composite to ~68°.
- Replacing the packing technique with a hydraulic model where the composites find their direction during the injection.

4.2.7.1 Working Technique

Injection-molded technique for class II cavities can be compared as a concept to an impression technique where we use fluid consistency silicone and putty silicone simultaneously—which we apply with pressure over the prosthetic field. Thus, this technique applied flowable composite (maximum 20% of the volume) to the base of the proximal cavity and preheated packable composite was injected over it. The two injected composites will then be simultaneously polymerized. Just as in the case of the modified oblique technique with flowable composite or the snowplow technique, the role of the flowable composite in this technique is to eliminate the risk of voids and to ensure better marginal sealing.

Review Questions

1. What are the specificities of the gingival margin area of class II cavities?
2. What are the variants of the centripetal technique by which the proximal wall of a class II cavity can be restored?
3. What does the centripetal oblique layering technique of the proximal wall consist of?
4. What is the centripetal technique for restoring the proximal wall using flowable composite on the gingival margin?
5. What is the centripetal snowplow technique for proximal wall restoration?
6. What is the bulk composite cavity depth reduction and marginal ridge restoration technique?
7. What does "open sandwich" technique consist of, and what are the recommendations for performing it?
8. What is the bulk-fill technique, and how is the occlusal morphology achieved in the case of this technique?
9. What does the class II cavity restoration technique by injection consist of and what are the characteristics of it?

Regardless of the type of layering chosen for the restoration of the proximal wall, the matrix must be well-adapted along the entire contour of the cavity. When necessary, additional means can be used (e.g., Teflon tape) (Fig. 4.27).

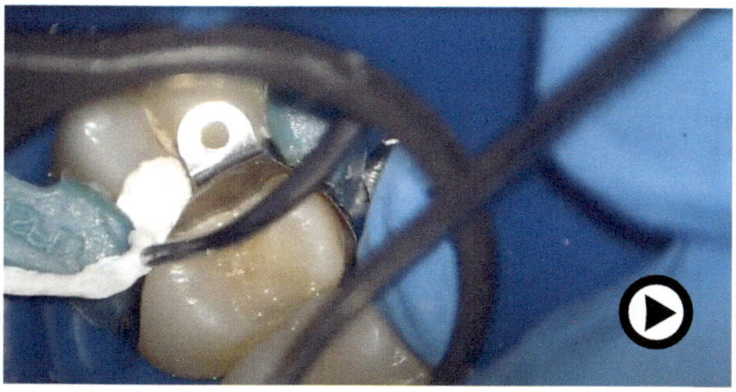

Fig. 4.27 Adaptation of a Palodent sectional matrix with Teflon tape (▶ https://doi.org/10.1007/000-bqn)

4.3 Techniques for Posterior Teeth Where Matrices Vary (Number, Type, and Manner of Mounting)

We will present some techniques that can be used to restore the proximal walls of simple or mirrored class II cavities in the purpose of transformation into class I cavities. The presented techniques mainly use sectional matrices, but also circular ones.

4.3.1 Saddle Matrix Technique

Main idea: The saddle matrix is a matrix with an intermediate design, between sectional and circular, which can be adapted to a wide variety of clinical cases.

This matrix exists in several variants of size but also of shapes, having different convexities (Fig. 4.28) (TOR VM Company). It is a highly versatile matrix type due to the possibility of fixing it regardless of the extent of the destruction (as long as at least one wall is present). The cavity adaptability of these matrices is limited compared to sectional matrices, given the extensive destructions that can be addressed. It can often provide a better solution than using circular matrices. The matrices are more contoured than standard or circular sectional matrices, helping to restore contact points when neighboring teeth are spaced (increased interproximal distances). Thus, among the possible indications for the use of these types of matrices, we mention:

- Class II cavities with a small, medium, and extended bucco-oral opening.
- Class II cavities when there is no adjacent tooth (Fig. 4.29a, b).
- Extensive destruction of the adjacent tooth so that it is not possible to mount a sectional matrix fixed with wedges and rings.

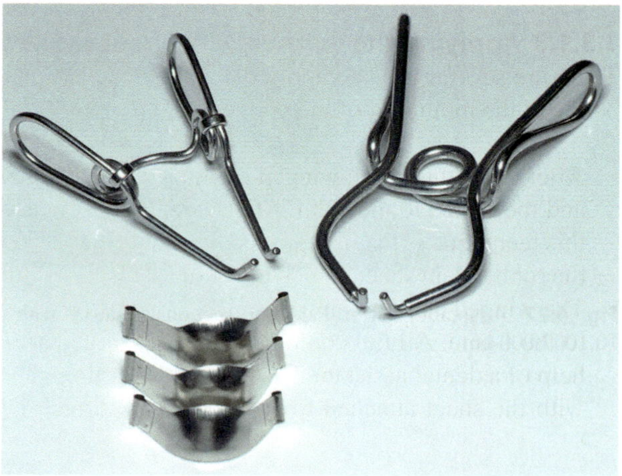

Fig. 4.28 Multi-size saddle matrices and applicator clamp

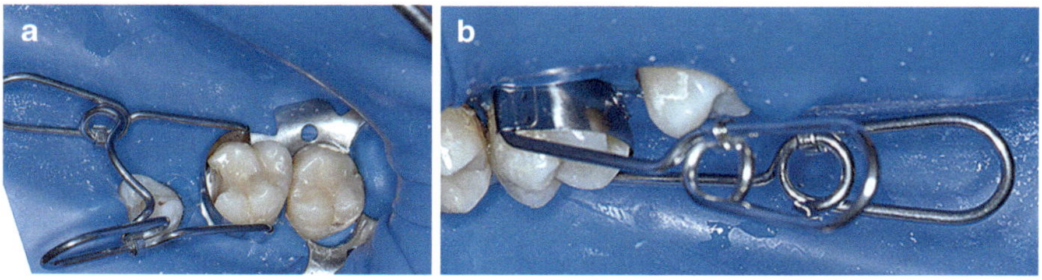

Fig. 4.29 Saddle matrix applied on a molar without mesial contact, occlusal view (**a**) and buccal view (**b**)

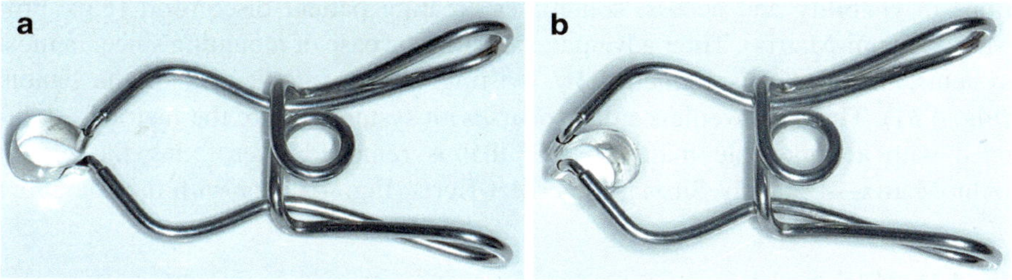

Fig. 4.30 Different ways of mounting the matrix in the applicator clamp for distal (**a**) or mesial (**b**) cavities

- Cavities on the distal surface of the last molar present on the arch.
- Small, medium, or extensive proximal cavities located on teeth in atypical positions that make it impossible to mount a sectional matrix.

4.3.1.1 Working Technique

The choice of matrix size and convexity is made according to the tooth and the individual clinical situation. They can be mounted by adaptation only with wedges, fixed with classic matrix rings (type Palodent, Garrison, etc.), or with a metal applicator clamp specially created for this brand of matrix. It is preferable to mount the matrix in the applicator clamp before inserting it into the oral cavity by fixing the two pins in the unique slots of the matrix. The clamp position will always be with the handles anterior/medial for actuation. The matrix can be mounted on a tooth's mesial and distal wall (Fig. 4.30a, b). At the level of the gingival margin, we recommend adapting the matrix with an interdental wedge.

Difficulties that may arise	Possible solutions
Difficulty in obtaining the point of contact of the matrix with the adjacent tooth	Modification of the insertion axis and fixation of the matrix during the application and polymerization of the composite until the contact point is obtained
Mounting difficulties due to the fact that the tips of the application clamp slide on the crown	Fixation with a liquid rubber dam

4.3.2 Circular Matrix Technique

Main idea: Circular matrices achieve a circumferential sealing of the crown when applied and tightened on the tooth, being recommended in specific clinical cases where sectional matrices cannot be fitted.

As also presented in Sect. 1.1.4, circular matrices come in various shapes, sizes, and mounting modes. Systems with a nonremovable long-handled matrix holder (retainer), which remains present in the oral cavity during treatment, have limitations in visibility and access, sometimes creating patient discomfort (e.g., Pro-Matrix; Omni-Matrix). Their advantage remains the ease of mounting since, in most systems, the matrix is tightened by twisting a drum at the end of the handle (Fig. 4.31). This inconvenience disappears with systems where the matrix is tightened with a removable matrix holder that is removed after fixing the matrix (AutoMatrix—Dentsply Sirona; SuperMat-Kerr) (Fig. 4.32) or with those that are

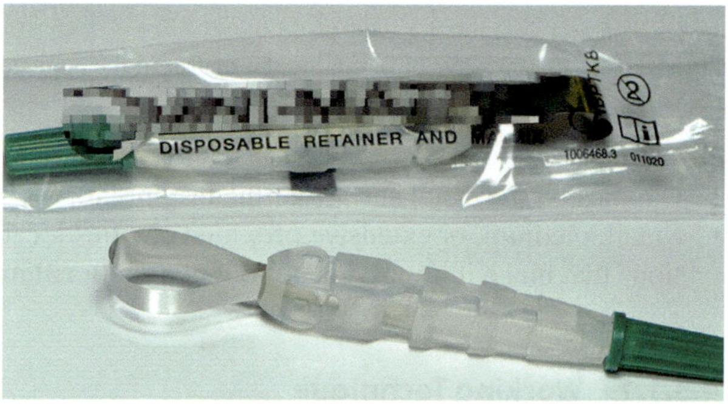

Fig. 4.31 Metal circular matrix with long plastic retainer

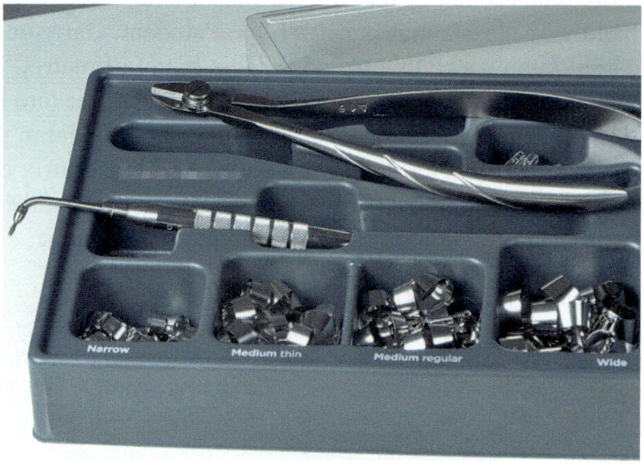

Fig. 4.32 Metal circular matrices with removable retainer

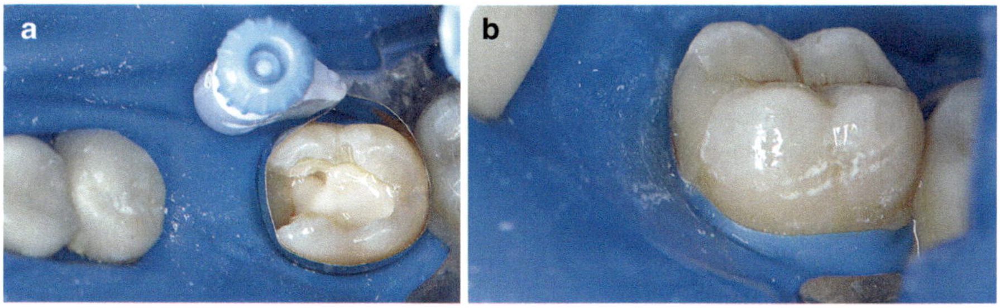

Fig. 4.33 Metal circular matrix without a retainer (**a**) and final restoration after matrix removal (**b**)

tightened directly by twisting it next to the matrix (Palodent 360, Dentsply Sirona; myQuickmat All-round, Polydentia) (Fig. 4.33).

These matrices can be indicated in some specific cases:

- Extensive destruction of the crown to restore abutments that will later be restored prosthetically.
- Extended proximal destructions toward the buccal or oral walls that exceed the indications of a sectional matrix.
- The absence of the adjacent tooth makes it impossible to fix a sectional matrix (edentations or the terminal area of the arch).
- Changes in position that make it impossible to fix a sectional matrix.

4.3.2.1 Working Technique

Regardless of the type of circular matrix used, upon tightening, it will shrink circumferentially equally in both its occlusal and cervical portions. Thus, if the taper of the matrix does not perfectly correspond to that of the crown (smaller cervical and larger occlusal diameter), the seal at the cervical level will be deficient. In the case of the presence of adjacent teeth, adaptation can be achieved relatively easily: by placing an interdental wedge. In order to create the necessary space for the matrix and achieve prewedging, the use of a full wedge or a matrix ring is indicated.

In the case of their absence or the case of distal cavities on the last molar, adapting these matrices to the cervical area can be a challenge for any clinician. However, the excess obtained in these cases can be easily removed, considering the easy access provided by the lack of the adjacent tooth.

Difficulties that may arise	Possible solutions
Adapting to the cervical area is impossible due to the lack of the adjacent tooth	Pressing with a spatula the matrix in the cervical area during the application and polymerization of the composite
Excess of the composite at the level of the gingival margin	If the lack of the adjacent tooth provides direct access, the excess can be removed with the bur; if there is no direct access, then an abrasive metal tape or curettes can be used to remove the excess

4.3.3 Single-Matrix Technique for Mirror Cavities

In clinical cases of mirror-symmetric caries (kissing cavities), preparation and obturation can be performed simultaneously in a single session for efficiency and workflow. Among the advantages of this approach, we can mention:

- Speed due to the use of the same instruments, passing from one tooth to another
- Decreasing difficulties by eliminating the requirement not to touch the adjacent tooth when preparing a single cavity
- The possibility of having an overall view of the case
- Speed due to the successive use of materials and instruments in the filling and finishing steps

The presence of matrices in restoring mirror cavities can influence the quality of the contact point between the two teeth. The primary objective is to obtain a close contact point that prevents food impact on the interdental papilla and a good distribution of forces.

4.3.3.1 Working Technique

Mirror cavity restoration requires the presence of two matrices, one on each tooth. Thus, it is recommended to avoid keeping both matrices in position until the restoration of the two cavities is completed to avoid doubling the space between the teeth imposed by the thickness of the two matrices. We, therefore, have the following possibilities:

1. Position a single matrix, restore the first tooth, and then continue with the second.
2. Position both matrices simultaneously, completely restore one tooth, remove the matrix from it, and only then restore the second tooth (Sect. 4.11.4).

> The main idea of the single-matrix technique for mirror cavities is to restore the cavities one at a time by fitting the matrix and completely restoring the first tooth, followed by repeating the procedure for the second tooth.

Applying the matrix to a single tooth when there are mirror-prepared cavities can create difficulties mainly related to positioning and stability:

- Its placement outside the contour of the tooth can generate an increase in the mesiodistal diameter of the restored crown at the expense of the remaining space available for the adjacent tooth. Invasion of the space of the adjacent tooth may prevent the achievement of adequate proximal anatomy and, therefore, a proper point of contact between the two teeth (Fig. 4.34).

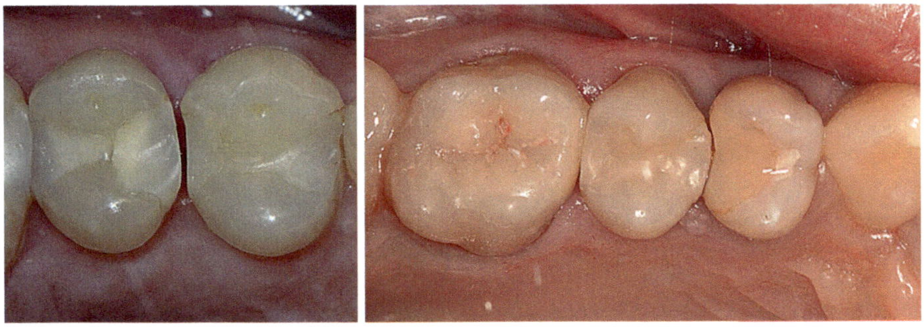

Fig. 4.34 Incorrectly restored interdental contacts on premolars

- The matrix may slide or bulge too much when positioning the matrix ring, or it may be inadvertently pushed into the adjacent cavity because it encounters no obstacle.
- Obtaining a too-accentuated proximal contour in cases of extensive destruction, considering that the matrix does not meet resistance to diminish its curvature.

This technique can be used successfully when there is reasonable control of the positioning and a certainty that the space intended for the adjacent restoration will not be invaded. After the restoration of the first tooth, the matrix will be mounted on the second tooth, which will also be restored (Fig. 4.35).

Difficulties that may arise	Possible solutions
Obtaining an over-contoured restoration, extended toward the adjacent tooth	Redoing or reducing size with rotary instruments
Matrix positioning instability	Additional fixation with fingers, liquid dam, and Teflon tape

4.3.4 Two-Matrix Technique for Mirror Cavities

Main idea: This technique involves the simultaneous mounting of the matrices (Fig. 4.36) to distribute the interdental space properly so that each matrix initially has a fixation point on the other matrix. Next comes the restoration of one tooth, removing the matrix from it to restore the second tooth with only one matrix in place (Fig. 4.37).

Overflowing old fillings that create interdental food retention can often lead to cavities on adjacent teeth. In these cases, it is necessary to remove the inadequate filling and to prepare the cavities on the two teeth. These are classic cases of mirror cavities. Mirror cavity preparation is most frequently performed simultaneously for efficiency and ergonomics of work with an interdentally placed wedge for pre-distancing and papilla protection (Fig. 4.38).

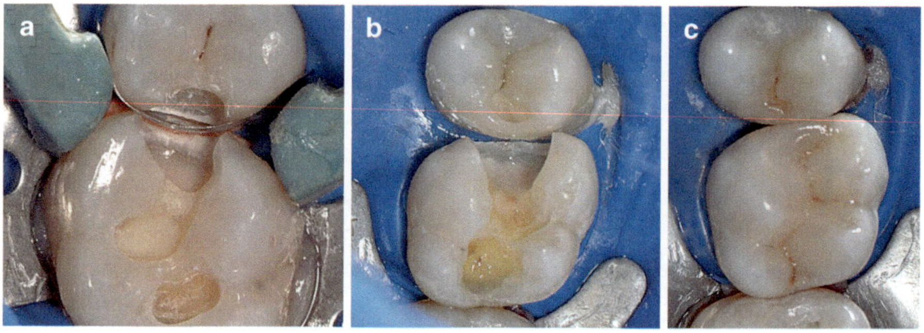

Fig. 4.35 Mounting the matrix on a single tooth (**a**) for the restoration of the proximal wall (**b**) in the case of mirror cavities; the final restorations (**c**)

Fig. 4.36 Simultaneous mounting of matrices to restore a mesial cavity on tooth 16 and mesial and distal cavities on tooth 15

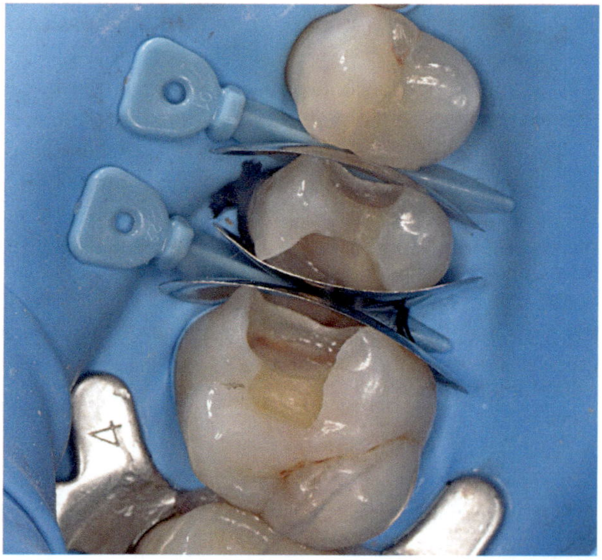

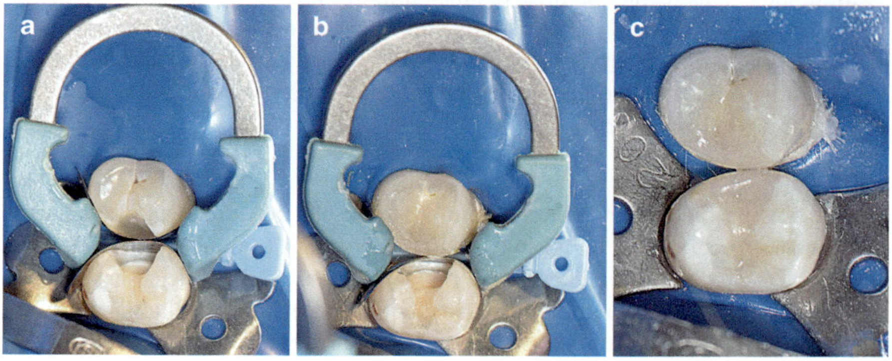

Fig. 4.37 Simultaneous application of sectional matrices in the case of two premolars on which mirror cavities were prepared (**a**); removing one of the matrices after restoration of one tooth (**b**) and restoration of the second premolar with only one matrix in place (**c**)

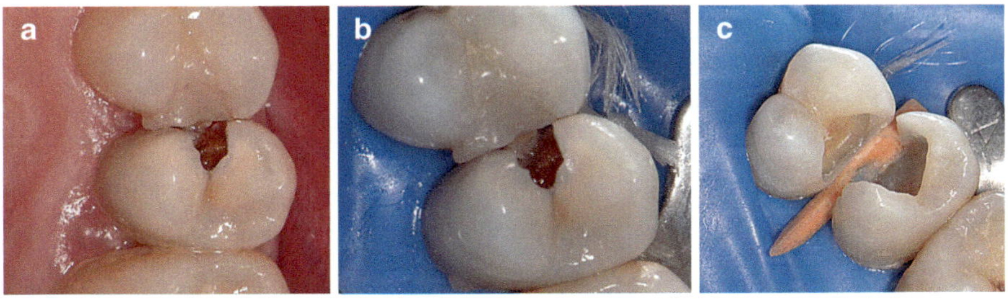

Fig. 4.38 Initial image of an old filling with composite excess on tooth 24 and deep mesial caries on tooth 25: before (**a**) and after rubber dam isolation (**b**); cavities prepared (**c**)

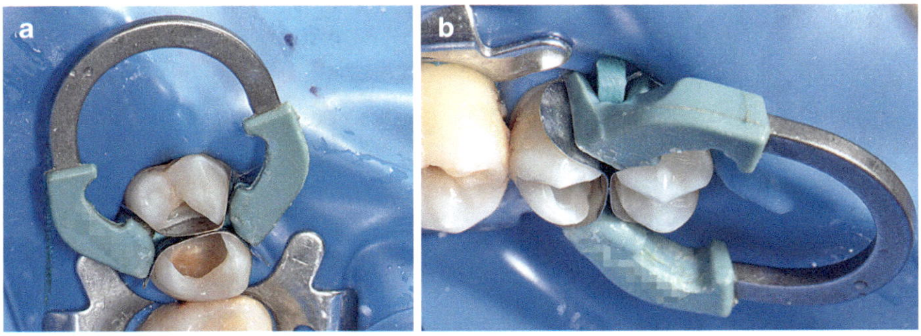

Fig. 4.39 Simultaneous mounting of sectional matrices on teeth 24 and 25 (**a**) fixed with Palodent ring and dental wedge (**b**)

4.3.4.1 Working Technique

After making and verifying the cavity preparation, two adapted sectional matrices with ring and wedge are mounted (Fig. 4.39). Due to easier access, the cavity disinfection and liner application can be performed prior to the matrix mounting step. After restoring a wall, the matrix will be removed after gently relaxing the matrix ring. The second wall will then be restored, thus obtaining two class I cavities (Fig. 4.40a).

Excess composite from the oral and buccal embrasures can be removed with a curette, and the interdental contact can be checked with dental floss [38] (Fig. 4.40b–d).

Amalgam fillings made in class II cavities are frequently the cause of caries appearing on the adjacent tooth (Fig. 4.41). This is due to food retention caused by excess amalgam [39] much more frequently than composite restorations [40]. Cavity preparation in such cases is carried out simultaneously and can be restored directly using sectional matrices fixed with wedges and matrix rings. It is possible to opt for one or two rings depending on the need for a tight fit of the matrices on the tooth (Fig. 4.42). However, the use of two matrix rings mounted simultaneously is to be avoided because they can mutually cancel each other's pre-distancing effect.

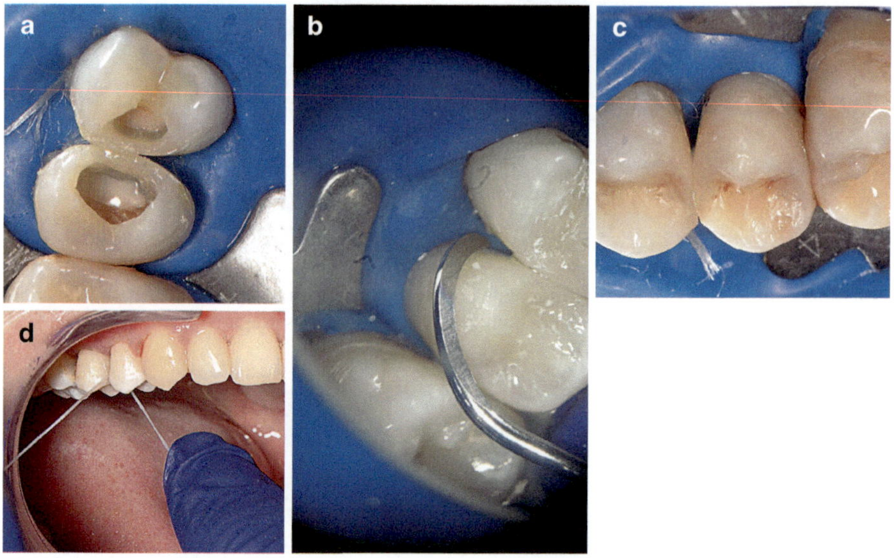

Fig. 4.40 Restoration of the proximal walls on teeth 24 and 25 (**a**); removal of excess proximal material with curette (**b**); the final restorations (**c**); checking the contact point with dental floss (**d**)

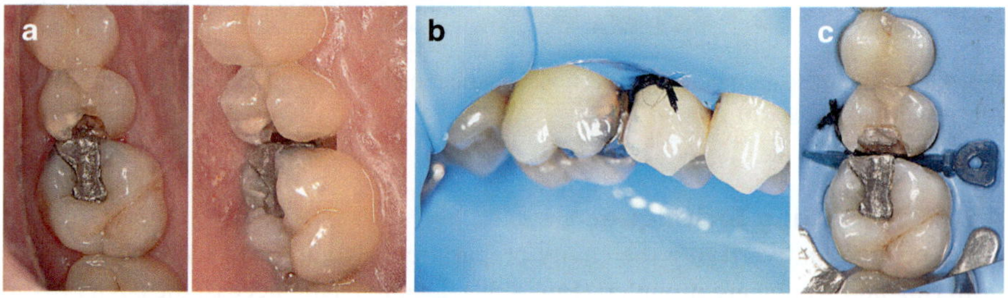

Fig. 4.41 Medium deepness ocluso-distal caries on tooth 15 and mesio-occlusal amalgam filling on tooth 16 (**a**); after the rubber dam isolation (**b**); during cavity preparation (**c**)

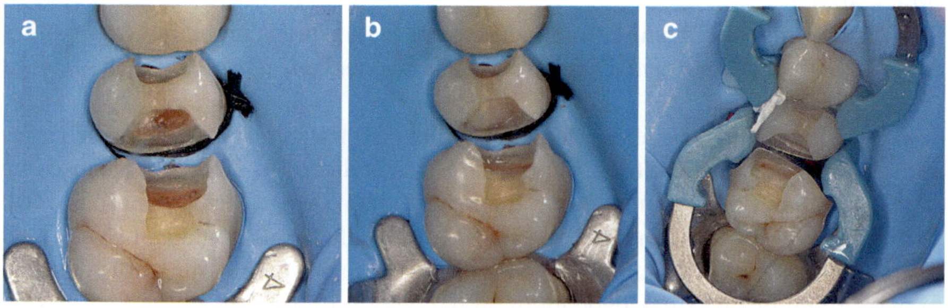

Fig. 4.42 Cavities prepared on teeth 25 and 26 (**a**); image after applying the liner on tooth 25 (**b**); matrices fixed with two Palodent rings (**c**)

The centripetal technique yields two class I cavities after the restoration of all proximal walls (Fig. 4.43).

Proximal mirror caries can occur on teeth without previous restorations, in which case the same protocol of simultaneous preparation of the two cavities can be followed using an interdental wedge for pre-distancing and protection (Figs. 4.44 and 4.45).

If another layering option is chosen, such as filling the cavity with flowable bulk (SDR, Dentsply Sirona) and restoring the marginal ridge with packable composite, the two adjacent proximal walls will be restored one by one, removing the first matrix after the complete restoration of the first wall (Figs. 4.46 and 4.47).

Difficulties that may arise	Possible solutions
Displacement of the matrices at the insertion of the wedge	The matrices can be fixed with the ring first and the wedge inserted later if the ring tines are V-shaped designed, with special slots, to accommodate the wedge
Bleeding at the time of removal of the first matrix	Wash, dry, and apply the adhesive system

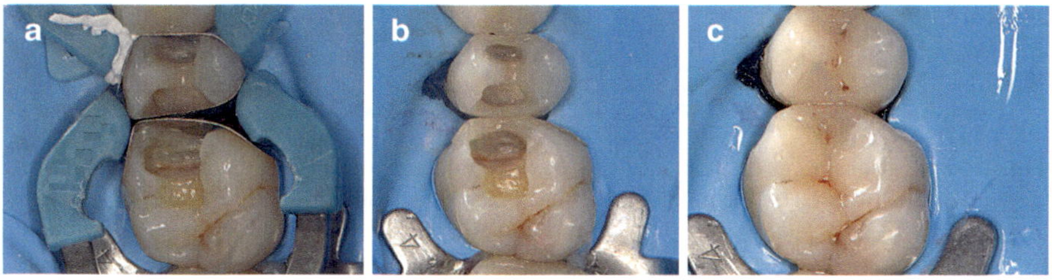

Fig. 4.43 Restoration of nonadjacent proximal walls by oblique layering (**a**); the image of the class I cavities obtained after the restoration of the proximal walls (**b**); the final restorations (**c**)

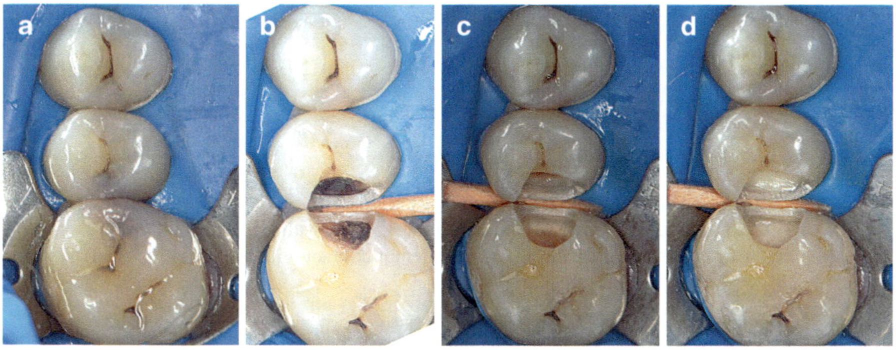

Fig. 4.44 Mirror caries on teeth 15 and 16 (**a**); image during cavity preparation (**b**); prepared cavities (**c**) and image after liner application (**d**)

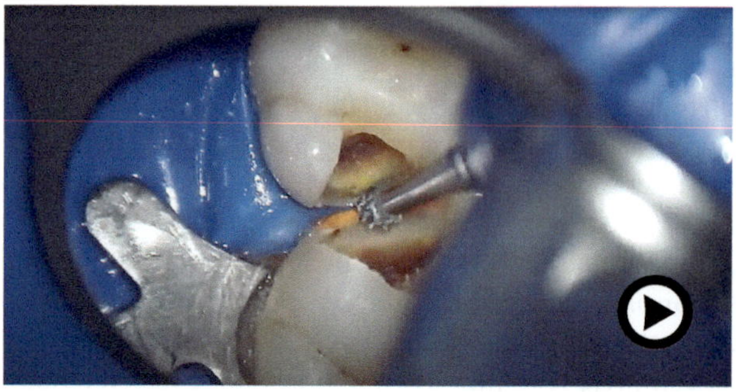

Fig. 4.45 Mirror proximal caries. Preparation. Restoration (▶ https://doi.org/10.1007/000-bqm)

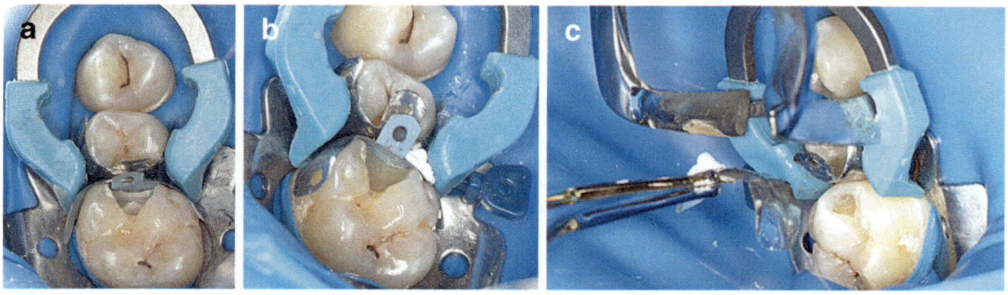

Fig. 4.46 Sectional matrices in place (**a**); flowable bulk composite in the cavity on the molar (**b**); marginal ridge restored on the molar and removal of matrix from this tooth (**c**)

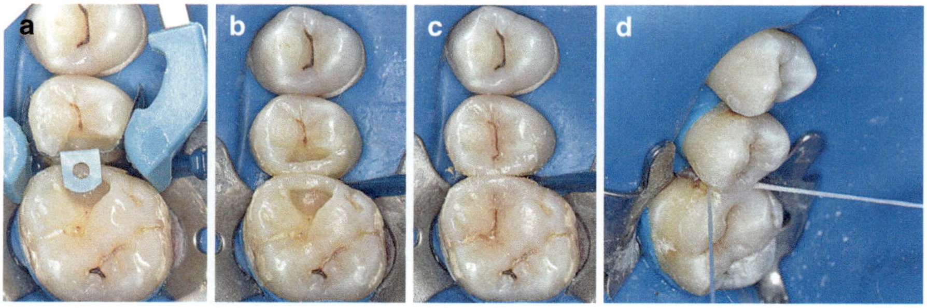

Fig. 4.47 Application of bulk composite and restoration of the marginal ridge on the premolar (**a**); the two class I cavities after the restoration of the proximal walls (**b**); the final restorations after the application of pigments (**c**); checking the interdental contact with the dental floss (**d**)

4.3.5 Matrix-in-Matrix Technique

The main idea: Sectional matrices can be fixed by clamping inside another circular matrix or in the saddle matrix for particular cases of direct restorations.

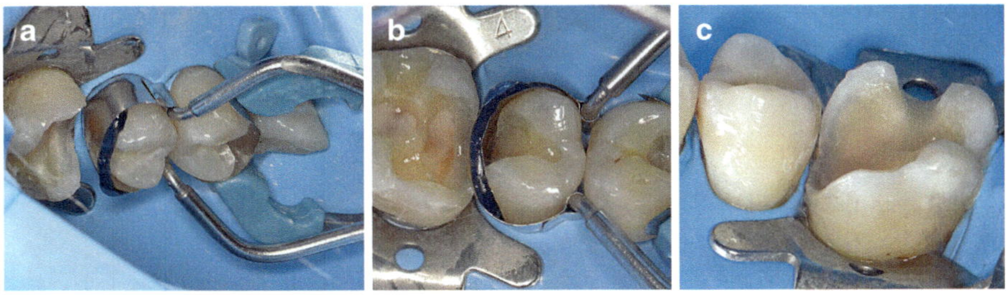

Fig. 4.48 Sectional matrix maintained in position with a saddle matrix (**a**); occlusal view (**b**); final restoration on premolar (**c**)

Different particular cases require the combination of several types of matrices, one of the situations being the placement of one inside the other. When adequate proximal anatomy is desired using a sectional matrix (but cannot be fixed with a matrix ring due to the lack of buccal and oral embrasures), using another circular- or saddle-shaped matrix may be helpful. One of the frequently encountered clinical situations is the restoration of ocluso-distal cavities located on the last molars.

4.3.5.1 Working Technique

The sectional matrix is placed in the appropriate position and fixed by applying a circular or saddle matrix. The two matrices can be in contact or, if the situation requires it, the space between them can be filled with Teflon or liquid dam (Fig. 4.48). Teflon inserted in the area of the gingival margin between the matrices can help adapt the sectional matrix to the cervical area.

Difficulties that may arise	Possible solutions
Deformation of the sectional matrix by compressing it with the second matrix	Replacing the sectional matrix with a new one, not distorted
Lack of tight marginal sealing	Tightening the matrix

4.3.6 Celluloid Transparent Anatomically Shaped Matrix Technique

Main idea: Transparent anatomically shaped sectional matrices made of celluloid can be successfully used to restore proximal walls and contact points in class II or MOD cavities.

The use of transparent matrices presents several advantages, among which we mention:

- Easy conformation of the contact area and being very flexible.
- Improving photopolymerization because they are transparent and allow the light beam to pass through.

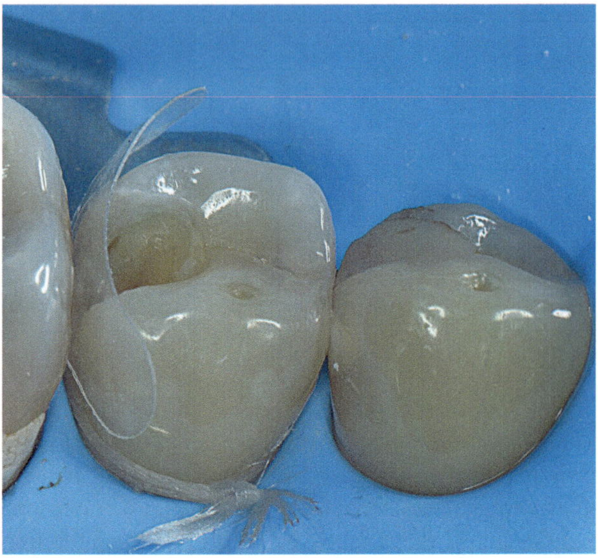

Fig. 4.49 Celluloid transparent sectional matrix

- Lead to obtaining particularly fine and glossy external surfaces.
- They allow an easy disinsertion after the polymerization of the composite, being non-adherent to the composite.

The difficulties introduced by using this type of matrices are especially associated with the fact that they are transparent and more difficult to identify visually (Fig. 4.49). Thus, modeling the composite and removing the excess in the vicinity of the matrix can sometimes be challenging. Choosing colored, semitransparent celluloid matrices can bring advantages related to their easier localization.

4.3.6.1 Working Technique

The installation of these matrices is done in the same way as the metal ones by placing them appropriately interdentally and fixing them with the help of the matrix wedges and rings (Fig. 4.50). Classic matrix rings and plastic or wooden wedges can be used. Checking the positioning of the matrix in contact with the adjacent tooth is done by pressing any tool with a round tip that avoids scratching the matrix. The shape of the matrix can be adjusted by inserting tweezers into the cavity to accentuate or decrease the proximal curvature of the matrix.

Difficulties that may arise	Possible solutions
The slipping of the matrix ring on the celluloid	Fiberglass tines matrix rings can slide more easily over the celluloid matrix, so fixation can be adjusted by supplementing with a liquid dam, or silicone tines rings can be used
Difficulties in visual identification of the matrix	Use of magnification or semitransparent matrices

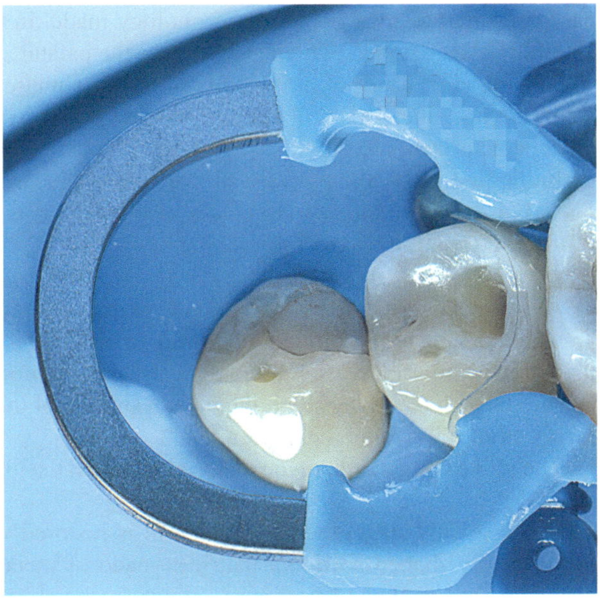

Fig. 4.50 Celluloid transparent sectional matrix fixed with Palodent ring

Did You Get It?

1. What are the possible indications for using a saddle matrix?
2. What are the possible indications for using a circular matrix?
3. What are the advantages of the simultaneous approach to symmetrical mirror cavities?
4. What is the working technique with simultaneous matrices mounting in the case of symmetric mirror cavities?
5. What is the matrix-in-matrix technique?
6. What are the possible advantages of using preformed transparent sectional matrices?

4.4 Techniques for Anterior Teeth

4.4.1 Centripetal Technique for Anterior Teeth

Full or partial restoration of proximal walls in the anterior area can be a clinical challenge in many cases. The difficulty of the case increases directly to the size of the proximal area to be restored. In the case of class IV cavities, obtaining satisfactory aesthetic results requires, in many cases, layering composites and applying biomimetic techniques. Therefore, the restoration of the proximal walls can be individualized as a separate stage of work, somewhat similar to the centripetal technique on posterior teeth.

Thus, by restoring the proximal wall of a posterior class II cavity, we aim to transform it into a class I cavity. This cavity opens on one side that can then be easily restored and the occlusal morphology made. In the case of extended fourth- and third-class cavities (which also involve the palatal and buccal surfaces), restoration of the palatal or proximal walls in the first phase leads to obtaining an open cavity on one side. This will later be restored by layering the desired dentin shades and characterizations.

In the first stage, the palatal walls are generally restored and then the proximal ones. For the restoration of the palatal wall, support is required for the application of the composite. It can be represented by:

- A pre-made silicone key. This leads to the best and most predictable results, which is why we recommend this way of working.
- A flexible matrix, most commonly a straight celluloid strip, fitted by finger pressure or with a cotton roll on the palatal surface of the tooth.
- A cotton roll wrapped in Teflon tape.
- The gloved finger, where the material of which the glove is made acts as a matrix.

In the second stage, the proximal wall is restored with the help of, preferably, anatomically shaped sectional matrices made of metal or celluloid, but there are also cases where wide, free access allows freehand modeling with manual instruments (e.g., with a spatula).

The palatal and proximal walls can also be restored simultaneously in a single stage by applying a single matrix (e.g., straight transparent celluloid strip) or an anatomically shaped or straight sectional matrix fixed in a slot of the silicone key). Using such a construction of a matrix fixed in the silicone key, the restoration can also be achieved by applying bulk composite, or by simplified stratification in horizontal layers from palatal to buccal (see Sect. 5.3.2). Applying this layering strategy will automatically generate the proximal wall as the cavity fills and not as a distinct anatomical entity.

Clear celluloid strips are widely used to restore class III cavities and the proximal walls of class IV cavities. In most cases of extended class III and class IV cavities, obtaining a convex cervico-incisal proximal anatomy and a good interdental contact is impossible using straight strips of clear celluloid. Only anatomically shaped matrices can lead to the restoration of correct interdental contacts. For this reason, we do not recommend using straight celluloid strips.

4.4.2 Technique with Metallic Anatomically Shaped Sectional Matrix

> Main idea: Metal anatomically shaped sectional matrices for posterior teeth can be successfully used to restore the proximal walls of anterior teeth but positioned vertically.

Restoration of an adequate proximal morphology requires interdentally placed and properly fixed anatomically shaped matrices. Manufacturers do not offer as varied range of matrices as in the case of posterior teeth. Thus, some of the most used matrices used in the case of anterior teeth are even the metal sectional matrices intended for posterior teeth. Clinicians prefer them due to their ease of handling, appropriate anatomical shape, and relatively easy fixation in the frontal area.

Among the main indications for the use of metal sectional matrices for anterior teeth we can mention:

- Restoration of class III cavities involving a larger area of the proximal wall.
- Restoration of class IV cavities obtained by removing carious processes, removing inadequate old fillings, and fracturing or dislocating previous restorations.
- Coronal fractures involving the proximal wall and incisal edge.
- Closing or reducing of diastemas.

4.4.2.1 Working Technique

In the case of proximal frontal cavities that do not involve the angle and the incisal edge (Fig. 4.51), anesthesia is performed and, subsequently, isolation with a rubber dam of the entire frontal group (Fig. 4.52). Minimally invasive class III cavities are prepared (Fig. 4.53). If these cavities involve a larger wall surface that requires anatomical restoration of the proximal morphology, metal sectional matrices can be used, mounted vertically and fixed with interdental wedges (Fig. 4.54). The working sequence can continue in several ways, among which we mention:

- The bilaminar centripetal technique using dentin and enamel composite for frontals: restoration of the proximal enamel composite wall by the centripetal technique (Fig. 4.55) and filling of the cavity obtained by layering one or more shades

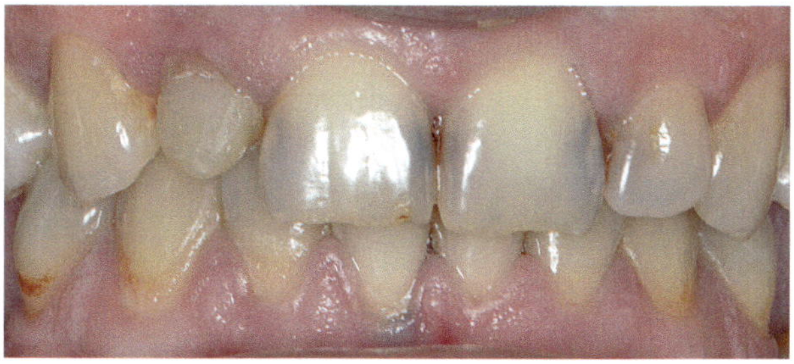

Fig. 4.51 Mesial and distal proximal caries—upper central incisors

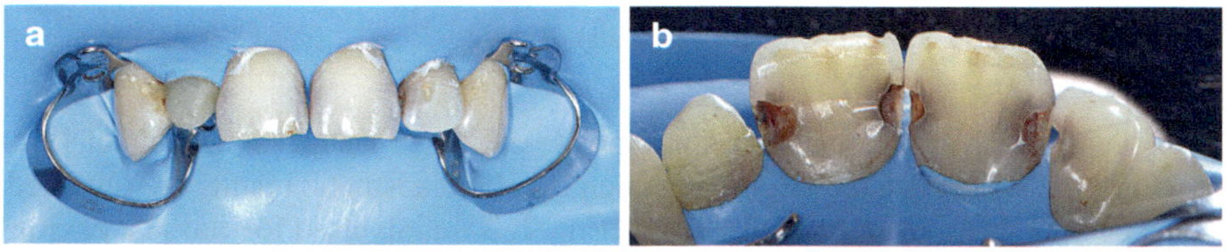

Fig. 4.52 Group isolation with rubber dam and dental floss ligatures in place (**a**); palatal view of proximal caries on 11, 21, and 22 (**b**)

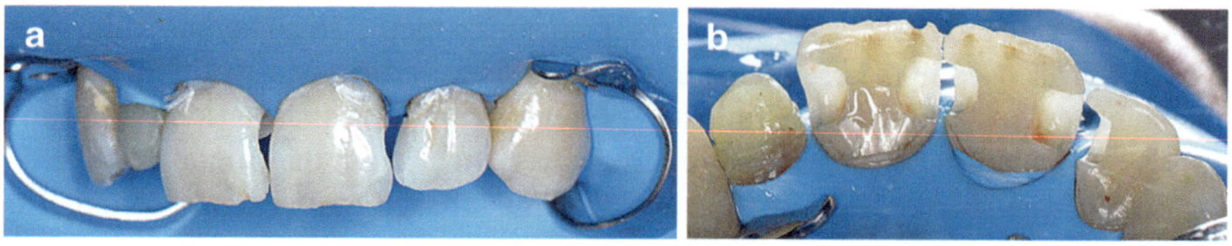

Fig. 4.53 Cavity preparation: buccal (**a**) and palatal (**b**) view

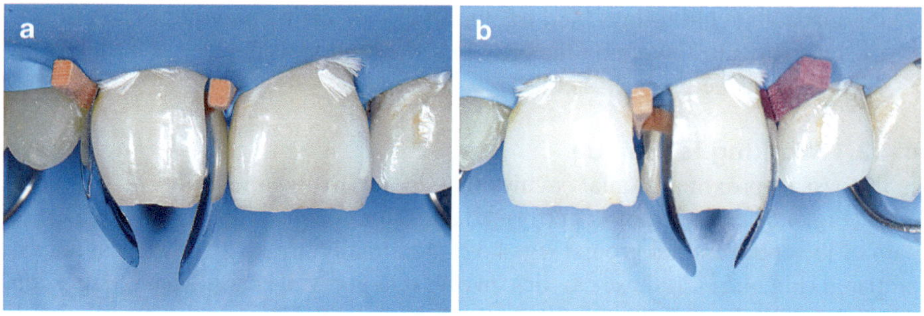

Fig. 4.54 Sectional matrices applied in a vertical position on tooth 11 (**a**) and on tooth 21 (**b**)

Fig. 4.55 Cavities after restoration of the proximal walls

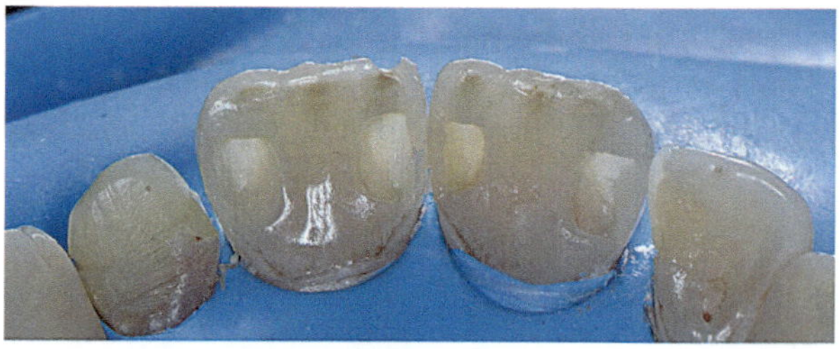

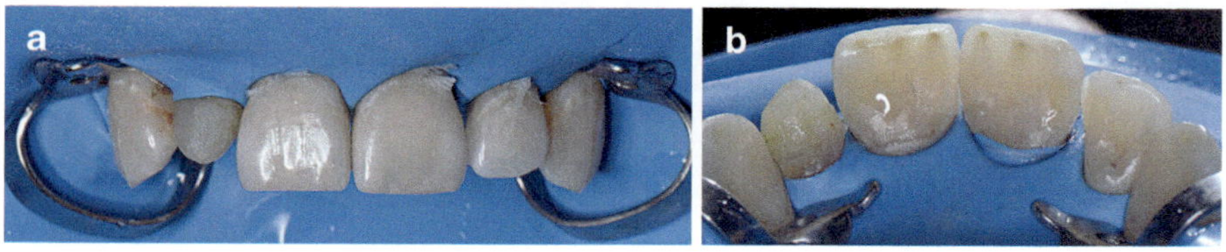

Fig. 4.56 Final restorations, buccal (**a**) and palatal (**b**) view

of dentin and applying enamel composite as the last superficial palatal layer (Fig. 4.56). This is a technique by which excellent aesthetic results are obtained, respecting the rules of biomimetic layering. It is mainly used for class IV cavities that also involve the incisal angle and the buccal surface of the crown. Restoration of class III cavities may be considered an overly elaborate technique that is generally unnecessary.

- Centripetal monoshade technique with a single shade of universal composite: restoration of the proximal wall by the centripetal technique, followed by layering of the resulting cavity.
- Oblique layering technique from palatal to buccal using universal composite. This is a widely used technique, simple, fast, and with good aesthetic results for restoring small and medium class III cavities.
- Bulk technique.
- Injection molding.

In the case of class IV cavities, the technique of applying metal matrices is similar (see Sect. 5.3) (Fig. 4.57).

Difficulties that may arise	Possible solutions
Matrix instability	This can be fixed in the incisal part with the tip of the finger (Fig. 4.58). The matrix can be applied at the cervical level between the dam sheet and the tooth for a better fit
The matrix can limit visibility and easy access for composite layering	Changing the matrix position to free the for easier instrument access and composite application

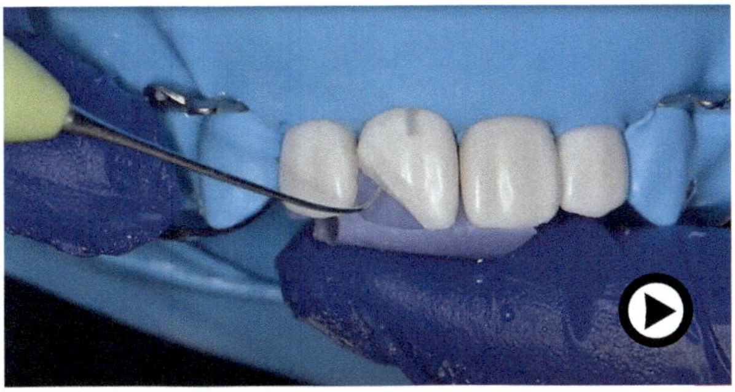

Fig. 4.57 Technique with metallic anatomically shaped sectional matrix, simplified layering (▶ https://doi.org/10.1007/000-bqq)

Fig. 4.58 Fixing the matrix with the finger allows it to be positioned in contact or at a distance from the adjacent tooth

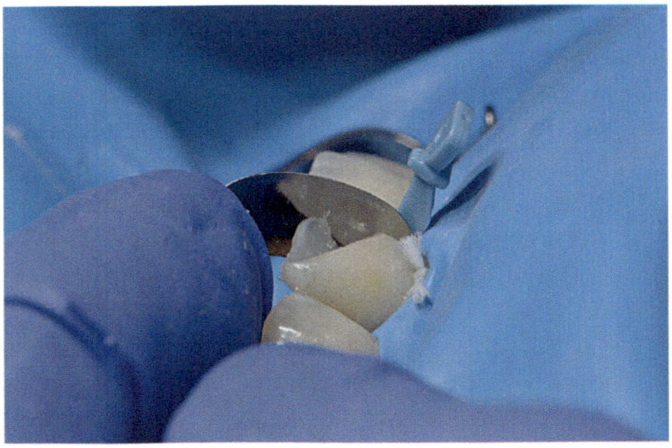

4.4.3 Celluloid Anatomically Shaped Sectoral Matrix Technique

Main idea: Proximal walls of anterior teeth can be restored using celluloid-contoured anatomically shaped matrices for anterior teeth.

These matrices can be used in the following cases:

- For the restoration of class III and class IV cavities.
- For reducing or closing diastemas.
- For closing the black triangles generated by gingival retraction.
- For restoring the crown shape (Figs. 4.59 and 4.60).

4.4.3.1 Working Technique

One of the most complex anatomically shaped celluloid anterior matrix kits is "Bioclear Complete Anterior," which contains nine different matrices and several sizes of interdental wedges. These varied forms allow for choosing the optimal

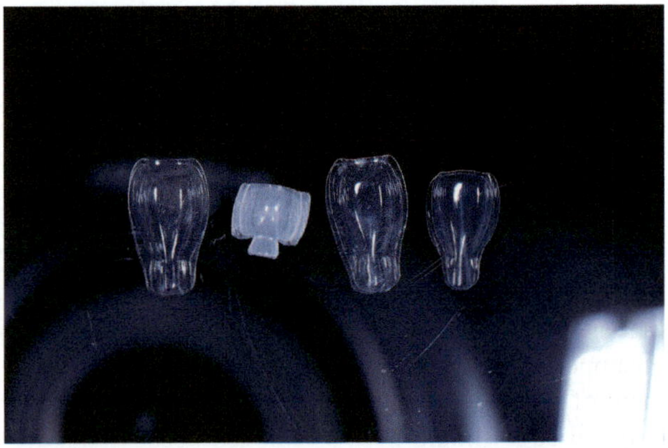

Fig. 4.59 Bioclear matrix for anteriors

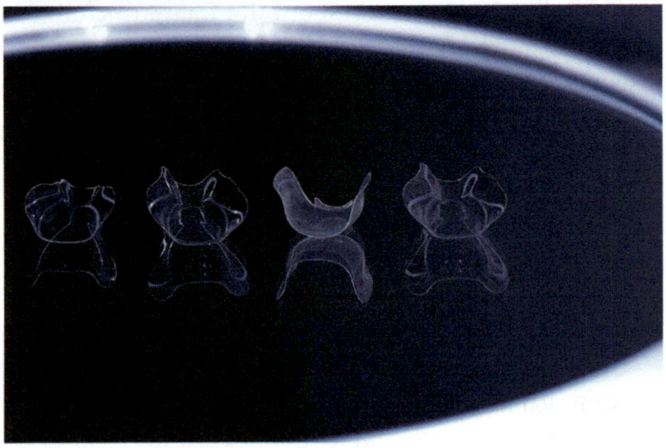

Fig. 4.60 Bioclear matrix for posteriors

variant adapted to the case. Fixation of the matrices is done with wedges at the gingival level and with the help of fingers for incisal and palatal.

Restoring the interdental contact between the canine and the premolar is always a challenge for the dentist, because this is the transition zone from the frontal teeth to the lateral, cuspidated ones with a larger volume. Furthermore, in these cases, the use of matrices is necessary, but there is difficulty in positioning the ring due to the different proximal morphology of the canine, which does not provide sufficient support. It can exercise its role of effectively adapting the matrix only on the premolar because on the canine; the ring comes into contact with the tooth only in the cervical area (Fig. 4.61a, b). If the matrix is mounted only on the premolar, adding a liquid dam between the tines of the matrix ring and the oral surface of the canine can help better stabilize the ring. Given the difficulty of mounting and fitting matrices for this particular clinical situation, the use of a rapid injection technique may be helpful. After injecting the heated composite into the canine, the morphology is performed, and the two types of flowable and heated packable composite are light-cured simultaneously. Remove the matrix from the canine and continue in the same way on the premolar (Fig. 4.62a, b).

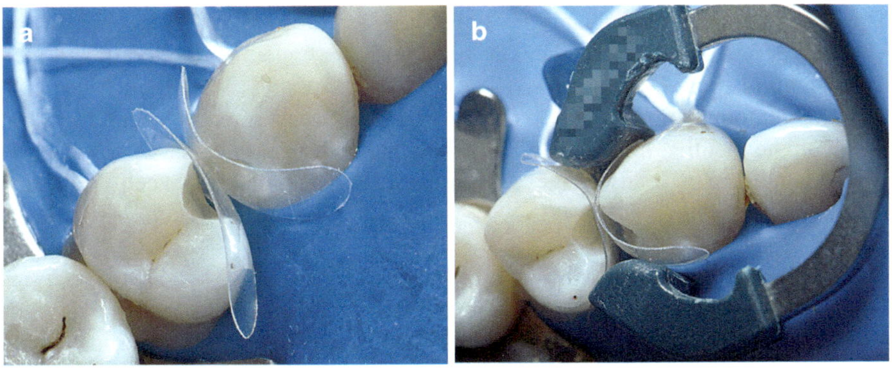

Fig. 4.61 Clear celluloid matrices mounted on teeth 13 and 14 (**a**), fixed with a Palodent ring (**b**)

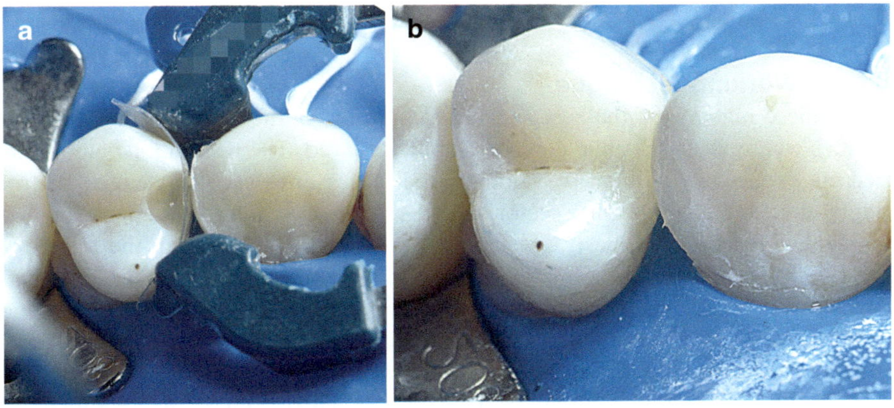

Fig. 4.62 Removal of first matrix after restoration of the first tooth (**a**) and final restorations of both teeth (**b**)

Difficulties that may arise	Possible solutions
Matrix stabilization	Additional fastening with fingers
Slippage of plastic wedges because they do not stick well to celluloid	Using wooden wedges instead of plastic ones

4.4.4 Straight Celluloid Tape Technique

Main idea: Clear straight celluloid strips are often used as matrices for restoring anterior teeth palatal or proximal walls.

Often used successfully for small class III cavities, straight transparent celluloid strips can also be used for class IV cavities. With their help, the palatal and proximal walls can be restored simultaneously or sequentially to obtain a cavity in which one or more shades of dentin will be layered. Their popularity among dentists can be due to several positive aspects, among which we can mention:
They are accessible, cheap, and easy to procure.
They are easy to use because they are fixed with the fingers on the tooth, and they do not require special accessories.
Lead to obtaining smooth and glossy composite surfaces, often associated by dentists with the fact that finishing and polishing are no longer necessary.

Among the main disadvantages associated with the use of straight celluloid strips we can mention:

- The straight conformation of the proximal wall.
- Moving the point of contact with the adjacent tooth toward the incisal.
- Fitting difficulties, such as the tendency to pull the band toward the tooth with the fingers for a good fit, can lead to it moving away from the adjacent tooth. Thus, an interdental contact will be difficult or impossible to achieve.
- The fact that they are transparent makes them more challenging to identify and work with them.

4.4.4.1 Working Technique

Using these matrices is the best and fastest solution in the case of small class III cavities where the interdental contact is still preserved. The restoration can be carried out exclusively with strips, without other accessories such as wedges, matrix rings, silicone keys, and other sector matrices. After their interdental insertion and the application of the adhesive system and the composite material, the matrix is fixed with the fingers by its traction toward the working tooth, both palatally and buccally. For more extensive class III cavities or conventional class IV cavities, the celluloid strips are mounted by fixing them with wedges at the gingival level (Fig. 4.63), followed by fitting them on the palatal surface.

Palatally, the celluloid tape can be fixed directly with the finger by pressure or by placing a cotton roll between the finger and the tooth (Fig. 4.64).

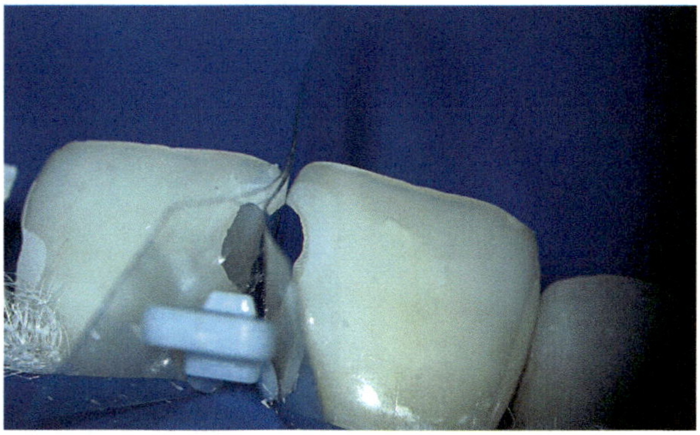

Fig. 4.63 Flat celluloid strip on tooth 21

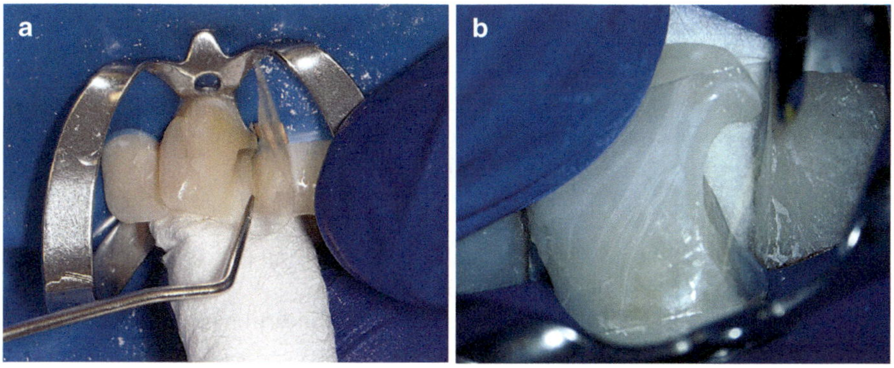

Fig. 4.64 Restoration of a class IV cavity using celluloid strip fitted palatally by cotton roll (**a**) and (**b**)

These strips can be associated with a silicone key to restore the palatal wall, in which case the celluloid strip will only serve to restore the proximal wall. The silicone key and celluloid tape can also be used simultaneously by scalpel sectioning the silicone key and passing the celluloid tape through this slit (Fig. 4.65).

However, the celluloid strip can also be associated with a metallic or contoured anatomically shaped sectional matrix, so the celluloid strip will only be used for palatal wall reconstruction and the anatomically shaped matrix for proximal wall reconstruction.

Difficulties that may arise	Possible solutions
Adaptation difficulties on the palatal surface to obtain the appropriate morphology	Since the band is flat, a proper fit is difficult to achieve on the concave palatal surface
Difficulties in obtaining the contact point	Fixing with a wedge at the gingival level and pressing it in contact with the adjacent tooth at the level of the contact point. If this fails, replacement with an anatomically shaped matrix can be helpful

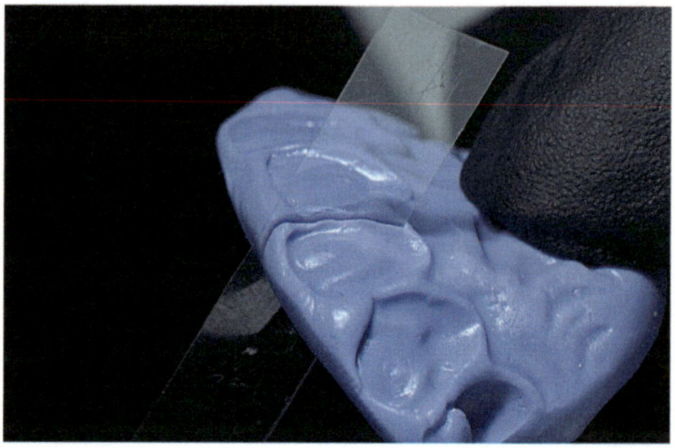

Fig. 4.65 Celluloid strip fixed directly into the palatal silicone key to allow simultaneous restoration of the palatal and proximal walls, or layering from the palatal side without prior restoration of the proximal wall

4.4.5 Free Modeling Technique

Main idea: The use of matrices can be avoided in cases where it is not necessary to restore interdental contacts, so that the proximal morphology can be easily conformed by free modeling with hand tools.

Free modeling of the proximal walls in the case of front teeth can be achieved in several clinical cases, among which we mention:

The existence of diastemas that allow the interdental insertion of modeling tools

Missing of adjacent tooth

The existence of cavities prepared on the adjacent tooth which will be later restored and temporarily allow interdental access to modeling tools

4.4.5.1 Working Technique

After isolation with the rubber dam and fixing the sheet with ligatures or gingival retractor clamps on the treated tooth, the cavity is prepared. The adhesive system is applied, and then the composite is shaped with the spatula or other tools from the modeling kit, restoring the proximal convex shape.

Difficulties that may arise	Possible solutions
Conformation of proximal convexities	Using matrices
The generation of excess material at the gingival area	Removal in the finishing and polishing step

4.4.6 Cotton Roll and Teflon Tape Technique

Main idea: In the absence of a silicone key to restoring the palatal wall, it can be applied directly to a cotton roll wrapped in Teflon tape.

A cotton roll can support the application of the palatal composite if it is applied and held with palatal pressure on the crown of the tooth. Its Teflon coating prevents the composite from being applied directly to the wadding, which acts as a flexible matrix supported by the cotton roll. A medium or thick Teflon tape leads to better results by preventing the cotton from the roll from entering the cavity. The flexibility of the cotton roll allows its proper conformation in the anatomical concavity of the palatal surface of the upper incisors. The technique is easy to perform, but the results are not as predictable as using a silicone key.

4.4.6.1 Working Technique

A cotton roll is wrapped with medium or thick Teflon tape. After preparing the cavity and applying the adhesive system, the roller is positioned palatally and pressed with the index finger of the left hand to seal the cavity palatally (Fig. 4.66). The first layer of composite is applied with an obturator, which will be uniform in thickness of a maximum of 1 mm to restore the palatal wall, after which it is polymerized (Fig. 4.67a–c). Next, an anatomically shaped sectional matrix will be mounted, and the proximal wall/cavity will be restored. This can be achieved either by prior restoration of the proximal wall, directly by anatomical layering with several shades of dentin and enamel, or by simplified layering.

Difficulties that may arise	Possible solutions
Applying too much pressure on the cotton roll can push the cotton into the palatal cavity, creating an overly concave aspect of the palatal surface	Carefully check the aspect of the roll inside the cavity
Movement of the roller during polymerization of the composite applied over it can lead to its dislocation due to lack of adhesion after polymerization	Removing the wall and repeating the application procedure

4.4.7 Closing or Reduction of Diastemas

Main idea: Diastema can be considered a personal characteristic, sometimes associated with a person's personality or, in some cultures, even a sign of beauty. Closing or reduction of diastemas can be successfully achieved by direct restorations in various layering modes, using (or not) silicone keys or matrices.

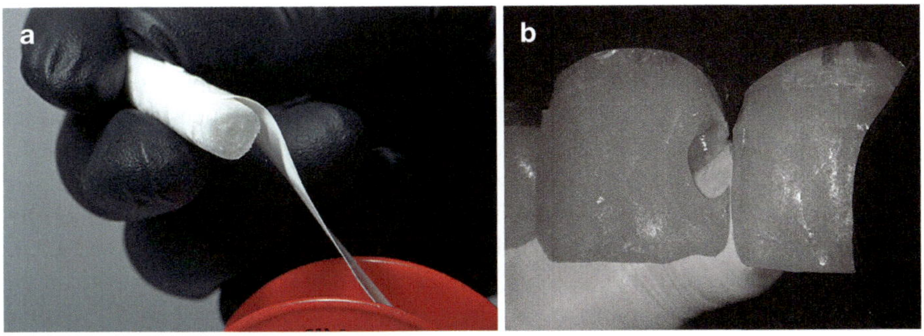

Fig. 4.66 Wrapping a cotton roll with Teflon tape (**a**); the cotton roll wrapped in Teflon fixed palatally (**b**)

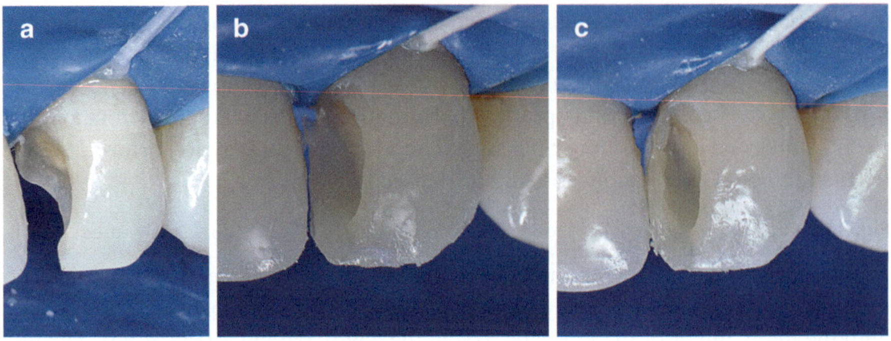

Fig. 4.67 Anterior restoration involving the incisal angle: initial image of the class IV cavity (**a**); restoration of the palatal wall (**b**) and the proximal wall (**c**)

When the mesiodistal dimension of the teeth is less than the normal value, or when this is normal, but patients refuse orthodontic treatments to close diastemas, aesthetic improvement may be possible by adding composite resins. Depending on the proposed result (closing or just reducing the diastema) and depending on the dentist's experience, these procedures can be performed in different ways. The most common and predictable working protocol involves using a silicone key. The dentist can choose between the classic protocol (impression, models, wax-up, silicone impression of the wax-up), or he can make a digital plan (Digital Smile Design) to analyze with the patient the desired final result. Afterward, the final design can be printed and the dentist makes a silicone impression to obtain the silicone key. A clear stent and an additive injection adhesive technique may also be considered.

The major challenge lies in identifying the optimal size so that adding material does not result in disproportionate, unsightly size of the new teeth. When complete closing of the diastema and achievement of an interdental contact is intended, the use of anatomically shaped sectional matrices leads to the best result. In cases where only diastema reduction is intended, matrices can be omitted as the space preserved between the crowns allows hand instruments to free-shape the proximal morphology.

4.4.7.1 Working Technique

Since an adhesive technique is used, good isolation of the working field with rubber dam is recommended (Fig. 4.68). A silicone key is made either based on a model with the proposed version (conventional wax-up or printed model of a digital design) or by direct impression of the clinical situation and then cutting with a bur or a scalpel until the desired final situation is obtained (Fig. 4.69). In this case, the complete sealing of the diastema would have led to an unaesthetically large mesiodistal dimension of the lower central incisors. That is why in this case, only a reduction of the diastema was made by addition of composite and free shaping with the spatula (Fig. 4.70) to half its original size (Fig. 4.71). Occlusal adjustments, finishing, and polishing are performed conventionally. Aesthetic result was acceptable to both the patient and the dentist (Figs. 4.72 and 4.73).

Another way to solve this case can be the addition of packable composite on the bucco-mesial transition line to widen the buccal surface, followed by the vertical fixation of a sectional metal matrix and the addition of flowable composite from the lingual side (front wing technique) [41].

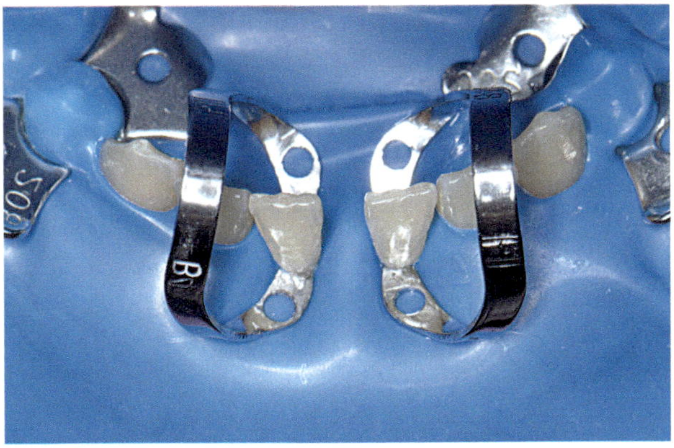

Fig. 4.68 Rubber dam isolation of the inferior anterior group with diastema

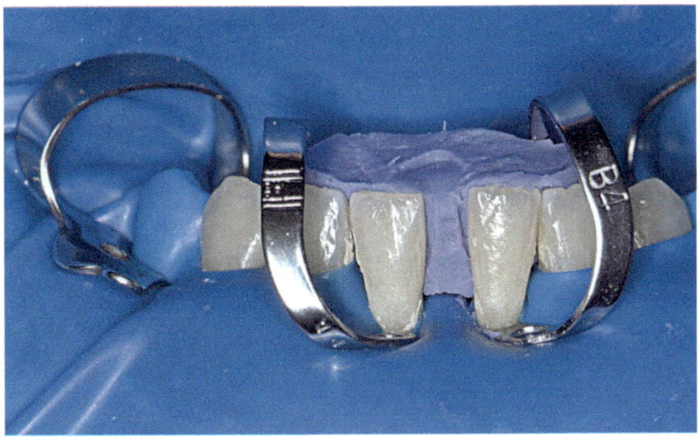

Fig. 4.69 Lingual silicone key individualized and fixed on the teeth

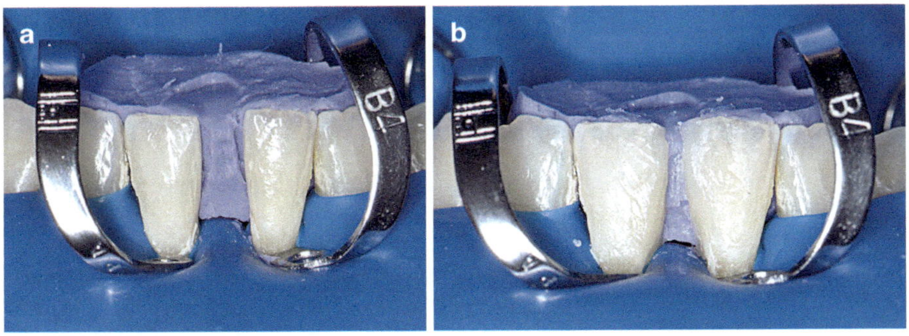

Fig. 4.70 The image before (**a**) and after the addition of composite resin to the tooth (b)

Difficulties that may arise	Possible solutions
Increased mesiodistal dimensions give an unaesthetic result	They appear especially in the absence of planning through wax-up/mockup or DSD. Orthodontic treatment can be a solution
Unaesthetic asymmetric proximal morphologies or asymmetric enlargement of the crowns	Redoing the restoration on one or both of the affected teeth

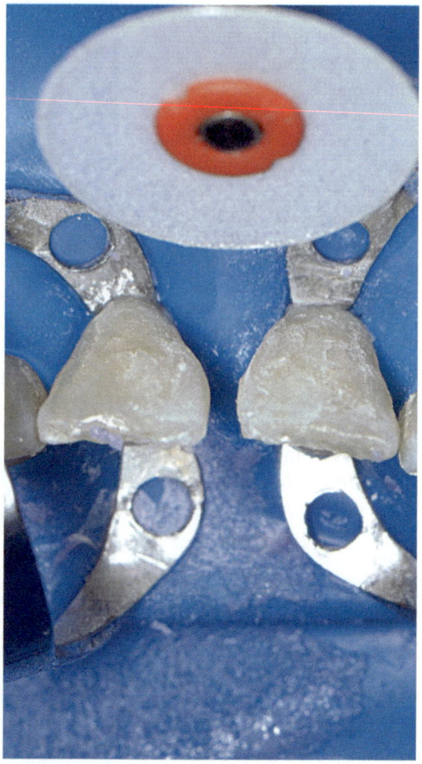

Fig. 4.71 Finishing with silicone abrasive disks

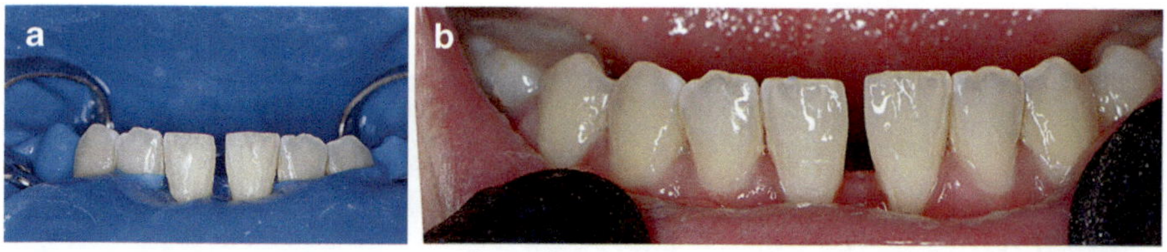

Fig. 4.72 The final restorations after finishing (**a**) and after removing the rubber dam sheet (**b**)

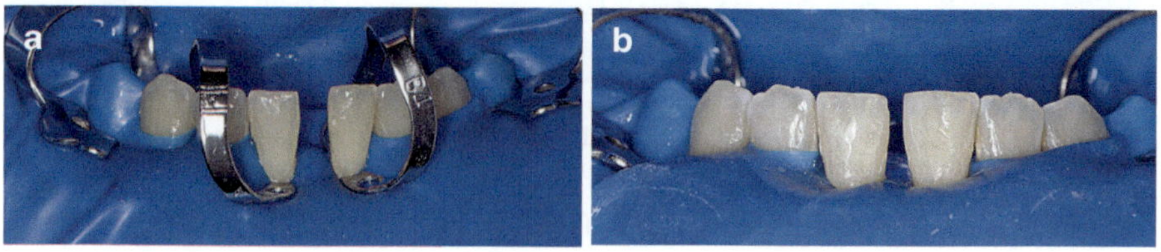

Fig. 4.73 Evaluation of diastema size change before (**a**) and after treatment (**b**)

Did You Get It?

1. What are the main indications for using posterior metal sectional matrices for anterior teeth?
2. What are the main disadvantages of using straight celluloid strips in frontal restorations involving proximal areas?
3. What are the possible restorative techniques for closing or reducing diastemas, and what do they consist of?

References

1. Kinoshita S, Wen CR. Kinoshita's color atlas of periodontics. St Louis: Ishiyaku EuroAmerica; 1985.
2. Bichacho N. The centripetal build-up for composite resin posterior restorations. Pract Periodontics Aesthet Dent. 1994;6:17–23.
3. Chuang SF, Su KC, Wang CH, Chang CH. Morphological analysis of proximal contacts in class II direct restorations with 3D image reconstruction. J Dent. 2011;39:448–56.
4. LM-Dental™. LM-ARTE™ Posterior Misura. https://lm-dental.com/products/hand-instrumentation/restoration/lm-arte/lm-arte-posterior-misura/. Accessed 10 Mar 2022.
5. Li F, Weir MD, Fouad AF, Xu HH. Effect of salivary pellicle on antibacterial activity of novel antibacterial dental adhesives using a dental plaque microcosm biofilm model. Dent Mater. 2014;30(2):182–91.
6. Lutz F, Krejci I, Barbakow F. The importance of proximal curing in posterior composite resin restorations. Quintessence Int. 1992;23:605–7.
7. Paolone G, Scolavino S, Bichacho N. The split centripetal build-up technique for large class II composite restorations. J Cosmetic Dent. 2020;36(1):78–84.
8. Ozel E, Soyman M. Effect of fiber nets, application techniques and flowable composites on microleakage and the effect of fiber nets on polymerization shrinkage in class II MOD cavities. Oper Dent. 2009;34(2):174–80.
9. Radhika M, Sajjan GS, Kumaraswamy BN, Mittal N. Effect of different placement techniques on marginal microleakage of deep class-II cavities restored with two composite resin formulations. J Conserv Dent. 2010;13(1):9–15.
10. Oliveira KM, Lancellotti AC, Ccahuana-Vasquez RA, Consani S. Influence of filling techniques on shrinkage stress in dental composite restorations. J Dent Sci. 2013;8:53–60.
11. Kwon Y, Ferracane J, Lee IB. Effect of layering methods, composite type, and flowable liner on the polymerization shrinkage stress of light cured composites. Dent Mater. 2012;28(7):801–9.
12. Lotfi N, Esmaeili B, Ahmadizenouz G, Bijani A, Khadem H. Gingival microleakage in class II composite restorations using different flowable composites as liner: an in vitro evaluation. Caspian J Dent Res. 2015;4(1):10–6.
13. Reddy SN, Jayashankar DN, Nainan M, Shivanna V. The effect of flowable composite lining thickness with various curing techniques on microleakage in class II composite restorations: an in vitro study. J Contemp Dent Pract. 2013;14(1):56–60.
14. Sood A, Munjal S, Sharma K, Malik M. An in vitro evaluation of voids and posities at different sites in class II composite resin restorations using different consistencies and placement techniques: a stereomicroscope study. Indian J Dent Sci. 2013;5:28.
15. Opdam N, Roeters J, Deborri T, Peschier D, Bronkhorst E. Voids inside restored micropreparations using various resin composites and applications techniques. J Dent Res. 2002;81:389.
16. Bore Gowda V, Sreenivasa Murthy BV, Hegde S, Venkataramanaswamy SD, Pai VS, Krishna R. Evaluation of Gingival Microleakage in Class II Composite Restorations with Different Lining Techniques: An In Vitro Study. Scientifica (Cairo). 2015;2015:896507.
17. Jeffcoat MK, Howell TH. Alveolar bone destruction due to overhanging amalgam in periodontal disease. J Periodontol. 1980;51(10):599–602.

18. Boruziniat A, Gharaee S, Sarraf Shirazi A, Majidinia S, Vatanpour M. Evaluation of the efficacy of flowable composite as lining material on microleakage of composite resin restorations: A systematic review and meta-analysis. Quintessence Int. 2016;47(2):93–101. https://doi.org/10.3290/j.qi.a35260. PMID: 26665259.
19. Ferracane JL, Lawson NC. Probing the hierarchy of evidence to identify the best strategy for placing class II dental composite restorations using current materials. J Esthet Restor Dent. 2021;33(1):39–50. https://doi.org/10.1111/jerd.12686. Epub 2020 Nov 18. PMID: 33206440.
20. Chuang SF, Jin YT, Tsai PF, Wong TY. Effect of various surface protections on the marginal microleakage of resin modified glass ionomer cements. J Prosthet Dent. 2001;86(3):309–14.
21. Arslan S, Demirbuga S, Ustun Y, Dincer AN, Canakci BC, Zorba YO. The effect of a new-generation flowable composite resin on microleakage in class V composite restorations as an intermediate layer. J Conserv Dent. 2013;16:189–93.
22. Natasha V. Efek Penggunaan Resin Komposit Flowable Pengganti Dentin Terhadap Kebocoran Tepi Dinding Gingiva Tumpatan Resin Komposit Proksimal. Jakarta: Universitas Indonesia; 2013.
23. Czasch P, Ilie N. In vitro comparison of mechanical properties and degree of cure of bulk fill composites. Clin Oral Investig. 2013;17(1):227–35.
24. Suzuki M, Jordan RE. Glass ionomer-composite sandwich technique. J Am Dent Assoc. 1990;120(1):55–7.
25. Liebenberg W. Return to the resin-modified glass-ionomer cement sandwich technique. J Can Dent Assoc. 2005;71(10):743–7.
26. Loguercio AD, Alessandra R, Mazzocco KC, et al. Microleakage in class II composite resin restorations: total bonding and open sandwich technique. J Adhes Dent. 2002;4(2):137–44.
27. van Dijken JW. A 6-year evaluation of a direct composite resin inlay/onlay system and glass ionomer cement-composite resin sandwich restorations. Acta Odontol Scand. 1994;52(6):368–76.
28. Mount JG, Hume WR, Wolff SM, Hien CN. Preservation and restoration of tooth structure. Wiley Blackwell. 2016;200.
29. Pereira LC, Nunes MC, Dibb RG, et al. Mechanical properties and bond strength of glass-ionomer cements. J Adhes Dent. 2002;4:73–80.
30. Taher NM, Ateyah NZ. Shear bond strength of resin modified glass ionomer cement bonded to different tooth-colored restorative materials. J Contemp Dent Pract. 2007;8(2):25–34.
31. Hate WH, Friedl KH, Powers JM. Bond strength of composites to hybrid ionomers. Oper Dent. 1996;21(4):147–52.
32. Kasraie S, Shokripour M, Safari MJ. Evaluation of micro-shear bond strength of resin modified glass-ionomer to composite resins using various bonding systems. Conserv Dent. 2013;16(6):550–4.
33. Woolford MJ, Grieve AR. The use of intermediary resins when bonding glass polyalkenoate (ionomer) cement to composite resin. J Oral Rehabil. 1993;20(3):249–55.
34. Koubi S, Raskin A, Dejou J, About I, Tassery H, Camps J, Proust JP. Effect of dual cure composite as dentin substitute on the marginal integrity of class II open-sandwich restorations. Oper Dent. 2010;35:165–71.
35. Moorthy A, Hogg CH, Dowling AH, et al. Cuspal deflection and microleakage in premolar teeth restored with bulk-fill flowable resin-based composite base materials. J Dent. 2012;40(6):500–5.
36. Kim RJ, Son SA, Hwang JY, et al. Comparison of photopolymerization temperature increases in internal and external positions of composite and tooth cavities in real time: incremental fillings of microhybrid composite vs. bulk filling of bulk fill composite. J Dent. 2015;43:1093–8.
37. Yasa E, Atalayin C, Karacolak G, Sari T, Turkun LS. Intrapulpal temperature changes during curing of different bulk-fill restorative materials. Dent Mater J. 2017;36(5):566–72.
38. Raghu R, Srinivasan R. Optimizing tooth form with direct posterior composite restorations. J Conserv Dent. 2011;14:330–6.
39. Sikri VK, Sikri P. Overhanging interproximal silver amalgam restorations. Prevalence and side-effects. Indian J Dent Res. 1993;4:13–6.
40. Fuks AB, Araujo FB, Osorio LB, Hadani PE, Pinto AS. Clinical and radiographic assessment of class II esthetic restorations in primary molars. Pediatr Dent. 2000;22(6):479–85.
41. Styleitaliano. The Front Wing Technique. https://www.styleitaliano.org/the-front-wing-technique/. Accessed 10 Mar 2022.

Layering Techniques and Morphology Modeling

5

Depending on the clinical case, the dentist's experience, and the manufacturers' instructions for different composite materials, the working techniques listed above can be combined or modified so that the final result is satisfactory and predictable. Common to all techniques is the application of a dentin composite to introduce an opaque area and a layer of buccal enamel. This enamel layer is an optional indication of specific composite materials. Different manufacturers may develop their layering recommendations, which is why applying a single technique to all materials available on the market is impossible. Moreover, the same kit of composite materials can be used by applying different layering techniques.

However, this multitude of options can also be a disadvantage, leading to unpredictable results if the appropriate layering technique is not chosen. This may cause dissatisfaction with the aesthetics of the results obtained both among dentist and patients.

This chapter will focus on some of the most frequently used layering techniques and the realization of the morphology of direct restorations on anterior and posterior teeth.

5.1 Munsell System

An important concept to remember while reading this chapter is the Munsell system. It is possible to have a restoration not turn out right even if following a specific technique to the letter. This is not necessarily the result of poor shade selection but a lack of understanding of the three color dimensions, which play an essential role in aesthetic dentistry today.

Supplementary Information The online version contains supplementary material available at https://doi.org/10.1007/978-3-031-55899-3_5. The videos can be accessed individually by clicking the DOI link in the accompanying figure caption or by scanning this link with the SN More Media App.

© The Author(s), under exclusive license to Springer Nature Switzerland AG 2024

M. Bud, *Direct Restorations*, https://doi.org/10.1007/978-3-031-55899-3_5

Munsell describes the three dimensions: hue, chroma, and value. It is not enough to select a shade and then find a single material that contributes only a single chroma and value to the restoration.

Hue is the family of color. In dentistry, the vita classic and other vita shade guides help us determine hue and chroma. On a vita classic shade guide, we have the following hues:

- A—red-brown
- B—red-yellow
- C—gray
- D—red-gray

Chroma is the strength of the hue. If someone were to edit a photo on their phone, they could change the saturation of a hue. In dentistry, chroma is the saturation of the hues established on the vita classic. Chroma is given a number designation after the letter designation of the hue. The lower the number, the weaker the saturation of the hue.

Now it should be easy to read a shade guide. For example, B1, B2, B3, and B4 are all on the vita classic. We know B is a designation to indicate a red-yellow hue, and B1 has a lower chroma than B4. This allows us to select the correct shade for a restoration if needed.

Value, however, is not as well represented on shade guides. Value describes the lightness or darkness of our materials. This is not black and white but much gray. This is because the value is the ability or lack of ability to reflect light. High value would be used for dentine where we do not want a light transfer. The lower value transfers light easier, which we would use to mimic enamel.

There is no perfect ratio for how much value to use for dentine and enamel to have pleasing esthetic restorations. To identify a rough value, manufacturers label their material now with an additional letter or description. For example, A2E or A2D exist, and the final designation means enamel and dentine. Manufacturers can have different designations to mark the value because there is no standard system yet.

After an experience with specific materials from different manufacturers, a dentist can judge the correct way to apply materials in all three color dimensions. Following the steps in this chapter and respecting the three color dimensions improves the aesthetic outcome of restorations.

5.2 Successive Layering

The application of conventional packable composite materials in successive layers was necessary for several reasons, the main ones being:

(A) Layering combines different shades and opacities of material to improve the aesthetic result, especially in the case of anterior teeth (see Sect. 5.3).

(B) Layering decreases shrinkage and improves marginal integrity, especially in posterior teeth, where cavities are larger in size and volume than anterior teeth (see Sect. 5.4).

5.3 For Anterior Teeth

Composite materials currently allow the successful restoration of anterior teeth to achieve aesthetic results close to the natural aesthetics of the tooth. This requires a good understanding of the notions related to the morphology, color, function, and natural optical properties of the teeth in order to be able to select the most suitable material and working technique [1].

In the case of small class III cavities, it is not necessary to use several shades of composite.

For extensive cavities on the buccal and oral surfaces of the anterior teeth, the use of a relatively translucent composite cannot completely block the dark background of the oral cavity [2]. Thus, an opaque composite followed by anatomical or simplified layering becomes necessary.

We, therefore, opt for layering using various techniques in most cases of cavity restorations that partially or fully involve the incisal edge and palatal wall.

In any of these cases, the layering of the composites must be done with palatal support (palatal shell), either using a silicone key or by fitting different types of matrices on the palatal and proximal surface, or even the gloved finger.

From the workflow point of view, there are a variety of work techniques:

(A) Centripetal technique with layering:
   (a) Anatomical shape: restoration of palatal and then proximal by enamel composite walls, followed by anatomical layering with multiple shades of dentin and buccal enamel (see Sect. 5.3.1).
   (b) Simplified: restoration of palatal wall in dentin and then proximal in universal composite—followed by filling the cavity thus obtained by simplified layering with one or more shades of dentin or universal composite (see Sect. 5.3.3). As the last layer, the enamel composite will be applied depending on the material used and the manufacturers' instructions.
(B) Direct layering technique (without prior restoration of proximal wall):
   (a) Anatomical shape: enamel composite palatal wall restoration followed by anatomical layering with multiple shades of dentin and buccal enamel.
   (b) Simplified: restoration of the dentin composite palatal wall that will fill approximately half of the bucco-palatal thickness of the crown, followed by the application of a layer of universal composite and, optionally, buccal enamel.

We will detail below some frequently used techniques:

- The centripetal technique with anatomical layering for the restoration of class IV cavities (Sect. 5.3.1)

- Additive restoration technique of incisal edges: anatomical and monoshade (Sect. 5.3.2)
- The simplified layering technique for the restoration of class IV cavities (Sect. 5.3.3)
- The monoshade technique (Sect. 5.3.4)

5.3.1 Centripetal Technique with Anatomical Layering for Class IV Cavities

Main idea: The centripetal technique with anatomical layering aims to follow the biomimetic principles. Biomimetics is the imitation of the natural model of the teeth to obtain an aesthetic result that imitates the natural appearance of the tooth as best as possible. The biomimetic anatomic technique involves replacing a certain type of absent tissue with materials with similar optical and strength characteristics. Thus, for restoring class IV cavities, we will use several shades of dentin and enamel composites, respecting the internal chromaticity of the crown of a tooth.

Direct anterior restorations involve several steps and are most predictably performed with a silicone palatal key:

1. Objective visual examination of the tooth and decision-making on whether making a silicone palatal key for a direct restoration is possible and appropriate (Fig. 5.1a). We recommend carrying out the treatment after anesthesia and isolation with a dam, choosing the color of the enamel and dentin composite before drying the tooth.
2. Making the silicone key with putty impression material and conforming it by cutting the excess material with a scalpel or a bur (Fig. 5.1b).
3. Removal of the old obturation and choosing a beveling option (Fig. 5.1c).
4. Disinfection, application of pulp protection if necessary, and adhesive system.
5. Restoration of the enamel palatal wall by applying a thin layer of enamel to the area marked on the silicone key. For ease of application, the silicone key can be held in hand to apply the palatal enamel layer and then attached to the tooth. After attachment, check the tightness of the enamel composite sealing on the palatal surface and polymerize according to the manufacturer's instructions (Fig. 5.2a, b). Brushes and special modeling instruments can manipulate and shape the composite material (Fig. 5.3a, b).
6. The restoration of the proximal wall is made of an enamel composite after applying an anatomically shaped sectional matrix for posterior teeth placed in a vertical position. This can be fixed gingivally with an interdental wedge, and the incisal part can be mobilized with the fingers to individualize the position of the matrix in relation to the adjacent tooth in each case. The wall is made of an

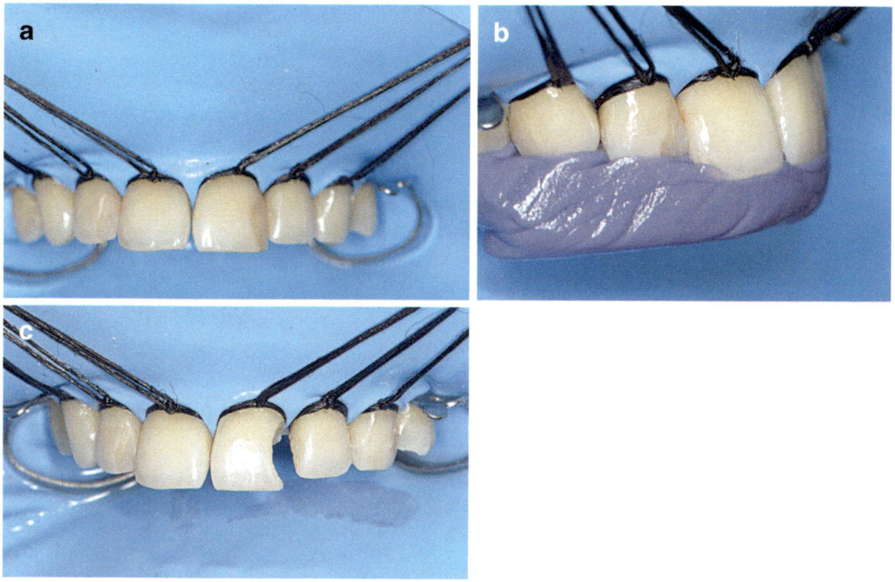

Fig. 5.1 The initial aspect after the isolation of the upper frontal group in order to replace some old restorations (**a**); impression of the palatal surfaces to make a silicone key (**b**); aspect after removal of the old restoration on tooth 21 (**c**)

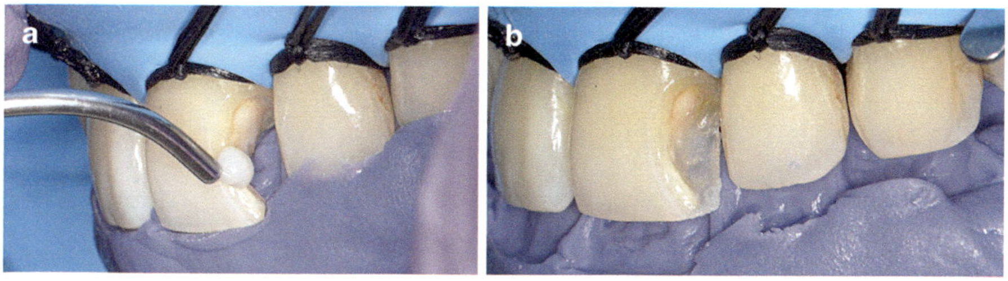

Fig. 5.2 Restoration of the palatal wall using the silicone key as a support on which the enamel composite is applied (**a**) avoiding its contact with the adjacent tooth (**b**)

enamel composite of the initially determined shade, and its thickness will be below 1 mm. The height of this wall will not exceed the level of the buccal surface (Fig. 5.4a, b). Thus, following the reconstruction of the palatal and proximal walls, a cavity or a "box" opened on one side, the buccal, will be obtained (Fig. 5.5). If we were to make an analogy between a class II cavity on the posterior teeth and a class IV cavity on the anterior teeth, we could consider that a centripetal technique is applied to obtain an open cavity on one side (occlusal in molars and buccal in frontals). In this cavity, we will layer the selected dentin shades.

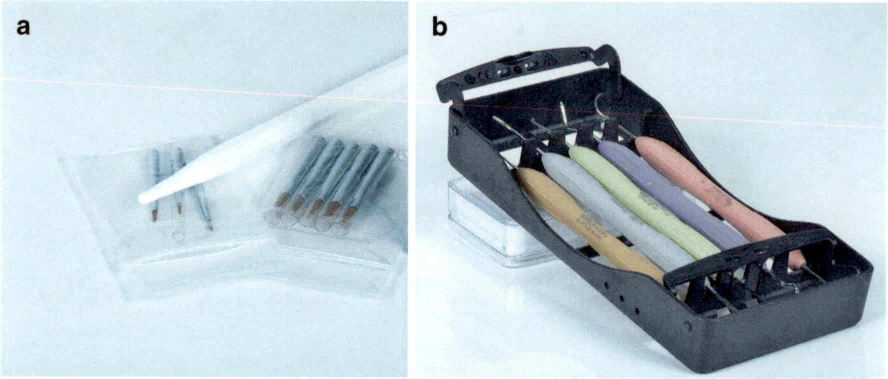

Fig. 5.3 Brushes for modeling composite resin (**a**); LM-Arte Composite Resin Modeling Kit (**b**)

Fig. 5.4 Restoration of the enamel composite proximal wall with a classic Palodent metallic sectional matrix (**a**) keeping its height at the level of the buccal surface (**b**)

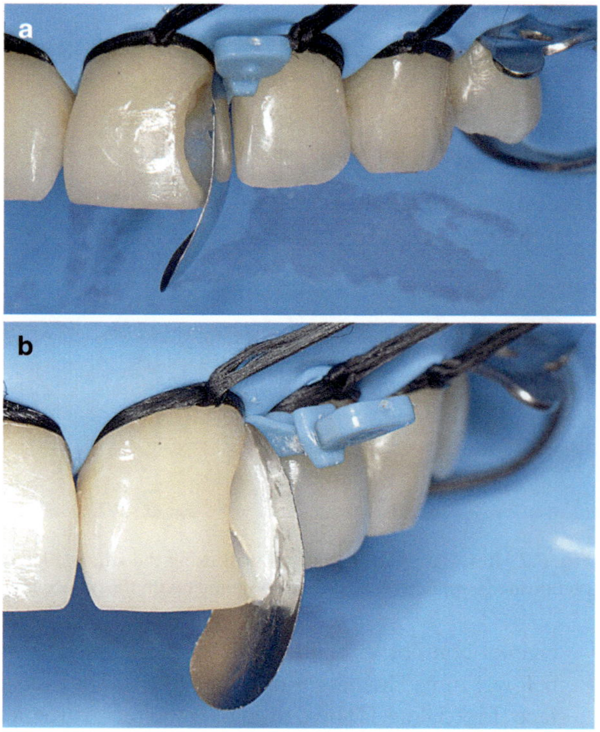

Fig. 5.5 The aspect after restoring the palatal and proximal enamel composite wall on tooth 21

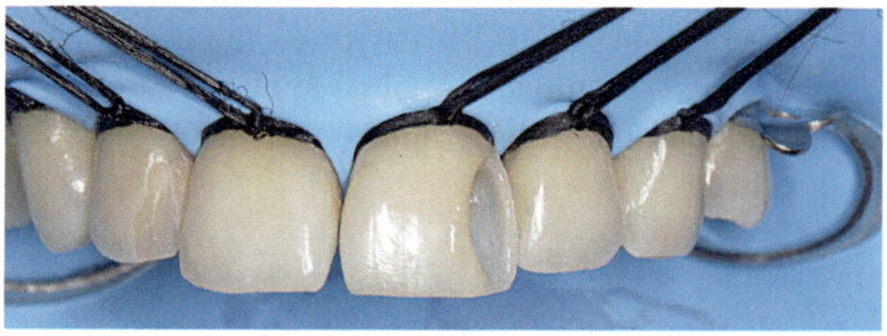

7. The layering of dentin shades according to the anatomical technique (described by Vanini [3]) begins with applying the first layer of dentin two shades darker than the initially determined color, the one we want to obtain at the end (Fig. 5.6). This layer will later be covered by the lighter shade of dentin, extending more incisally than the previous layer. The last layer of applied dentin will be placed approximately 0.5 mm below the level of the buccal surface to allow space for the enamel layer. We can calibrate the size of this space using the "Misura" instrument from the modeling kit (LM-Arte) (Fig. 5.7). The buccal enamel layer is applied superficially and reproduces the morphology with macro- and microtexture (Fig. 5.8).
8. Checking for proximal excess material, making macro- and microtexture elements, finishing and polishing the obturation (see Chap. 7).

Summarizing the stages of stratification, we could conclude that in the first stage, we aim to form an "enclosure" by restoring the palatal and proximal walls so that in the second stage, we fill this new created cavity by layering two or more shades of dentin (Fig. 5.9a–f).

For destructions that partially or fully involve the incisal edge, it is recommended to replicate the incisal morphology of the corresponding tooth in a symmetrical way. Thus, if the corresponding tooth presents dentinal lobes and transparent incisal areas, these elements will be replicated on the restored tooth as well (Fig. 5.10).

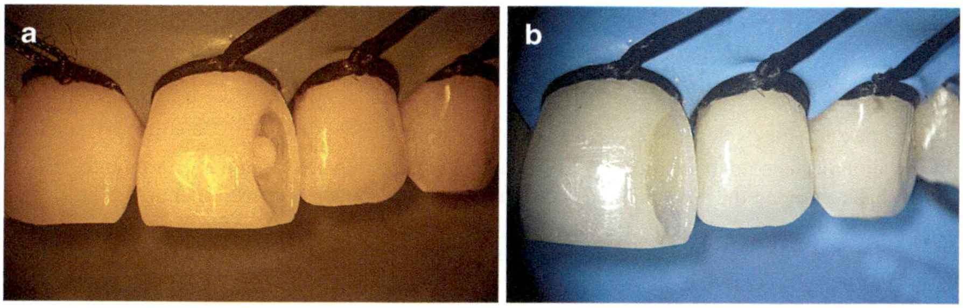

Fig. 5.6 Application of the first layer of dentin two shades darker than the determined final shade, 1.6× magnification under the dental operating microscope with the orange filter in place to prevent the polymerization of composite resins during working (**a**); first dentin layer (**b**)

Fig. 5.7 Application of the last layer of dentin that will attach to the enamel at the level of the bevel keeping the space free for the enamel composite layer by removing the excess with the Misura instrument

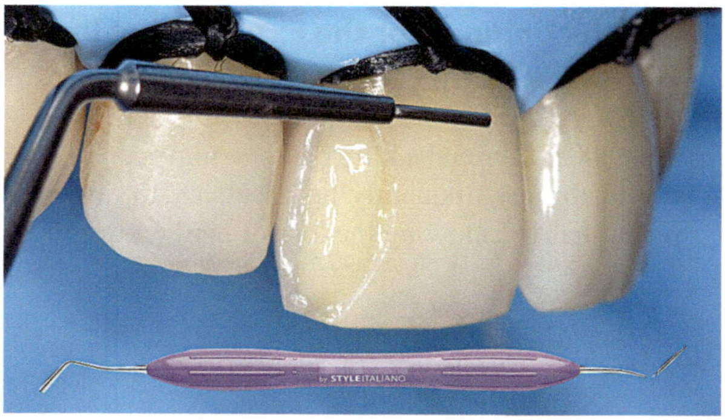

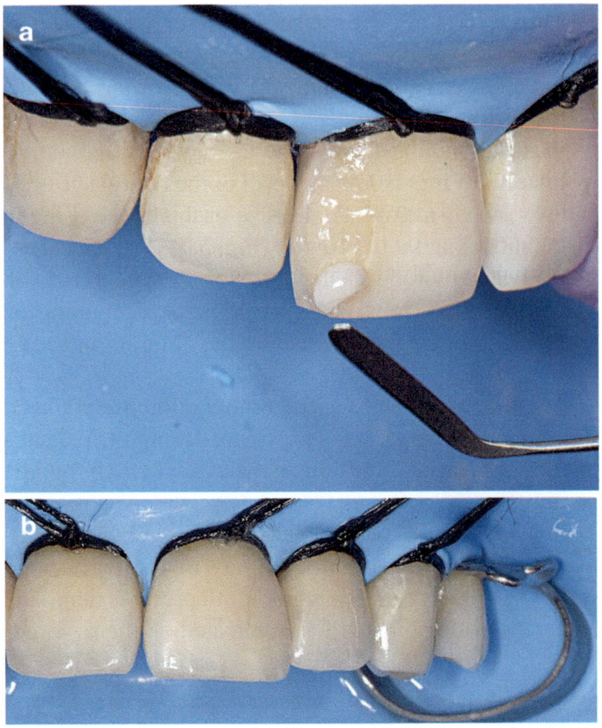

Fig. 5.8 Application of the superficial layer of enamel composite (**a**) and the aspect before finishing (**b**)

Difficulties that may arise	Possible solutions
Dislocation of the composite palatal wall when removing the silicone key	Its attachment with flowable composite or its integral restoration using a modeling brush to improve the sealing to the tooth (Fig. 5.11)
The restoration obtained immediately after polishing is darker in color than the tooth	Evaluation of the aesthetic result after rehydration of the tooth
The existence of a white line at the limit between the restoration and the tooth	Total or partial removal of the restoration in the superficial interface area and application of appropriate enamel and dentin. Redo restoration

5.3.2 Techniques for the Extension of Incisal Edges by Addition

Main idea: Minimal additive interventions on the incisal edges of certain anterior teeth may frequently be necessary to restore aesthetics, symmetry, and functionality following the loss of hard tooth substance in this area.

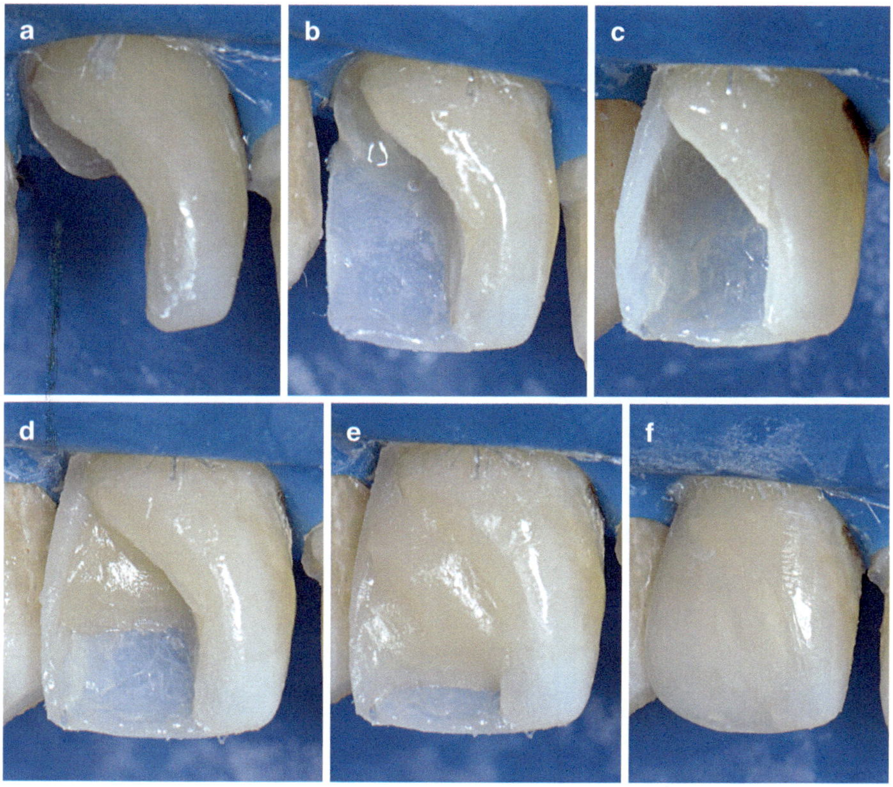

Fig. 5.9 Steps of a restoration in the case of an extended class IV cavity with the anatomical layering technique: initial aspect (**a**); the aspect after the restoration of the palatal wall with enamel composite (**b**); aspect after reconstruction of the palatal and proximal wall (**c**); aspect with the first layer of dentin two shades darker than the final shade (**d**); the aspect after the application of the second layer of dentin with a shade darker than the final shade (**e**); aspect after application of the last dentin layer of final shade and enamel layer (**f**)

There are several clinical situations of non-carious lesions where aesthetics and functionality can be resolved with minimal direct additive techniques:

- Mild uni-dental abnormalities of shape and position that do not require orthodontic treatment or are refused by the patient. Their treatment through direct additive restorations is achieved either by free modeling or by injection into a transparent stent obtained based on a wax-up (see Chap. 10).
- Wear processes associated (or not) with position changes of the teeth following orthodontic treatments. Often, following the derotation effect of the anterior teeth produced by the orthodontic treatment, unevenly modified incisal edges require minimally invasive restorations.
- Fractures or small chipping of the incisal edge. Most often, these are treated by adding a monoshade composite that does not require layering.

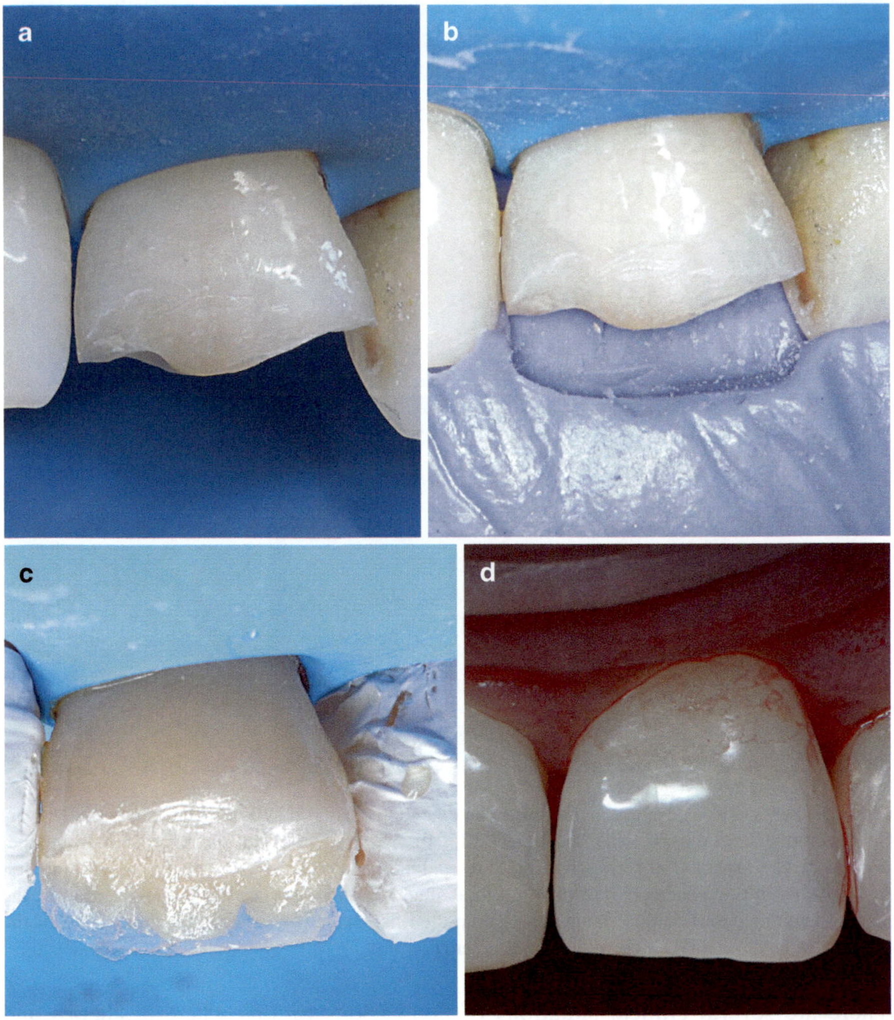

Fig. 5.10 Anatomical restoration of the incisal morphology: initial aspect (**a**); the use of an individualized silicone key as palatal support for the restoration of the palatal wall (**b**); making lobes from dentin composite (**c**); application of incisal enamel (**d**)

Depending on the clinical case, among the possible options we could mention:

- The additive anatomical technique using enamel and dentin to restore the internal incisal morphology with mamelons and characterizations (case 1 presented below).
- A monochrome additive technique (case 2 presented below).

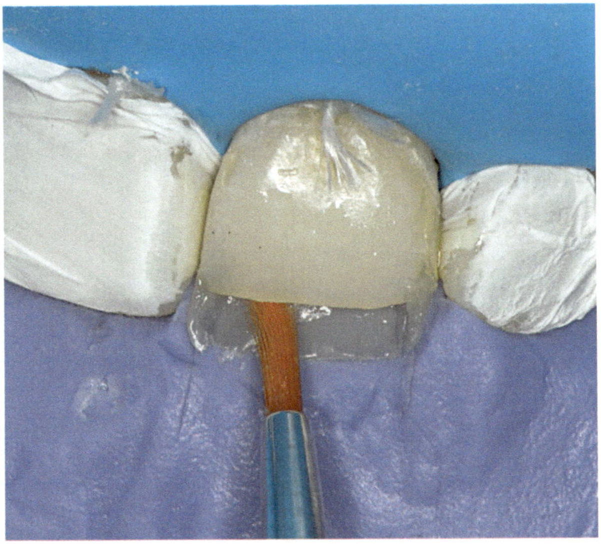

Fig. 5.11 Adapting the composite to the tooth using a brush when restoring the palatal wall with a silicone key

5.3.2.1 Working Technique

In the initial step, the shade of the composite will be determined. Then, the patient's static and dynamic occlusion is analyzed to identify the relationships of the tooth with the antagonists in maximum intercuspation, propulsion, and laterality. Rubber dam isolation of the entire frontal group and application of ligatures provides good isolation, visibility, and access (Fig. 5.12a). Any residual composite from previous restorations will be removed, and if the clinical situation requires it, the enamel margins can be beveled. A silicone key is made (through one of the techniques described in Sect. 3.1.2) that will be a shell for the composite's placement and palatal conformation (Fig. 5.12b, c).

Since the lack of substance is minimal in these cases, located above the points of contact with adjacent teeth (more incisal), the use of matrices, for conforming the proximal walls and contact area, is not imperative. Free modeling can shape the composite with the silicone key as shell. Adjacent teeth should, in all cases, be isolated by wrapping them with Teflon tape or placing a transparent celluloid strip interdentally. Thus, they will be protected during the application of the etching, the adhesive, and the composite during the procedure.

After the isolation of the adjacent teeth (e.g., Teflon tape), etching, adhesive application, and the first layer of a palatal composite can be performed (Fig. 5.13a–d). It aims to achieve a suitable attachment of the composite to the tooth by adapting it with the brush or by applying additional composite so that it remains in position after removing the silicone key (Fig. 5.14a).

When the length of the addition area does not exceed 1–2 mm of the crown height and when there is not enough space, layering several shades of dentin is

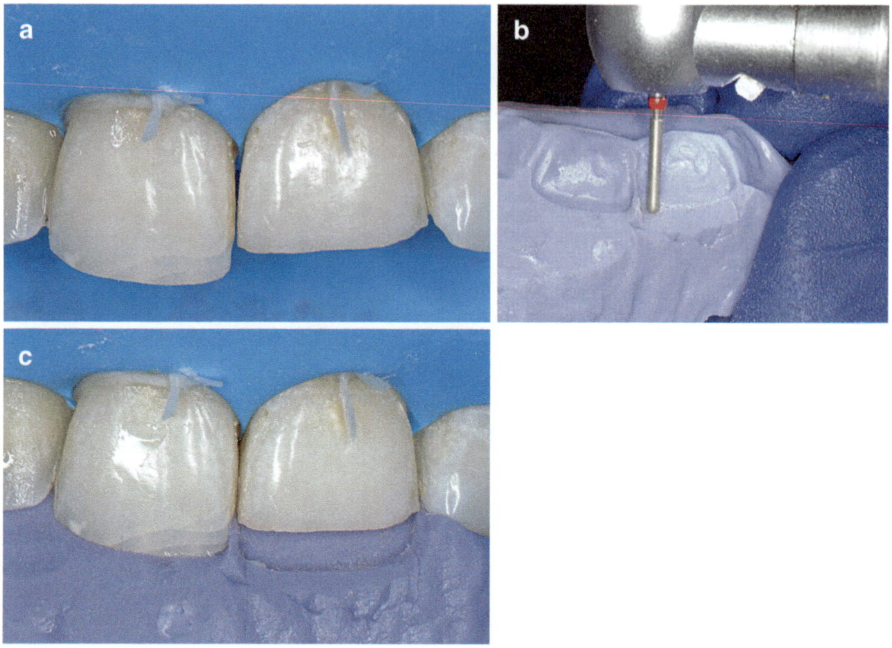

Fig. 5.12 Initial aspect after rubber dam isolation in order to restore tooth 21 where the old direct restoration has dislodged (**a**); palatal impression with putty silicone and individualization by cutting excess silicone with a diamond/multibladed bur (**b**); the aspect of the silicone key after individualization with a bur (**c**)

unnecessary. One shade of dentin and one of enamel is sufficient for most cases (Fig. 5.14b, c).

The mamelons' number, shape, and size will be dictated by the need to achieve symmetry with the adjacent or homologous tooth. The special characterizations (white, transparent, amber, etc.) are achieved by placing the pigments following the map of the adjacent teeth. The instruments that can be used are the spatula for coarse application and modeling, the microbrush for packing the composite, and the modeling brush for improving marginal sealing and fine modeling the composite (Fig. 5.15a–c).

Finishing may be done according to the standard protocol (see Chap. 7).

The incisal anatomy may sometimes be well-defined in the teeth of one arch and absent in the opposite arch (Fig. 5.16). The existence of some orthodontic treatments that have the effect of aligning the incisors may lead to the need for aesthetic restoration of the incisal edges. Careful evaluation on examination may indicate the presence or absence of an internal morphology with lobes and incisal transparencies (Fig. 5.17). The treatment begins with a silicone key, fitting it, and removing any remaining old composite areas from previous restorations (Fig. 5.18a–c). The

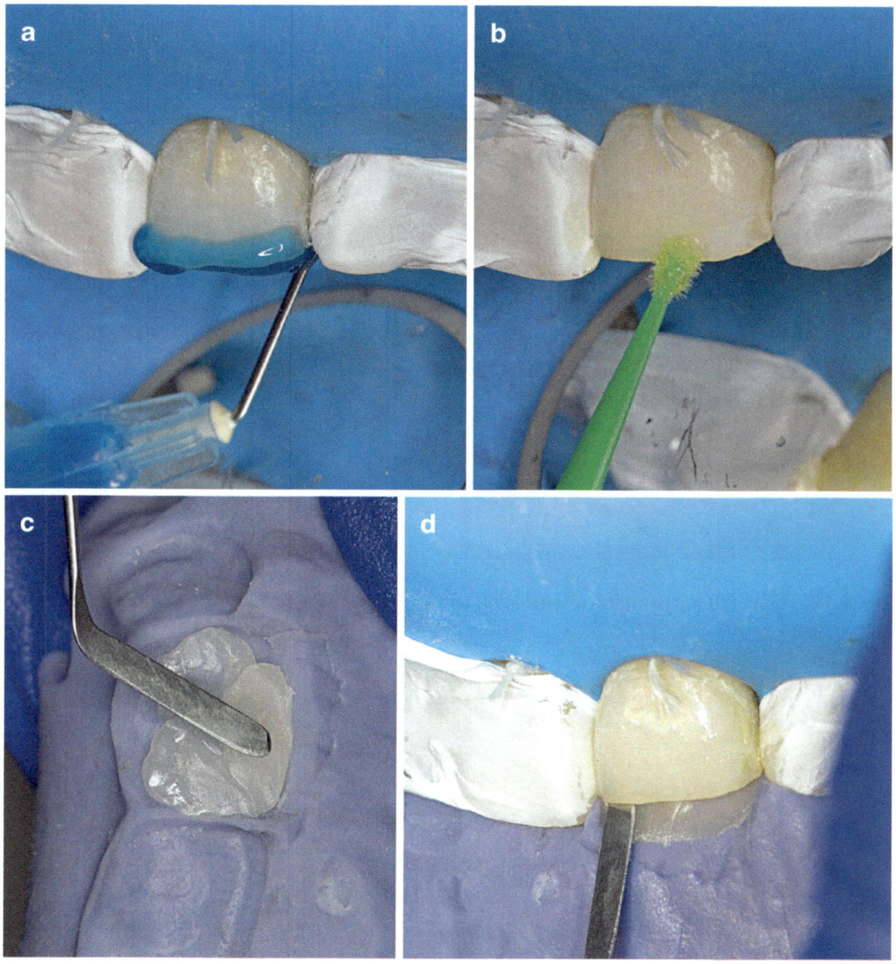

Fig. 5.13 Application of the etching (**a**); applying the adhesive (**b**); applying the composite on the silicone key to restore the palatal wall (**c**); removing excess composite from the silicone key before polymerization (**d**)

layering of the composite on the silicone key is done by one of the anatomical, simplified, monochrome techniques. Finishing follows the usual steps (see Chap. 7) (Fig. 5.19a–c).

Difficulties that may arise	Possible solutions
In the absence of a wax-up, the cutting out of the silicone key can lead to the improper conformation of the incisal edge	Shape adaptation with the help of rotary instruments (finishing burs, disks, etc.)
Inadequate integration of the restoration's aesthetics into the crown's overall chromaticity	Redo restoration

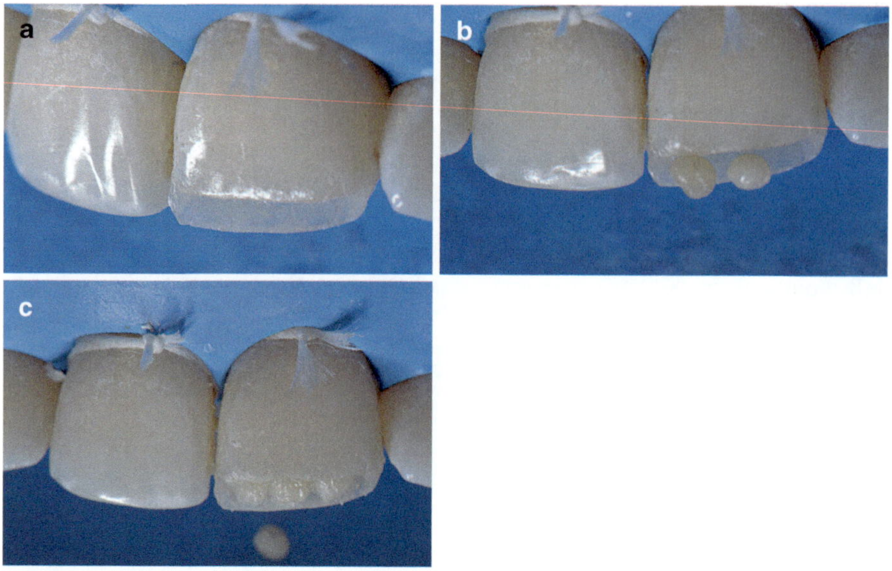

Fig. 5.14 Aspect of the palatal wall (**a**); application of dentin and enamel composite (**b**) to restore incisal anatomy (**c**)

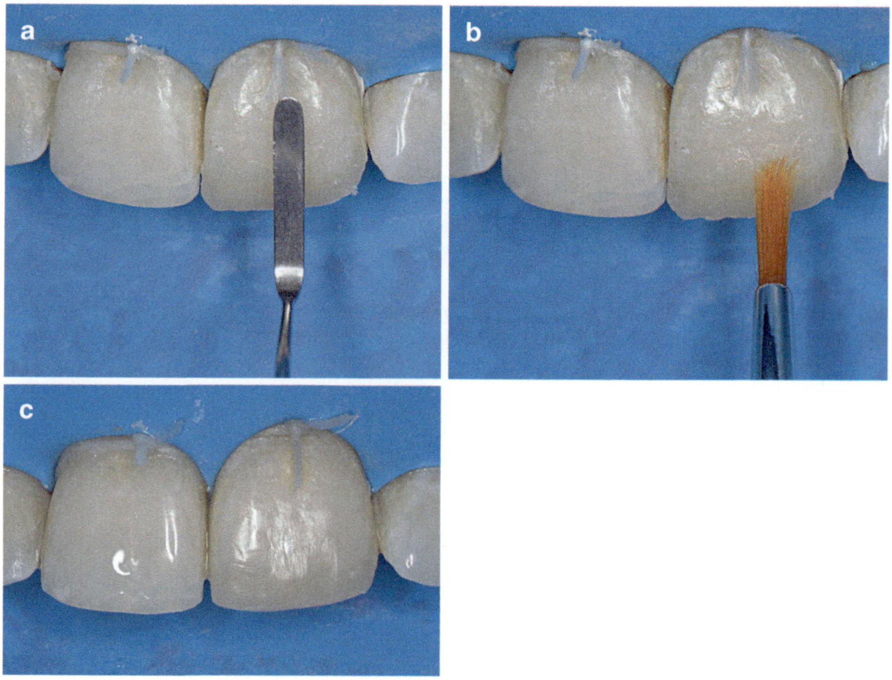

Fig. 5.15 Buccal modeling with a spatula (**a**), brush (**b**), and aspect before finishing and polishing (**c**)

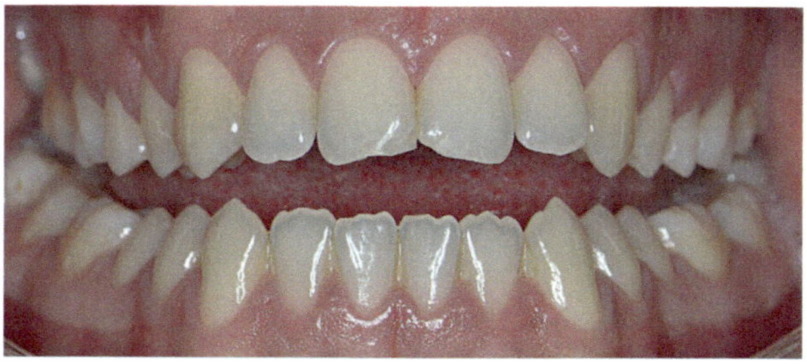

Fig. 5.16 Aspect of the incisal morphology of the lower and upper central incisors

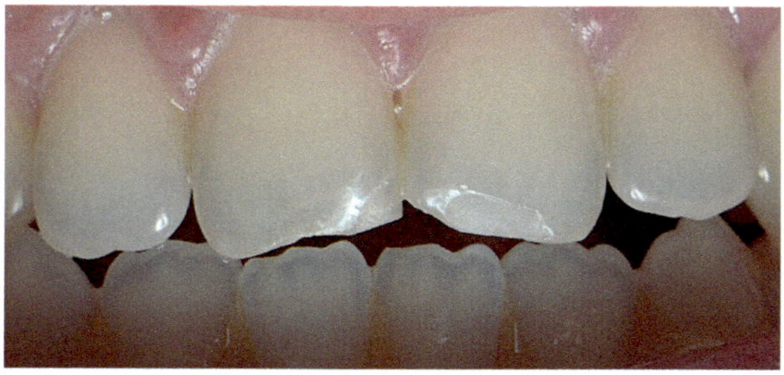

Fig. 5.17 Initial aspect of the incisal edge of the upper central incisors

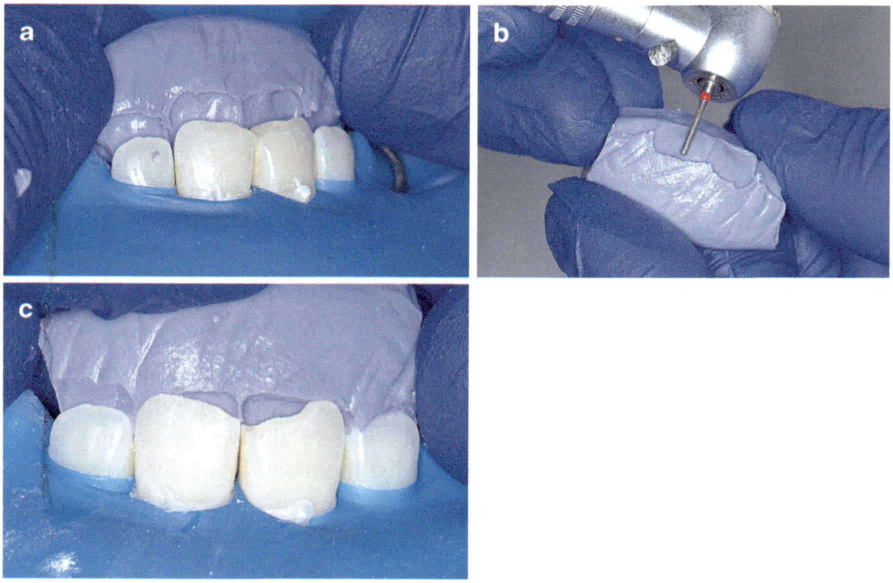

Fig. 5.18 Making a silicone palatal key (**a**); individualization of the silicone key by removing the excess (**b**); silicone key try-in (**c**)

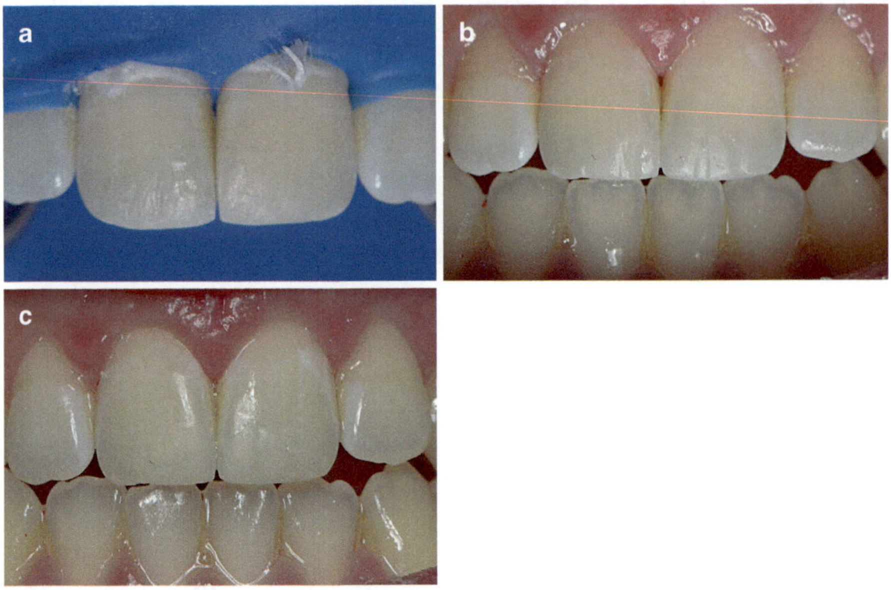

Fig. 5.19 Aspect after incisal edge restoration with universal composite A2 (**a**) before (**b**) and after finishing (**c**)

5.3.3 Simplified Layering Technique for Class III and Class IV Cavities

The main idea: In cases that do not require particular incisal anatomy, the layering technique can be simplified using only a universal composite combined with a dentin shade and an enamel shade.

Simplifying working protocols is a major concern in all areas of dentistry in terms of obtaining good clinical, aesthetic, and functional results. Regarding the direct restorations of the anterior teeth, their aesthetics are always conditioned by the chromatic and morphological complexity of the tooth and its neighbor/correspondent. In many clinical situations, specific incisal anatomy elements such as natural transparencies, dentin mamelons, and other chromatic elements may be absent or difficult to detect. In these cases, the layering protocol can be simplified so that combining a shade of dentin composite and one of universal composite or enamel composite can lead to good results. They can be directly layered from palatal to buccal or be layered centripetally after the prior restoration of the palatal and proximal walls. The layering technique always remains at the doctor's discretion.

5.3.3.1 Working Technique

The simplified layering technique involves omitting some steps, most frequently, the enamel composite as the first palatal layer. Thus, the restoration starts directly with the application of a palatal layer of dentine composite. The technique can be performed in a centripetal way, initially restoring the palatal wall in dentin and the proximal wall in universal composite (Fig. 5.20a–d) or directly by layering several

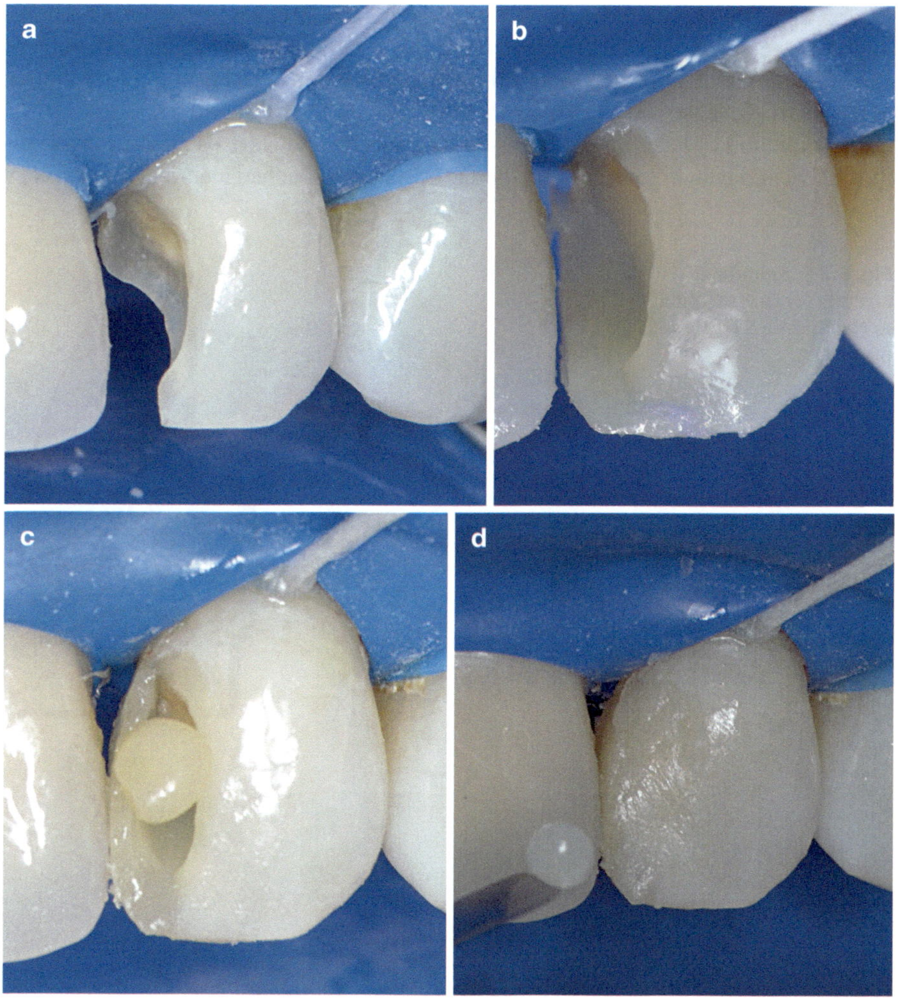

Fig. 5.20 Initial aspect after isolation and class IV cavity preparation on tooth 22 (**a**); the aspect after the restoration of the dentin composite palatal wall (**b**); aspect after the restoration of the proximal wall with universal NeoSpectra composite (**c**) and application of dentin and universal composite in approximately equal thicknesses; application of buccal enamel composite layer (**d**)

shades of dentin from the palatal to the buccal side, or the use of a universal composite over the first layer of palatal dentin.

A possible way of simplified layering (as indicated for NeoSpectra, Dentsply Sirona) can be the palatal application of a shade of dentin composite on approximately half of the crown's bucco-palatal thickness, followed by applying a layer of universal composite in the buccal half (Fig. 5.21). Enamel application may be optional in the incisal area. Depending on the incisal morphology, it can be applied incisally with or without dentin composite or universal composite support (Fig. 5.22). The simultaneous presence of the palatal silicone key and the sectional matrix placed proximally can help achieve this stratification. Thus, the silicone key can be sectioned to allow the matrix to be fixed, or it can even be completely cut out at the matrix level so as not to interfere.

This method of layering may be used for class IV and class III cavities involving the buccal and palatal surfaces. The latter must be approached identically to class IV

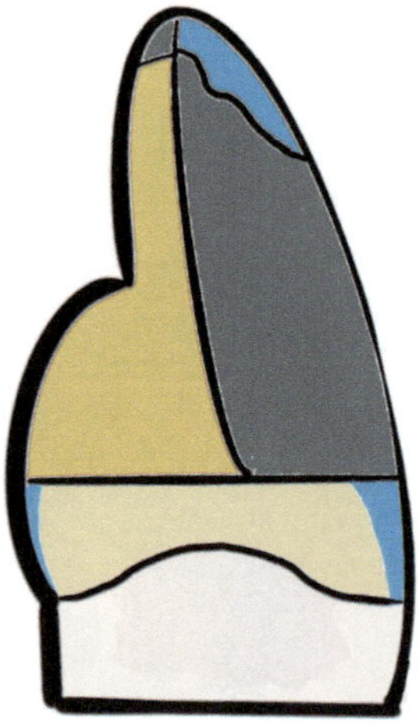

Fig. 5.21 Simplified layering scheme according to NeoSpectra ST Effects prospect

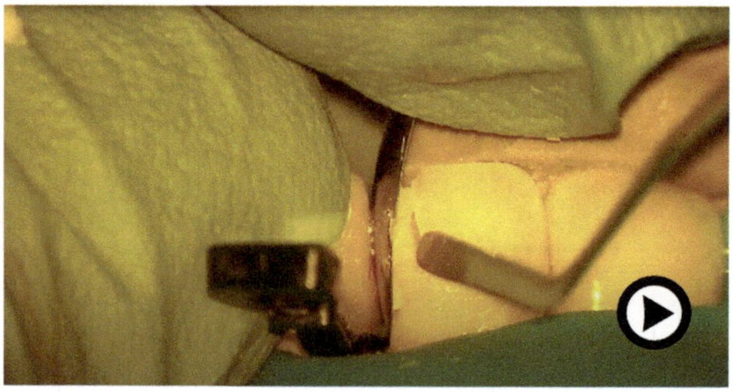

Fig. 5.22 Simplified layering technique using sectional matrix fixed in a palatal silicone key (neo spectra ST effects, Dentsply Sirona) (▶ https://doi.org/10.1007/000-bqs)

cavities regarding light transmission through the composite mass. Thus, introducing a blocker, the dentine/opaque composite, becomes essential to prevent the too-easy passage of the light coming from the outside, respectively, the "darkness" coming from inside the oral cavity.

Difficulties that may arise	Possible solutions
Appropriate case selection (e.g., proximal transparencies were not identified)	If it has been decided to perform a simplified stratification in a difficult case that requires a complex stratification, it is possible to opt for the correction or redo of the restoration following an anatomical stratification

The technique itself does not create specific difficulties different from other techniques; on the contrary, it is the easiest to achieve.

5.3.4 The Monochrome Technique (Monoshade) Using a Silicone Key

Main idea: In exceptional cases, frontal restorations can be successfully achieved by applying a single shade of universal composite.

Selecting a case to use the monochrome technique with universal composite would require evaluation of multiple aspects. Thus, following the coronal examination of the tooth that will be restored, the following should be found:

- The relatively constant shade of the dental crown in the area to be restored
- Lack of transparencies and incisal pigmentation
- The lack of an internal mamelons
- Relatively small size missing part (of lack of substance)

One can opt for simplified layering using a universal composite in these cases. Most frequently, this technique may be used for the restoration of crowns with the incisal edge or the incisal angle slightly chipped or abraded (Fig. 5.23a–c). These cases can be easily solved even without rubber dam isolation. A silicone key can be helpful, but free shaping using hand instruments leads to good results in most cases.

Difficulties that may arise	Possible solutions
Obtaining a restoration that is too dark, perceived as gray The lack of an opaque composite layer to block the passage of light associated with a medium/large size of the lack of substance can lead to restorations that light passes through easily, creating a restoration that feels too gray	The solution is to remove and restore it by adding an appropriate shade layer of dentin/opaque composite
The difficulties are particularly related to a good selection of cases that can lend themselves to this technique	Correct case selection

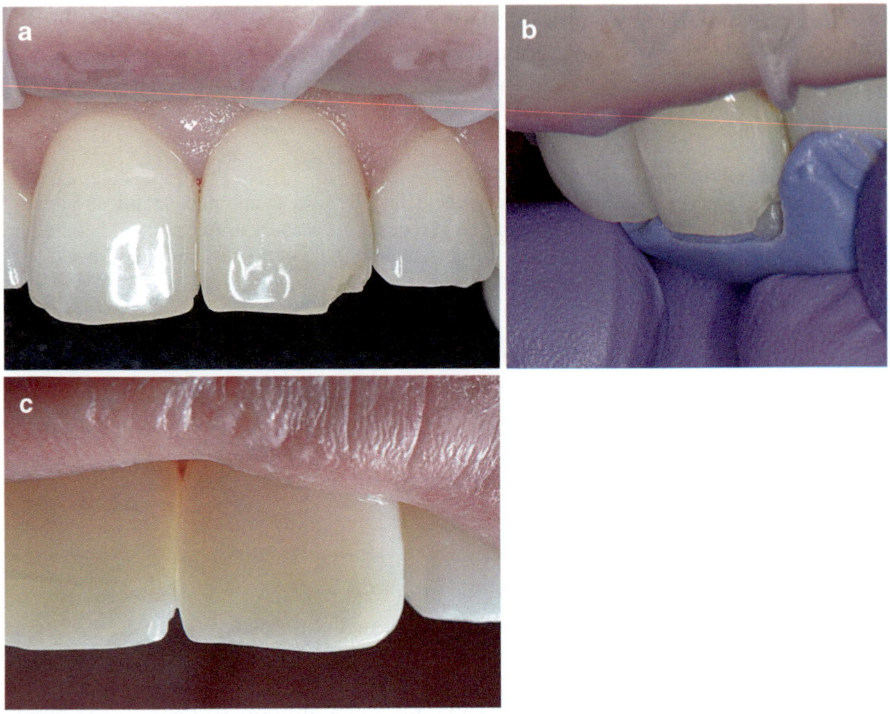

Fig. 5.23 Restoration of the disto-incisal angle on tooth 21 (**a**) using a silicone key individualized (**b**) and final aspect (**c**)

5.4 For Posterior Teeth

One of the main reasons the layering of conventional composites is carried out in the case of posterior teeth is the technical limitation imposed by the manufacturers. They recommend limiting the polymerization thickness to less than 2 mm to decrease the shrinkage coefficient, improve marginal sealing, and decrease cuspid deflection.

Factors affecting polymerization shrinkage include [4]:

- C-factor
- Filler content
- Conversion rate
- Modulus of elasticity
- Water absorption
- Photopolymerization variables
- The influence of the tooth substrate on which the composite material is applied

The techniques of application and layering of composite materials are universally recognized as a major factor influencing shrinkage. The stress from polymerization shrinkage can be reduced by using specific application techniques of composite resins in the cavities. Applying conventional composite resins in layers is recommended to reduce shrinkage stress [5]. No application techniques completely reduce the polymerization shrinkage of the composite.

Three main factors contribute to the reduction of the polymerization shrinkage:

- The use of a small volume of material
- A lower cavity configuration factor (C-factor)
- Minimal contact with the opposite walls of the cavity during polymerization

The use of liners with a low modulus of elasticity as stress absorber and soft-start polymerization is related to the reduction of the polymerization shrinkage.

It is widely accepted that incremental filling lowers shrinkage stress due to the reduced volume of the polymerizing material. Each newly added layer is offset by the next, and the resulting polymerization shrinkage is diminished [6].

More details about these properties of conventional and bulk composite materials can be found in Sect. 1.2.2.

5.4.1 Successive Cusp Technique

Main idea: This technique involves restoring the cusps by applying a portion of composite corresponding to the size of a cusp, shaping, and polymerizing it. It continues with restoring each cusp in an order chosen by the operator. The technique allows easy modeling of the occlusal morphology. There are recommended working sequences for different didactic or workflow advantages.

The successive cusp technique [7] is one of the most popular modeling techniques, representing the working protocol in many dental faculties due to its multiple advantages. Among the advantages of the technique of successive cusps, we can mention:

- Decreases the C-factor, the additions in small quantities that do not link two opposite walls.
- The polymerization stress decreases due to the small volumes of composite polymerized step by step and the amount of material being equivalent to the size of a cusp.
- The excess material is reduced and therefore, the finishing time decreases.
- A good marginal sealing is obtained [8].

- A good morphology can be obtained, thanks to focusing on a single cusp that will be polymerized immediately after modeling. Therefore, the possibility to change its morphology when modeling the adjacent cusp disappears.
- It reduces the operator's stress generated by the fact that it could modify the cusp morphology already achieved and not polymerized yet.
- It is a didactic technique and easy to learn and apply.
- The increased degree of standardization that increases ergonomics and efficiency.

5.4.1.1 Working Technique

Occlusal morphology can be done using universal conventional composite or bilaminar composites (enamel composite and dentin composite) by successive cusp technique. It is preferable to transform any type of cavity into a class I with a centripetal technique and then to fill it with composite resin (bulk or layered) to a depth of 1.5 mm from the occlusal surface.

To restore the first cusp, a portion of composite resin of relatively equal size to the size of the future cusp and spherical shape is prepared. This composite sphere can be applied to the cavity base with a basic modeling instrument (Fissura; a conventional explorer) (Fig. 5.24). The advantage of spherical pre-forming lies in the subsequent exploitation of convexities for cusp shaping, with most cusps having a convex shape. The composite resin is placed in the cavity and later distributed over the entire projection area of the cusp (Fig. 5.25a, b). The projection of each cusp onto the cavity base is relatively rectangular (Fig. 5.25b) and can be imaged or marked on the underlying composite layer for better orientation. Morphology modeling can be most conveniently and efficiently accomplished using thin modeling instruments or even the tip of a straight probe. One may apply pressure on composite with the instruments especially at the margin of the composite sphere, to partially maintain its convex shape (Fig. 5.26).

Using spatulas or obturators for modeling can lead to obtaining straight shapes. In addition, the shaping of grooves (Fig. 5.27a) can be more easily done with sharp-tipped instruments or even by slight pressure with the tip of a thin modeling brush (Fig. 5.27b).

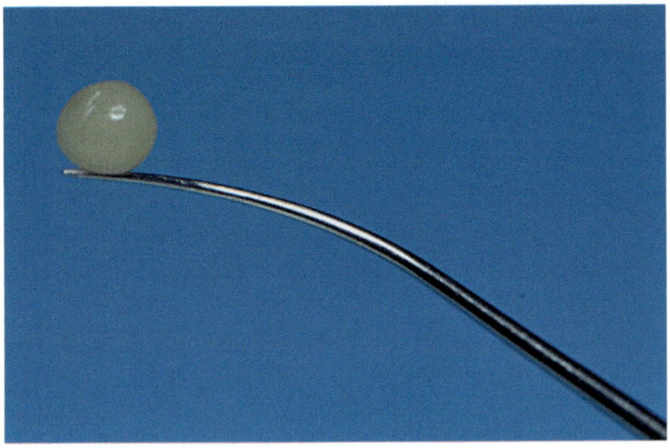

Fig. 5.24 Increment of composite resin prepared in a spherical shape on the tip of a sharp instrument from the modeling kit

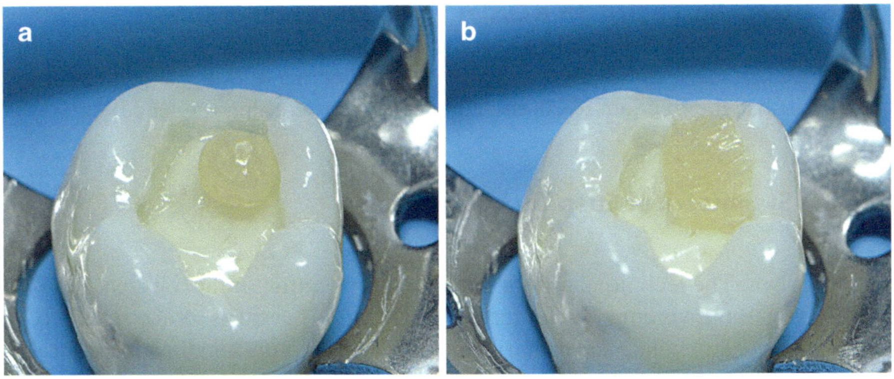

Fig. 5.25 Restoration of the first cusps by the successive cusp method: placing an increment of composite on the base of the cavity, in its projection area (**a**); spreading the composite over the entire surface corresponding to the cusp projection area and occlusal sculpting (**b**)

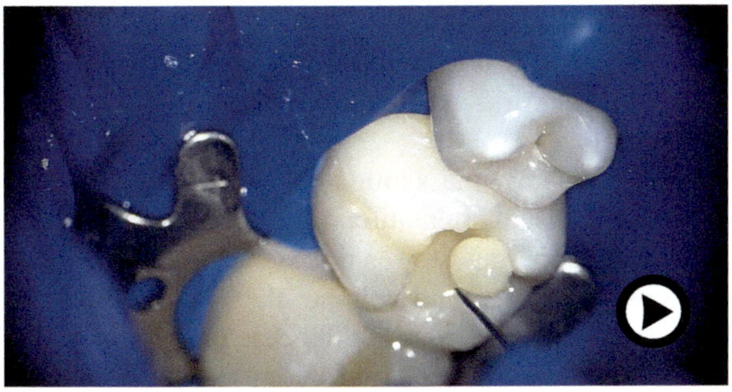

Fig. 5.26 Occlusal modeling using the successive cusp technique (▶ https://doi.org/10.1007/000-bqr)

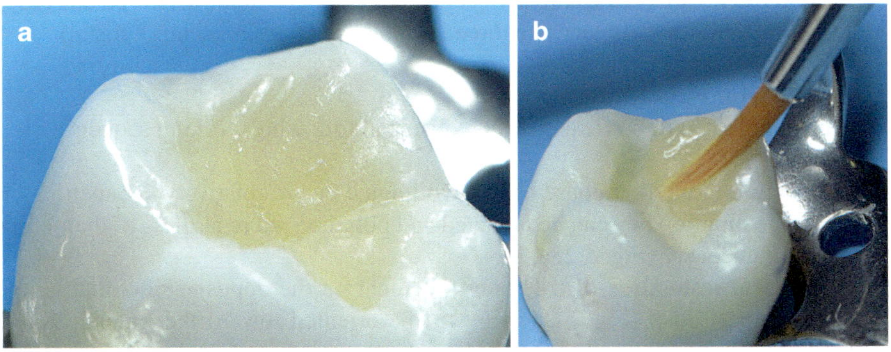

Fig. 5.27 Occlusal modeling of grooves on the cuspid slopes (**a**) using the sharp tip modeling brush (**b**)

5.4.1.2 Cusp Reconstruction Order

The literature does not indicate a specific sequence in which the cusps should be restored. Each clinician identifies advantages to specific working sequences. Thus, the dentist has the freedom to choose and apply their working sequence.

5.4.2 Symmetrical Cusp Technique

Main idea: The technique aims at the initial restoration of the adjacent cusps of comparable volume located on the same side (buccal or oral), relatively symmetrical, to create a necessary landmark for restoring and then the central anatomical structure located on the opposite side. The technique represents an easy-to-apply, didactic, and predictable way of restoring the occlusal morphology of upper and lower first molars.

When there is extensive destruction of the occlusal surface involving all cusps of a molar, much of the anatomical landmarks disappear. In these cases, it is more difficult to calibrate the size and positioning of the cusps with their anatomical elements. Their placement and the direction of orientation of the cusps can create difficulties.

To counter these problems, the symmetric cusp technique follows a working sequence based on easier visual orientation when evaluating symmetrical structures. Thus, in the case of the upper and lower first molars, we recommend first making relatively similar cusps in shape and volume: the buccal cusps in the case of the upper first molars and the lingual cusps in the case of the lower first molars. These will be significant landmarks for restoring the cusps on the opposite sides where there are three different anatomical structures:

- In the case of the upper first molar: the disto-palatal cusp, the oblique ridge, and the transverse ridge—the latter two being together parts of the mesio-palatal cusp;
- In the case of lower molars: the three buccal cusps (mesial, central, distal).

5.4.2.1 Lower First Molar

The technique of symmetrical cusps involves the following working sequence:

- Restoration in the first phase of the two lingual cusps, relatively symmetrical in size and volume. They can be modeled and polymerized regardless of their order or simultaneously (Fig. 5.28a, b).
- Subsequent restoration of the central element on the opposite side, that is, the centro-buccal cusp (Fig. 5.28c). It will be oriented toward the lingual groove between the lingual cusps restored in the previous step. The position of the

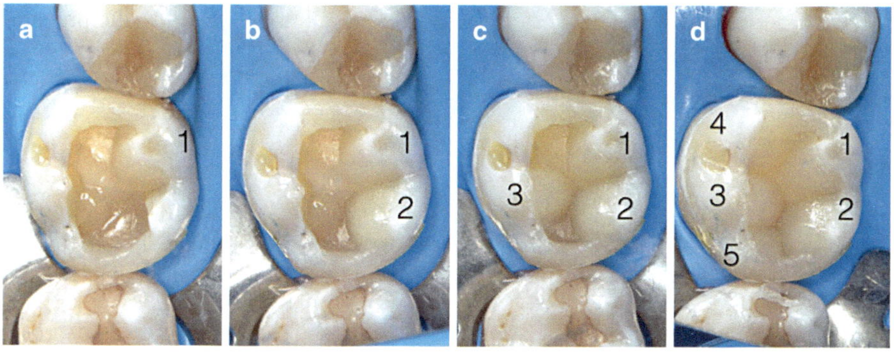

Fig. 5.28 Symmetrical cusp technique for occlusal modeling of the last layer of composite on a lower first molar: modeling of one of the lingual cusps (**a**); modeling of the second lingual cusp (**b**); creation of the centro-buccal cusp (**c**); rebuilding of mesial and distal buccal cusps (**d**)

central fossa will be determined by how far the centro-buccal cusp extends toward/into the lingual intercusp groove.

- Restoration of the mesio-buccal and disto-buccal cusps. They can be shaped and polymerized one by one or simultaneously, because they do not come into contact with each other (Fig. 5.28d).

5.4.2.2 Maxillary First Molar

An easy way of volumetric orientation for the restoration of the occlusal morphology of the upper first molars is based on splitting the occlusal surface into two halves, buccal and oral. The working sequence:

- The restoration in the first phase of the two buccal cusps, which are relatively symmetrical in size and volume. They can be shaped and polymerized one by one or simultaneously (Fig. 5.29a, b).
- Subsequent restoration of the central morphological element on the opposite side, i.e., the oblique ridge (Fig. 5.29c). The oblique ridge is a connecting bridge between the mesial-palatal cusp and the disto-buccal cusp (already restored), separating mesially and distally the following two anatomical elements that will be restored.
- Restoration of the transverse ridge, part of the mesio-palatal cusp (Fig. 5.29d).
- Restoration of the disto-palatal cusp (Fig. 5.29e).

This sequence of working provides good control of the restoration of the occlusal morphology, especially in the upper first molars. Shaping the mesio-palatal cusp of these molars can sometimes be challenging for a clinician due to the complex morphology consisting of two ridges that must connect with two cusps on the opposite side (Fig. 5.30a–d).

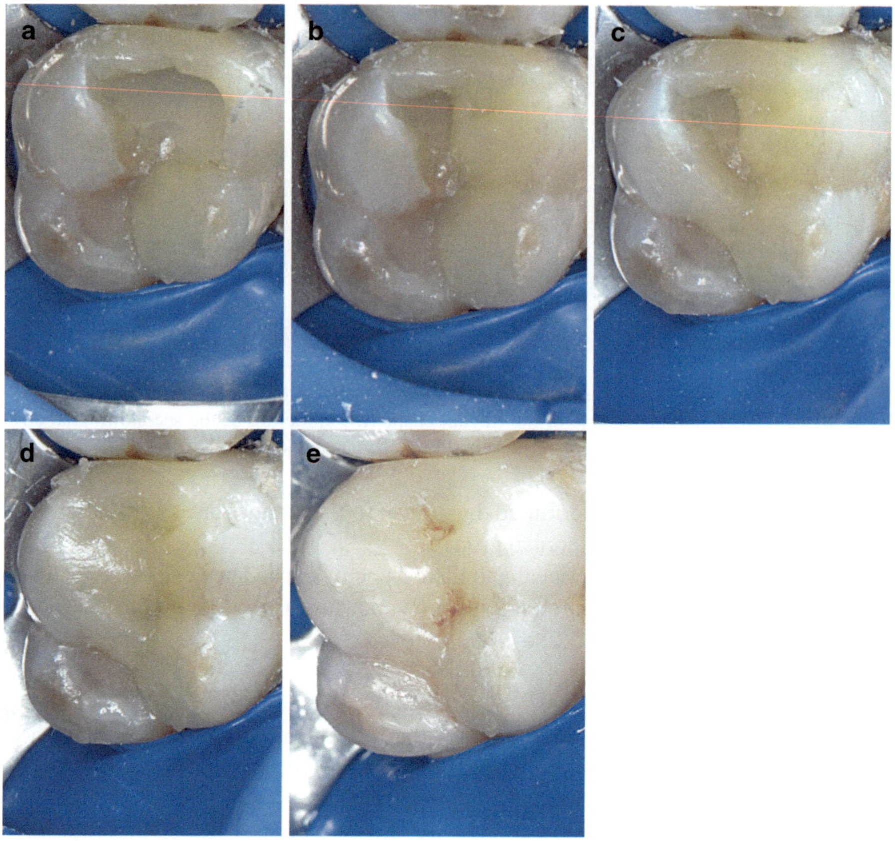

Fig. 5.29 Symmetric cusp technique for occlusal modeling of the last layer of composite on a first upper molar: the creation of one of the buccal cusps (**a**); making the other buccal cusp (**b**); making the oblique ridge (**c**); making the transverse ridge (**d**); rebuilding of the disto-palatinal cusp (**e**)

A diagram of this restoration sequence can be shown in Fig. 5.31.

Depending on the clinical aspect of the adjacent teeth and the patient's desire, pigments can be added in the grooves and pits, to better fit the restoration aesthetics in the full arch (Fig. 5.32a–e).

Difficulties that may arise	Possible solutions
Creating an anatomy that is too retentive	Adding a flowable composite to grooves and pits
Spacing too much the cusps and creating grooves too wide	Addition of packable composite

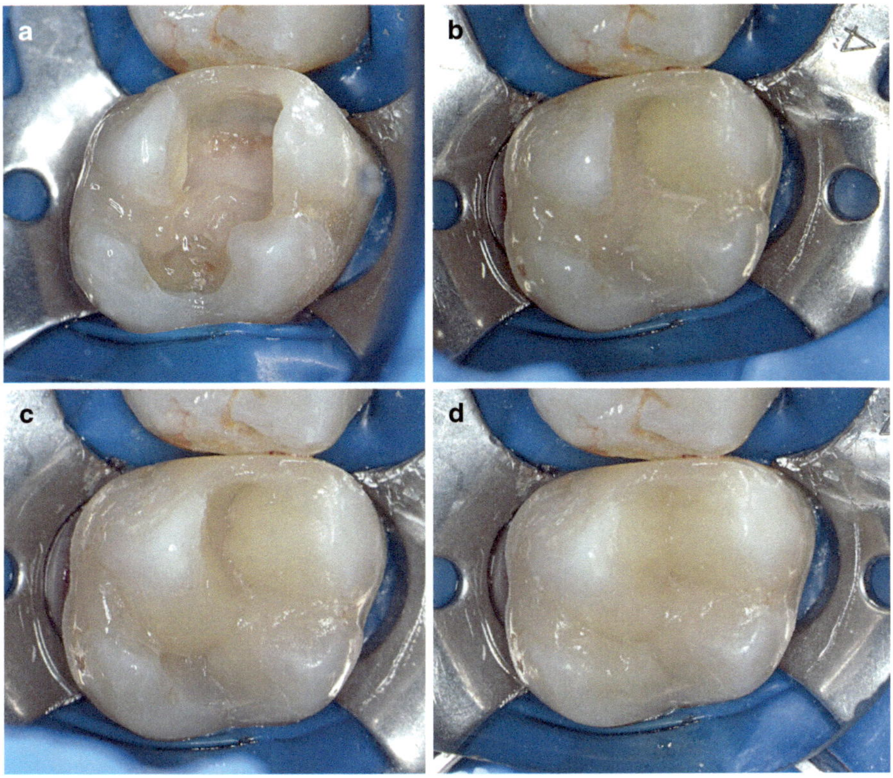

Fig. 5.30 Symmetric cusp technique for occlusal modeling of the last layer of composite in an upper first molar: the initial aspect of the cavity (**a**); successive buildup of the buccal cusps (**b**); buildup of the oblique ridge (**c**); buildup of the transverse ridge and disto-palatinal cusp (**d**)

5.4.3 The Simultaneous Cusp Technique

Main idea: This technique involves modeling the entire occlusal morphology and then polymerizing all cusps simultaneously. This technique presents several disadvantages, especially related to technical aspects (C-factor, shrinkage), and is used in the case of conventional and packable bulk composites. This modeling technique is primarily associated with bulk composite resins and self-curing materials.

This technique has been widely used to restore occlusal morphology in amalgam and composite resin restorations. The technique consists of modeling and then polymerizing all the cusps simultaneously.

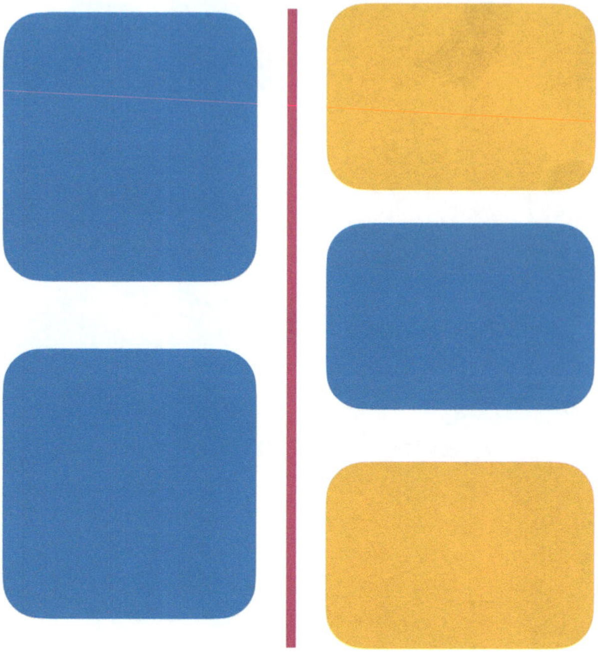

Fig. 5.31 Rebuilding the cusps in the order dictated by the main anatomical elements in the case of the symmetrical cusp technique

The advantages of this technique:

- Saving time, as only one polymerization is required for all cusps.
- The overview of all modeled but uncured cusps allows good evaluation and adjustments before curing.

The technique has several disadvantages, among which we can mention:

- It generates stress, the operator approaching the entire occlusal surface simultaneously with the risk of damaging the relief already modeled.
- Making it difficult to conform to the occlusal morphology. Applying pressure with the modeling instrument in a specific area can lead to the deformation of the composite in the vicinity.
- Through this technique, several opposite walls are linked, the polymerization being a global one at the end, increasing the C-factor, and the polymerization stress due to the large volume of composite.

Variants of this technique have been described, which avoid these drawbacks. Thus, Scolavino et al. propose an improved simultaneous technique variant [9]. In the first step, the class II or MOD cavity must be converted into a class I cavity and filled to a depth of 1.5 mm, conforming the base of the cavity to be approximately flat or slightly concave. Later, the cusps are made simultaneously by successive layering, but without touching each other, and are polymerized simultaneously. In the end, the composite is inserted into the free spaces between them and polymerized.

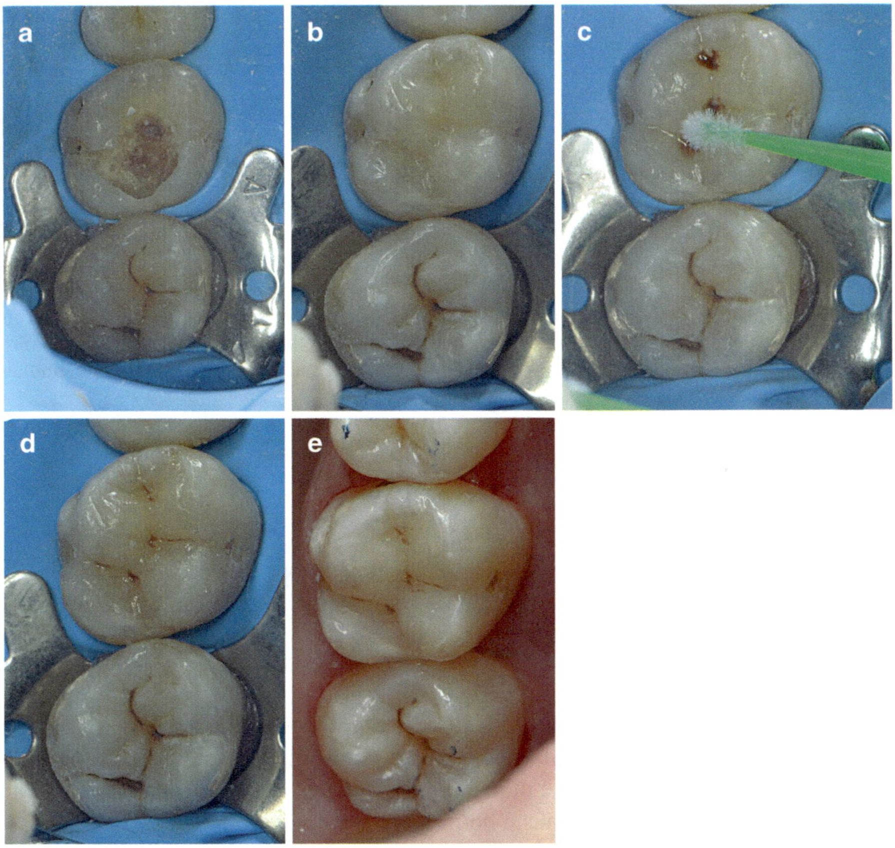

Fig. 5.32 Direct composite resin restoration of an upper first molar by the symmetrical cusp technique followed by characterization with brown pigment: the initial aspect of the prepared cavity (**a**); aspect after the restoration of all cusps (**b**); applying the pigment in the pits followed by removing off the excess with microbrush (**c**); the aspect of the restoration after the polymerization of the pigment (**d**) and, respectively, after the removal of the rubber dam (**e**)

5.4.3.1 Working Technique

After applying the last layer of occlusal composite, the occlusal morphology is modeled with modeling instruments. The negative relief (grooves, pits) is shaped by pressure and the positive by reflow or addition of composite (Fig. 5.33).

Difficulties that may arise	Possible solutions
Extending the time of occlusal modeling	Changing the technique to the sequential one, cusp to cusp, or essential line technique
Obtaining areas of excess material when pressure is applied to the composite to express occlusal relief. These will be identified when examining static and dynamic occlusion	Removal of reflowed composite following occlusal modeling before its polymerization

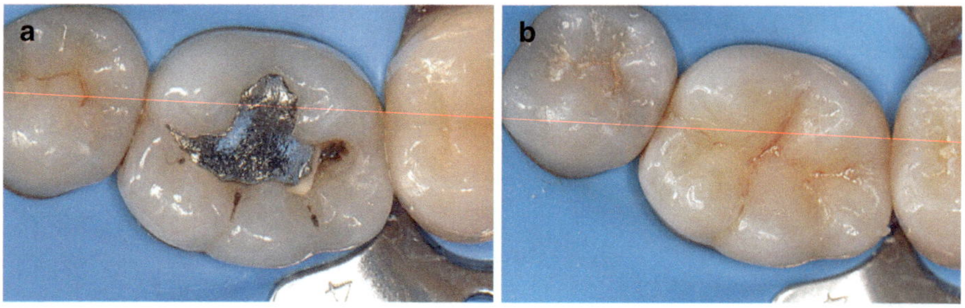

Fig. 5.33 Replacement of an amalgam occlusal filling, partially fractured and inadequate in terms of marginal sealing and occlusal morphology: initial aspect (**a**); the new restoration made of composite resin by applying the last layer of composite resin bulk and modeling all the cusps simultaneously (**b**)

5.4.4 Stamp Technique with Occlusal Key

Main idea: In the case of occlusal cavities with a minor lack of substance, the occlusal morphology can be copied, this key serving to conform the composite resin used in the direct restoration of the cavity.

The time to make a direct composite restoration has been estimated to be twice that of amalgam fillings [10]. One of the most time-consuming phases is occlusal modeling, which requires knowledge of anatomy, precision, dexterity, and maybe some artistical skills. All this is to achieve both aesthetics and functionality [11].

For these reasons, a technique was developed to allow the replication of the original morphology of the tooth, saving modeling time in cases where the occlusal morphology was minimally or moderately affected by the carious process. The "stamp technique" (or the occlusal key technique) consists in making a copy of the initial occlusal morphology before its destruction by cavity preparation [12, 13].

This occlusal key, most commonly made of a liquid dam, will shape the last layer of the composite before its polymerization. The key can also be made of silicone-based impression material, but most of these materials does not allow the initial polymerization of the composite through the key.

The advantages of this technique are reproducing the natural morphology, obtaining a fine composite surface, and reducing the occlusal adjustments time, even if the total time of making the obturation may not be majorly changed due to the additional step of making the occlusal key.

The occlusal key method is recommended in the following situations:

- Relatively preserved occlusal anatomy (superficial caries in grooves and pits, small cavities)
- Class I Black cavities or class II cavities with transformation into class I [14]
- Posterior teeth with relatively well-preserved occlusal morphology

The major disadvantage of this technique, as with the simultaneous cusp technique, lies in the bulk polymerization of the entire thickness of the occlusally applied composite.

The polymerization stress seems to be more related to the polymerized composite volume than to the C-factor [15], so in this polymerization situation, we encounter the biggest cusp deflection [16].

5.4.4.1 Working Technique

1. Evaluation of occlusal morphology and caries size

   Before cavity preparation, its size and occlusal relief are assessed (Fig. 5.34). Highly retentive morphologies with multiple deep primary and accessory grooves will be difficult to copy to make an occlusal key.
2. Remove retentive areas of the occlusal surface

   If the occlusal opening of the cavity exceeds 0.5 mm, we recommend quick covering the decay with a material (cement, composite, liquid dam, etc.) to smooth out the occlusal surface slightly. Lubrication is most commonly done with glycerin, but any oily substance can be used. Furthermore, wetting the occlusal surface with water spray may be sufficient. Both removing retentions and lubricating are necessary to be able to easily remove the key.
3. Impression of the occlusal surface (Fig. 5.35a, b)

   A thin layer of a liquid dam (or similar photopolymerizable material) is applied over the entire occlusal surface (maximum thickness 1 mm), and then the tip of a microbrush is placed on top of it and approximately in the middle of the occlusal surface. A new amount of liquid dam will continue to be applied until the tip is completely covered with the liquid dam, followed by its polymerization. The thickness of the occlusal key must provide sufficient resistance to press the composite in order to transfer the shape. It will be avoided that the tip

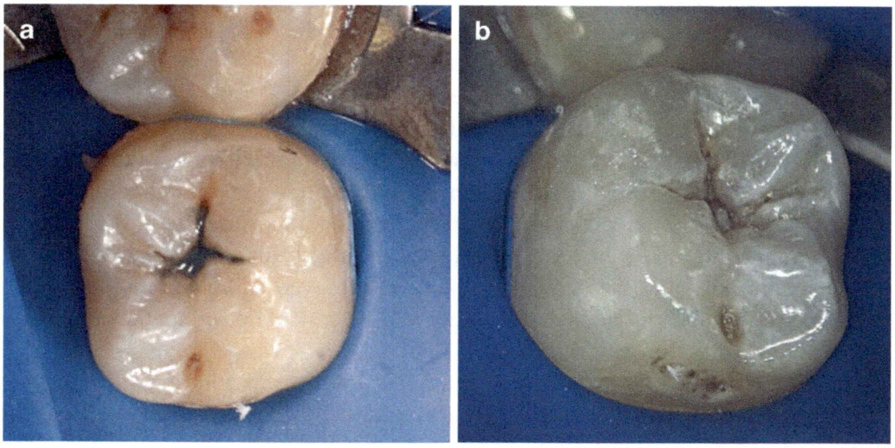

Fig. 5.34 Initial aspect of some occlusal carious lesions with relatively preserved occlusal morphology (**a**) and (**b**)

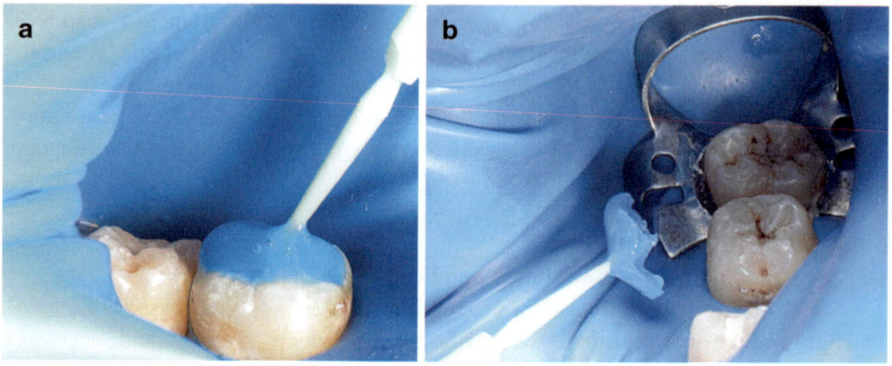

Fig. 5.35 Making the occlusal key by liquid rubber dam, centered fixation of a microbrush (**a**); removing the occlusal key from the tooth (**b**)

of the microbrush is in contact with the tooth, thus causing perforation of the impression material and affecting the proper conformation of the composite. The position of the handle of the microbrush can be a beneficial guideline for correctly positioning the key when using it to shape the composite. Instead of a microbrush, any other instrument can be used on the tip of which the liquid dam can be fixed and which functions as a handle for applying pressure over the composite (e.g., obturator). Removing the key should be easy. If this does not happen, it can be removed with the help of an explorer, the tip of which is inserted between the liquid dam and the occlusal surface at its edge.

4. Cavity preparation and filling to within 1.5 mm of the occlusal surface (Fig. 5.36)

   The class I cavity is filled in such a way as to obtain a superficial cavity that allows the application of the last layer of composite in a maximum thickness of 1.5 mm, for conventional packable composites. This thickness can be increased if bulk composites are used instead of conventional composites. If the depth of the prepared cavity does not exceed 1.5 mm, then the cavity can be filled with a single layer of conventional composite.

5. Application of the last composite layer and the occlusal key

   This layer will be applied bulk in the cavity, and a rough morphology will be quickly achieved with the spatula or with the obturator without polymerization. A Teflon strip is inserted between them to prevent adhesion of the composite to the occlusal key. Then press the key to shape the composite (Fig. 5.3).

6. The composite can be cured through the occlusal key for a few seconds

   (maximum 5), or the occlusal key can be removed without completely light curing the composite. In the latter case, there is a risk of detaching the composite when removing the occlusal key.

   Teflon tape can be substituted by applying a layer of adhesive or modeling resin over the occlusal key as a lubricant. It does not have to be polymerized. Even short polymerization time through the occlusal key would bond the

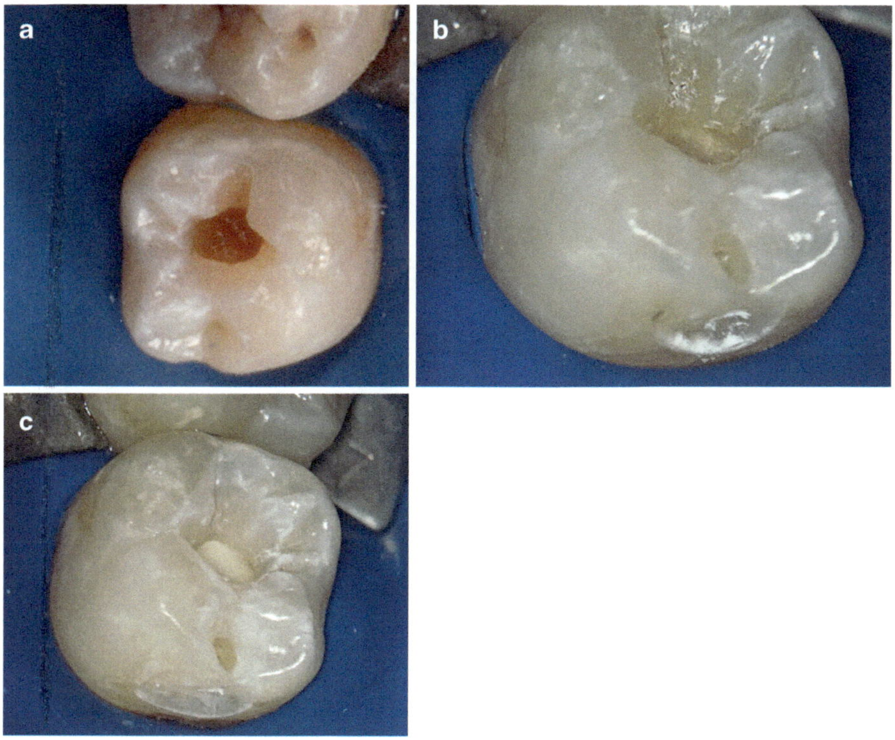

Fig. 5.36 Aspect of the cavity during preparation (**a**) and after finishing the cavity preparation (**b**), respectively, after applying the liner (**c**)

occlusal key to the composite. After stamping the morphology by pressing the key over the composite, the key and the excess are removed, and only then the composite will be polymerized.

The transfer of the initial morphology copied in the first phase will be done by placing the occlusal key in the same position and applying sufficient pressure to impregnate the initial morphology. The key can be pressed using a tweezer (Fig. 5.37b). This can prevent the key from breaking or the microbrush handle from bending. This allows pressure to be applied without bending the tip of the applicator.

Removal of occlusal key and excess material

After removing the occlusal key, the Teflon tape and excess composite reflowed from the cavity over the occlusal surface are also removed. This can be done with the tip of an explorer or with a spatula, and then polymerization is completed.

7. Occlusal adjustments, finishing, and polishing (Fig. 5.38)

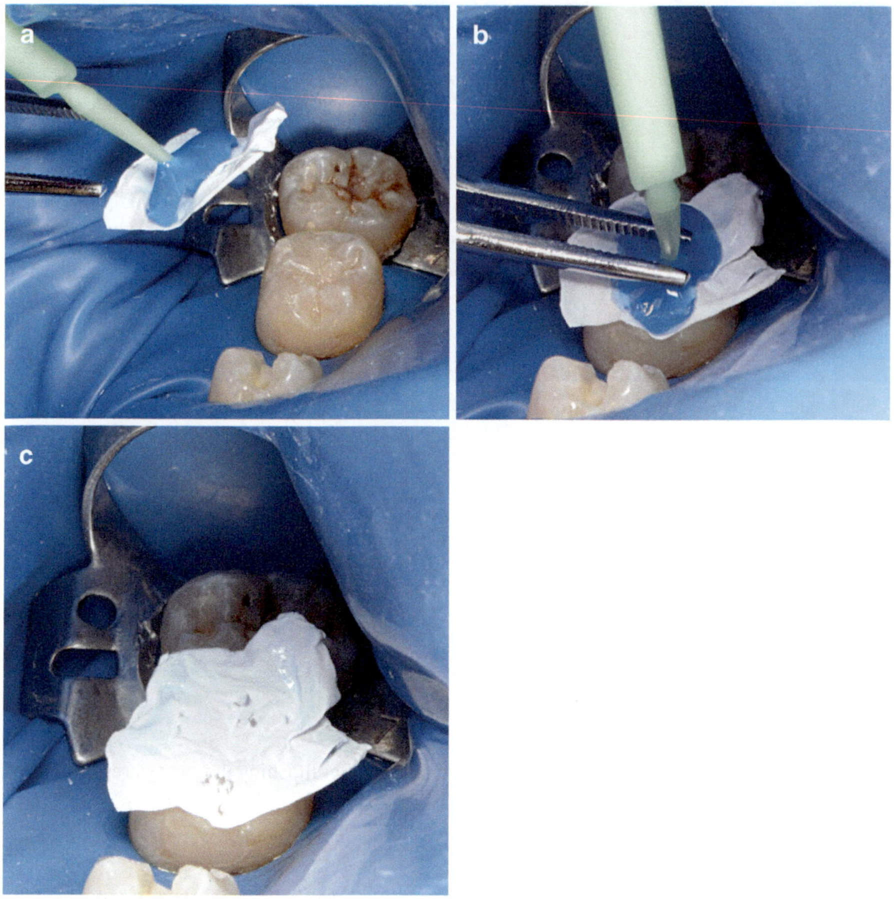

Fig. 5.37 Preparing the occlusal key by covering it with Teflon tape (**a**), applying it with pressure over the last layer of uncured composite resin (**b**), and removing the occlusal key from the tooth (**c**)

Fig. 5.38 Occlusal adjustments, finishing, and polishing

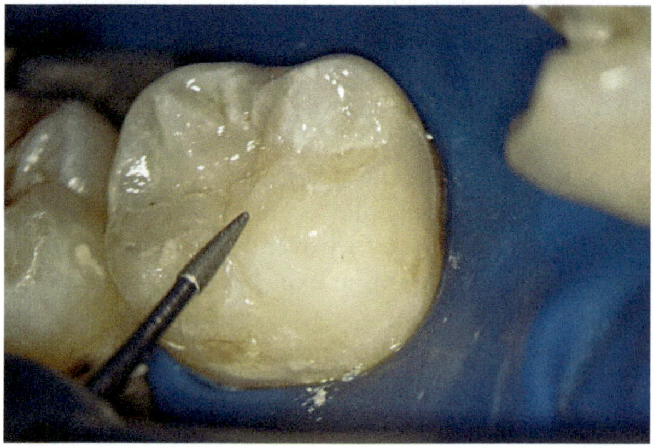

Difficulties that may arise	Possible solutions
The tip of the microbrush is in contact with the occlusal surface	Making another occlusal key
Fracture of the occlusal key at the time of applying pressure or bending of the handle of the microbrush	Pressing with the tip of a tweezer with the jaws placed on the occlusal key
Detachment of the uncured composite when removing the occlusal key	Press the composite and allow the composite to polymerize for a few seconds (maximum 5) through the occlusal key before removing it

5.4.5 Essential Line Technique

Main idea: The occlusal morphology of the posterior teeth can be done by drawing the main lines corresponding to the grooves and pits on the surface of the last composite layer. The "essential line technique" summarizes a natural anatomical relief by rendering the main elements.

Reproducing the natural occlusal anatomy is one of the most challenging and decisive steps in restoring posterior teeth. Lines can be a powerful tool to conform to an appropriate occlusal morphology. Thus, the main lines represented by the grooves and pits on the occlusal surfaces of each posterior tooth were identified. They form a universal pattern, an "occlusal map," for each type of posterior tooth, both in the upper teeth (Fig. 5.39) and in the lower ones (Fig. 5.40). By tracing them in the composite, an occlusal design can be obtained that respects the restoration's anatomy and a natural aspect (Fig. 5.41). Pigments can be added to the pits and grooves for a more natural result.

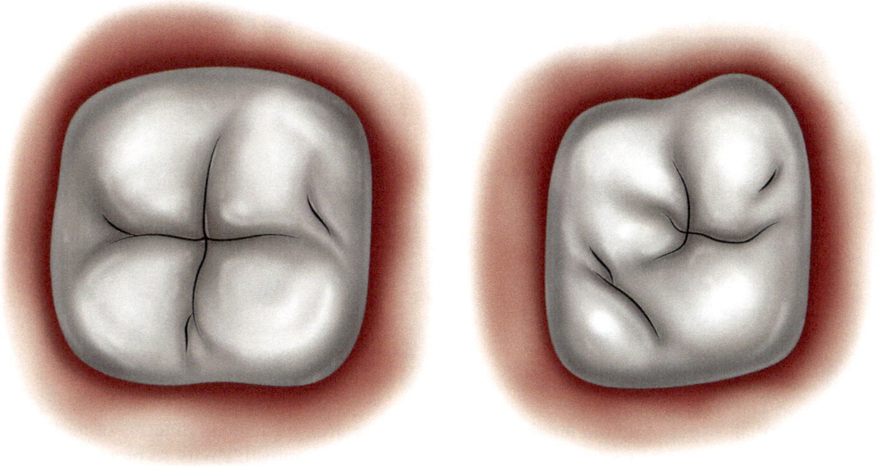

Fig. 5.39 Map of essential lines for a posterior maxillary teeth

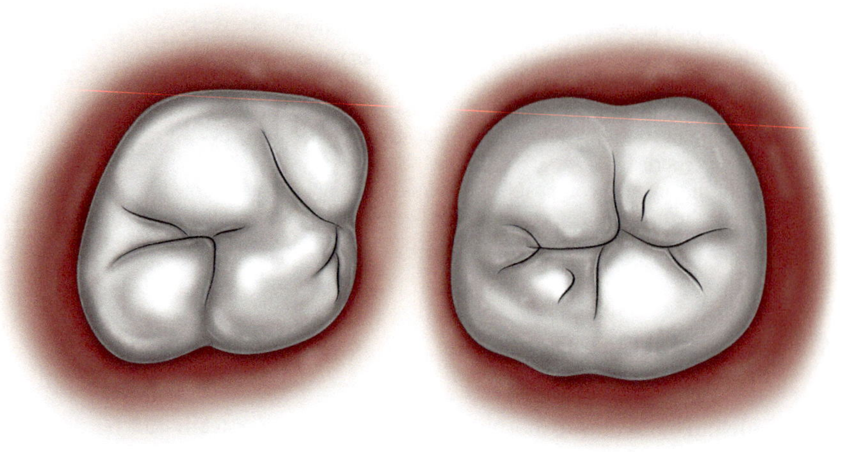

Fig. 5.40 Map of essential lines for mandibular posterior teeth

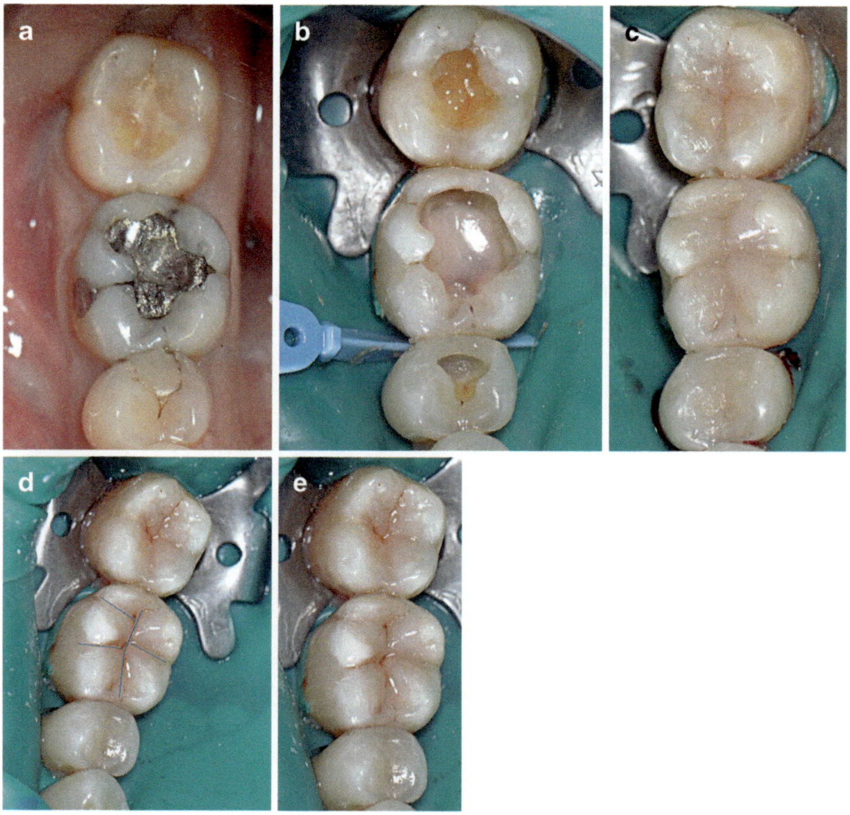

Fig. 5.41 Initial aspect of an old amalgam occlusal restoration inadequate in terms of aesthetics, morphology, and marginal sealing (**a**); aspect after amalgam removal, cavity re-preparation, and liner application (**b**); applying composite resin and drawing essential lines (**c**, **d**); final aspect after applying of pigments (**e**)

Among the advantages of this technique, we can mention the following:

- It is a simple technique.
- It leads to satisfactory aesthetic results.
- It is a quick technique, and it saves time.
- It allows a good calibration of the proportions of the different anatomical elements because the modeling is done simultaneously for all the cusps.
- It can be successfully applied for universal composites applied in layers and bulk composites.

Thus, this technique combines the advantages of the bulk filling technique with a modeling technique that uses the so-called minimal topographic lines to restore the tooth anatomy [17]. Essentially, the technique improves the simultaneous modeling technique by adding essential line tracing.

5.4.5.1 Working Technique

After anesthesia, isolation, and cavity preparation, it is filled with bulk or by stratification up to 1.5 mm from the occlusal surface. In the case of proximal cavities or MOD, the proximal walls are restored first by applying the centripetal technique. Thus, the first-class cavity of 1.5 mm depth is obtained, in which the last layer of composite will be applied. The location of the remaining intercuspid grooves is carefully identified (Fig. 5.42), and with the aid of an obturator or spatula, the morphology is roughly sculpted (Fig. 5.42). The appropriate cusp inclination is rendered according to the remaining cusp portions. With the help of a sharp instrument (the Fissura modeling instrument or an explorer), the intercuspid grooves are drawn, continuing the existing ones, and the central pit and the secondary pits are marked, these being important landmarks for drawing the lines. Thus, the essential lines will link these points (Fig. 5.42).

Difficulties that may arise	Possible solutions
Improper drawing of essential lines	Repeating the step
Composite stretch when drawing lines	Using a modeling resin

5.4.6 Bilaminar Technique for Posteriors

The main idea: Although the most common universal composite is used for direct restorations in the posterior area, the bilaminar layering technique of dentine and enamel composites aims to obtain functional and aesthetic direct restorations.

The bilaminar technique combines different shades of dentin and enamel and particular shades of achromatic enamel or pigments [18] of different colors (white, brown, amber, etc.). Dentin with a higher opacity is placed inside the cavity, while enamel is placed outside [19]. The application is carried out with any sequential

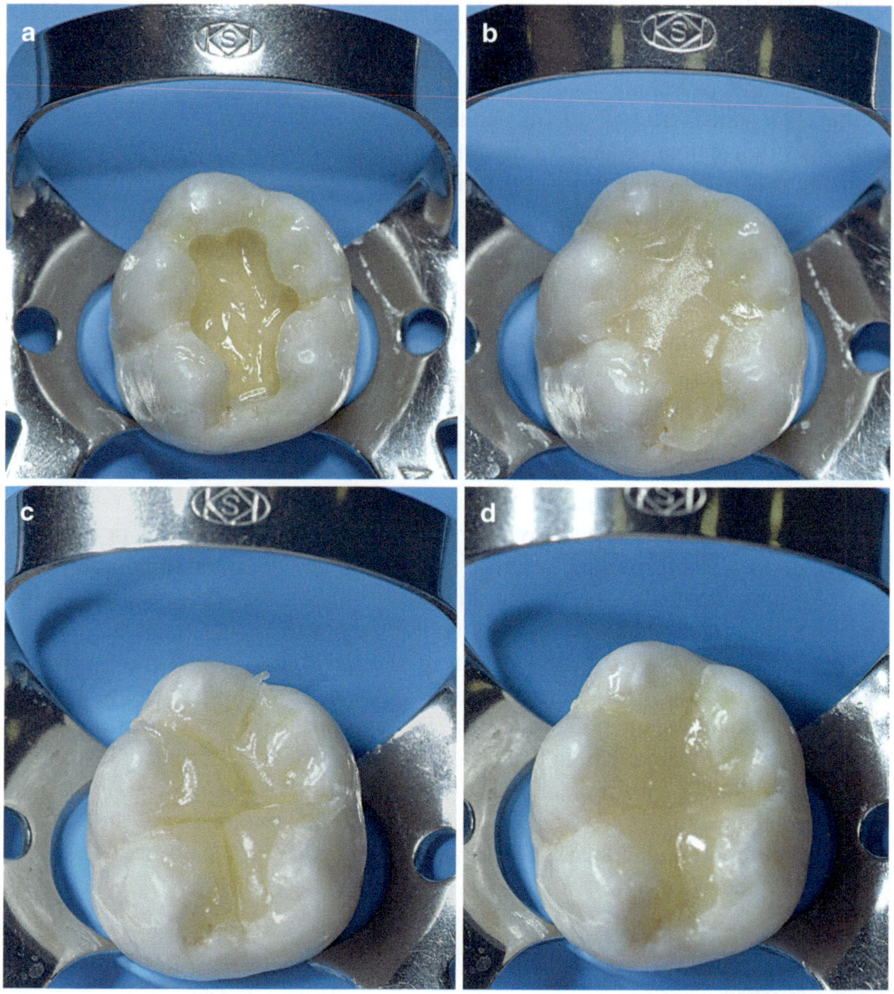

Fig. 5.42 Steps of a direct restoration using essential line technique: the initial aspect of the prepared cavity (**a**); composite application and a summary shaping of the composite (**b**); drawing essential lines (**c**); removing the excess, finalizing the occlusal morphology with the modeling brush (**d**)

technique (successive, symmetrical cusps, oblique layering). The restoration of the cusps will respect the internal anatomy of the teeth. Thus, the dentin layer will have a concave shape corresponding to the anatomy of natural teeth, and the enamel layer covering the dentin will have a convex shape [20].

5.4.6.1 Working Technique

The first layer of dentin is applied (in many cases, two shades darker than the desired color). After placing the dentin composite in the cavity, an obturator or a microbrush may be used to compact it (Fig. 5.43a–c). After light-curing, continue with the

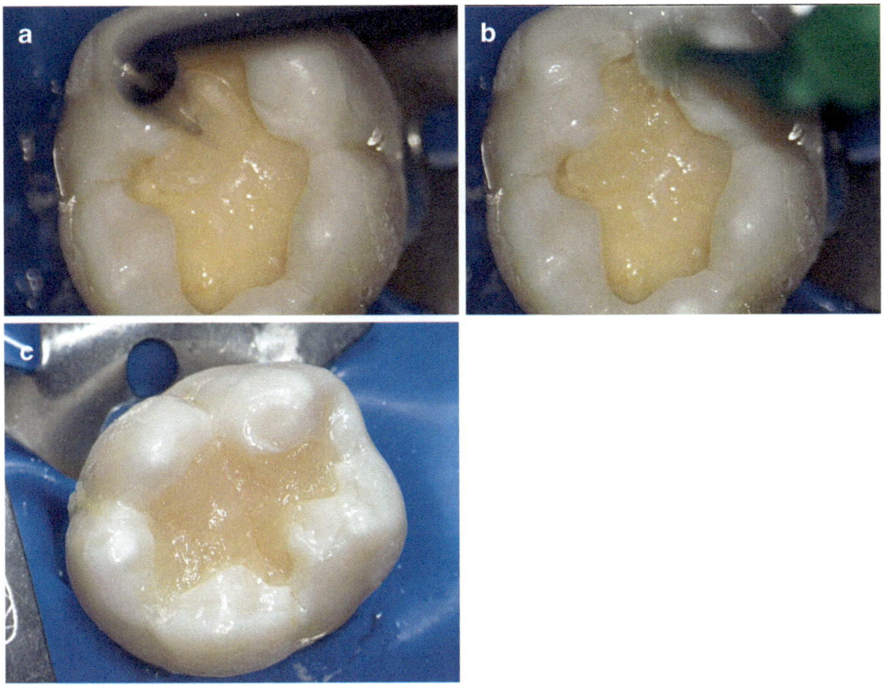

Fig. 5.43 Applying the dentin composite layer successively, starting with the first cusp (**a**) by compacting with the microbrush (**b**) to obtain a concave morphology of the cusp slopes (**c**)

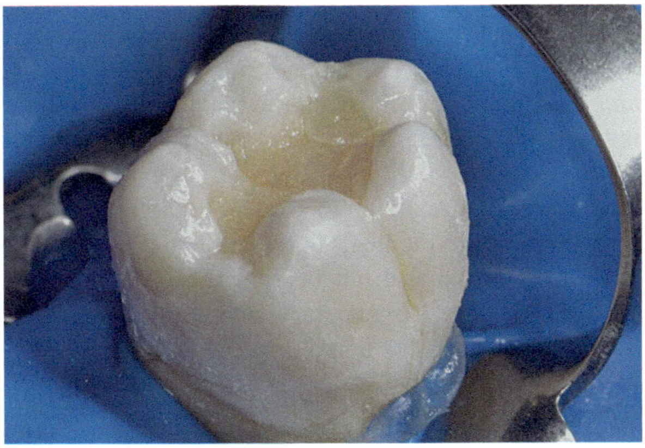

Fig. 5.44 Aspect after applying the dentin composite layer

following increments, keeping enough space for the last layer of enamel that will be applied. The application technique can be oblique layering or successive cusp technique. At the end of this step, a concave morphology of all the cusps will be obtained (Fig. 5.44), over which the enamel layer will be applied. This last layer will ensure the final conformation of the occlusal morphology. The recommended application technique is successive cusps, starting with the cusps on the one side (Fig. 5.45a–d)

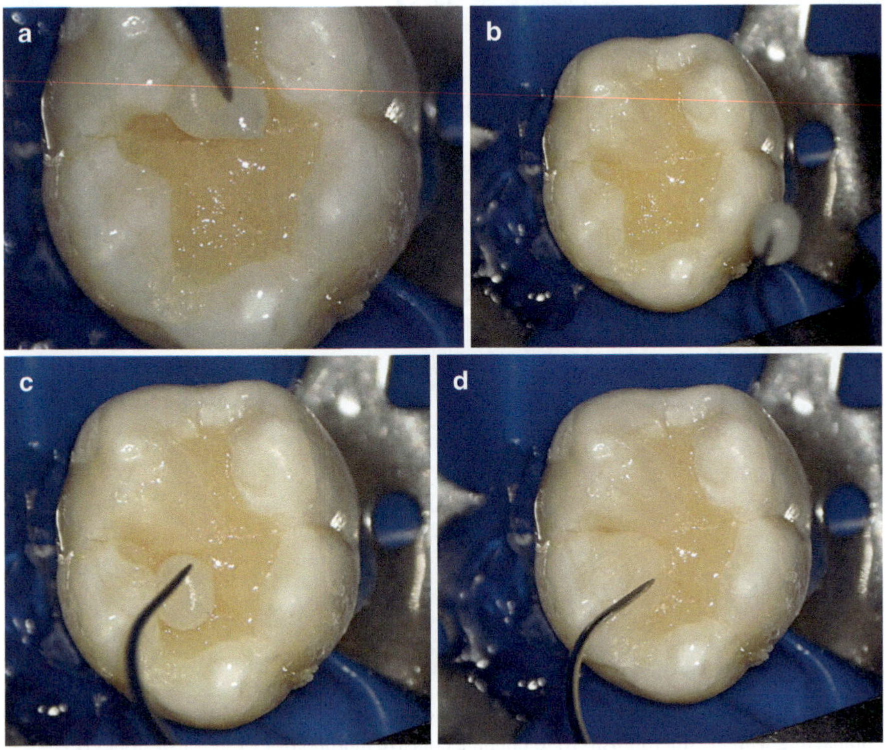

Fig. 5.45 Applying the enamel composite layer using the successive cusp technique (lingual cusps): buildup of the first lingual cusp (**a**); preparation of a new spherical increment of composite (**b**) for rebuilding the second lingual cusp (**c**) and modeling the cusp (**d**)

and continuing with those on the opposite side (Fig. 5.46a–c). The Fissura instrument and the modeling brush can be used or any other modeling instrument that the dentist considers helpful in obtaining appropriate occlusal relief. In situations of generalized pigmentation in grooves and pits, if the patient accepts, the dentist can apply dark brown pigments to restore a more natural aspect. Pigments can be applied with the tip of thin instruments (probe, fissure, endodontic files) or directly from the syringe. The excess pigment can be removed with a microbrush (Fig. 5.47a–d) until the desired shade is obtained (Fig. 5.48).

Difficulties that may arise	Possible solutions
Keeping insufficient space for the final layer of enamel	Removing a layer of dentin with a diamond bur, without water, air cleaning, and applying a new layer of adhesive followed by the enamel layer
Complete removal of the enamel layer in certain areas during occlusal adjustments	Additional finishing of exposed dentin composite areas

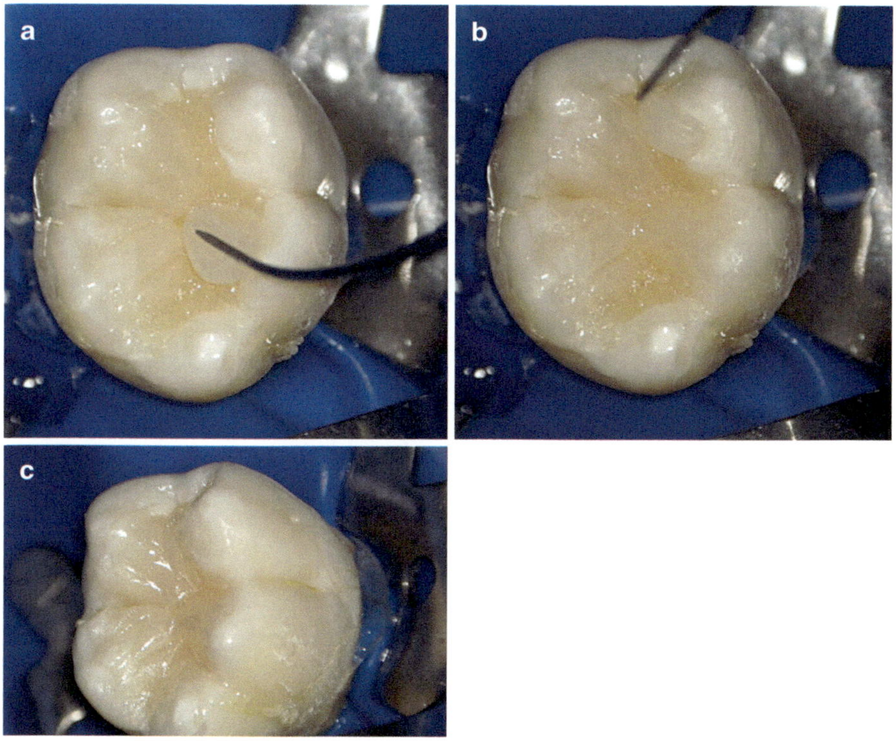

Fig. 5.46 Modeling the centro-buccal cusp (**a**) followed by the mesial (**b**) and distal (**c**) cusp

Conclusion

The restoration of posterior teeth can be achieved using several techniques, each of which has advantages and disadvantages that indicate their choice in certain cases. The dentist has the freedom to decide which technique to apply in each individual case to achieve the expected results. Furthermore, no statistically significant differences were found in marginal sealing using the stamp technique, bulk, successive cusp, modeling brushes, or magnification. This proves that clinicians can take the liberty of safely using multiple direct restoration techniques with similar results in marginal sealing/infiltration, one of the most common problems with direct restorations. None of the different incremental layering techniques (oblique, horizontal, vertical) seems superior to the others [21–24].

Review Questions

1. What is the biomimetic anatomical technique for class IV cavities?
2. What is the additive restoration techniques for incisal edges?
3. What is the simplified layering technique for classes III and IV cavities?
4. What is the monoshade technique?
5. What is the successive cusp technique?
6. What is the symmetrical cusp technique?

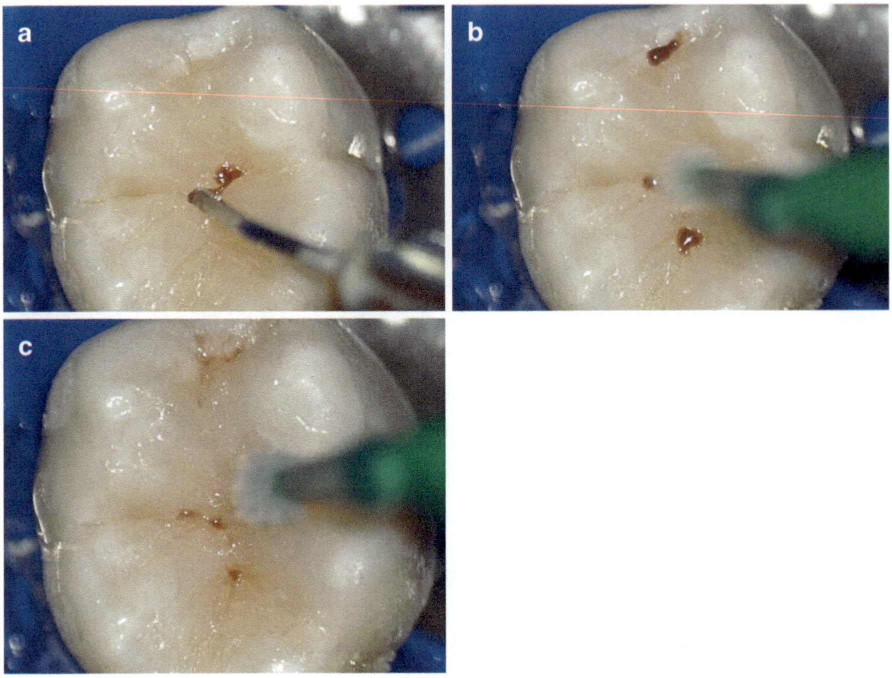

Fig. 5.47 Applying the brown pigment in the pits (**a**) and removing the excess with microbrush (**b**) until the desired result is achieved (**c**)

Fig. 5.48 Final aspect of the direct restoration

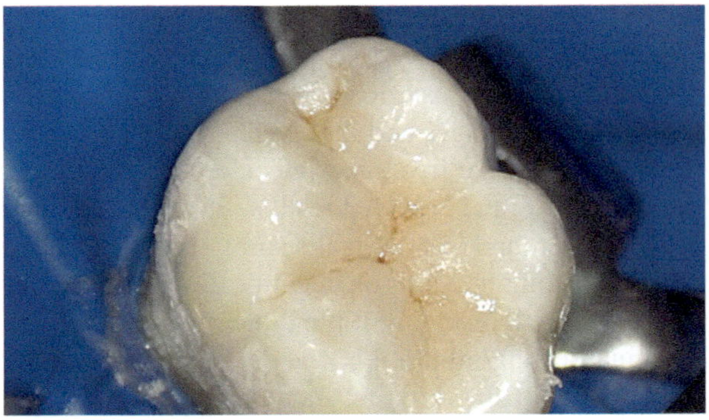

7. What is the simultaneous cusp technique?
8. What does the occlusal key stamp technique consist of?
9. What is the essential line technique?
10. What is the bilaminar technique for posteriors?

References

1. Fahl N Jr. Single-shaded direct anterior composite restorations: a simplified technique for enhanced results. Compend Contin Educ Dent. 2012;33(2):150–4.
2. Ikeda T, Murata Y, Sano H. Translucency of opaque-shade resin composites. Am J Dent. 2004;17(2):127–30.
3. Vanini L, Mangani F, Klimovskaia O. Conservative restoration of anterior teeth. Viterbo: ACME; 2007.
4. Chandrasekhar V, Rudrapati L, Badami V, Tummala M. Incremental techniques in direct composite restoration. J Conserv Dent. 2017;20(6):386–91.
5. Donly KJ, Jensen ME. Posterior composite polymerization shrinkage in primary teeth: an *in vitro* comparison of three techniques. Pediatr Dent. 1986;8:209–12.
6. Giachetti L, Scaminaci Russo D, Bambi C, Grandini R. A review of polymerization shrinkage stress: current techniques for posterior direct resin restorations. J Contemp Dent Pract. 2006;7:79–88.
7. Liebenberg WH. Successive cusp build-up: an improved placement technique for posterior direct resin restorations. J Can Dent Assoc. 1996;62(6):501–7.
8. Mackenzie L, Shortall AC, Burke FJ. Direct posterior composites: a practical guide. Dent Update. 2009;36(2):71–2, 74–6, 79–80 passim.
9. Scolavino S, Paolone G, Orsini G, Devoto W, Putignano A. The simultaneous modeling technique: closing gaps in posteriors. Int J Esthet Dent. 2016;11(1):58–81.
10. Dilley DC, Vann WF Jr, Oldenburg TR, Crisp RM. Time required for placement of composite versus amalgam restorations. ASDC J Dent Child. 1990;57:177–83.
11. Duque C, da Silva RC, dos Santos-Pinto L. Treatment options for the occlusal surface of first permanent molars. J Clin Pediatr Dent. 2004;29:5–9.
12. Attin T, Wegehaupt FJ. Impact of erosive conditions on tooth-colored restorative materials. Dent Mater. 2014;30:43–9.
13. Ramseyer ST, Helbling C, Lussi A. Posterior vertical bite reconstructions of erosively worn dentitions and the "stamp technique"—a case series with a mean observation time of 40 months. J Adhes Dent. 2015;17:283–9.
14. Alshehadat SA, Halim MS, Carmen K, Fung CS. The stamp technique for direct class II composite restorations: a case series. J Conserv Dent. 2016;19(5):490–3.
15. Rodrigues FP, Silikas N, Watts DC, Ballester RY. Finite element analysis of bonded model class I 'restorations' after shrinkage. Dent Mater. 2012;28:123–32.
16. González-López S, LucenaMartín C, de Haro-Gasquet F, Vilchez-Díaz MA, de Haro-Muñoz C. Influence of different composite restoration techniques on cuspal deflection: an in vitro study. Oper Dent. 2004;29:656–60.
17. Styleitaliano. Essential lines. https://www.styleitaliano.org/essential-lines/. Accessed 10 Mar 2022.
18. Vanini L. Light and color in anterior composite restorations. Pract Periodontics Aesthet Dent. 1996;8:673–82.
19. Ritter AV. Posterior resin-based composite restorations: clinical recommendations for optimal success. J Esthet Restor Dent. 2001;13:88–99.
20. Klaff D. Blending incremental and stratified layering techniques to produce an esthetic posterior composite resin restoration with a predictable prognosis. J Esthet Restor Dent. 2001;13:101–13.
21. Ferracane JL, Hilton TJ. Polymerization stress—is it clinically meaningful? Dent Mater. 2016;32:1–10.
22. Soares CJ, Faria-E-Silva AL, Rodrigues MP, Vilela ABF, Pfeifer CS, Tantbirojn D, Versluis A. Polymerization shrinkage stress of composite resins and resin cements—what do we need to know? Braz Oral Res. 2017;31:e62.

23. Dietschi D, Argente A, Krecji I, Mandikos M. In vitro performance of class I and class II composite restorations: a literature review on nondestructive laboratory trials: Part II. Oper Dent. 2013;38:182–200.
24. Bud MG, Pop RC, Pricope R, Mesaros A, Voina A, Delean A, Lucaciu O, Cîmpean S. Comparative microleakage outcomes of different techniques used for creating the occlusal anatomy in occlusal direct restorations using the dental operating microscope. Clin Exp Dent Res. 2022;8(6):1623–9. https://doi.org/10.1002/cre2.664.

6 Restoration Techniques in the Cervical Area

Cervical lesions benefit from minimally invasive preparations and can be restored with materials based on glass ionomers, giomers, composite resins, or combinations thereof. This chapter will focus on some key features of the cervical area, isolation, cavity preparation and choice of materials, and presentation of the working technique.

Cervical lesions can be carious and non-carious. The non-carious ones have a multifactorial etiology, and a single causal factor cannot always be blamed [1]. These are mainly represented by abrasion, abfraction, and erosion injuries. Their causes are mainly related to occlusion, bad habits, diet, poor hygiene, etc. [2]. Their presence causes sensitivity, and plaque retention affects the integrity and vitality of the tooth [3].

6.1 Peculiarities of the Cervical Area

The aspect of non-carious cervical lesions may be straight or curved, following the gingival edge, having a triangular shape in section (like a watermelon slice) and a glossy inner surface (Figs. 6.1 and 6.2).

The most cited etiological factor of non-carious cervical lesions is mechanical abrasion. Thus, in a survey conducted among dentists, 94% diagnosed non-carious cervical lesions as abrasions generated by tooth brushing in 66% of cases. Regarding the treatment, there was no single therapeutic preference [4]. Other authors, however, incriminate premature contacts and alcohol consumption [5] as the main reasons for the appearance of non-carious lesions of the cervical area.

Most frequently, these lesions cause sensitivity to cold and pressure, but over time, after the dentinal tubules' obliteration and the dentin's sclerosing, they become asymptomatic [6].

© The Author(s), under exclusive license to Springer Nature Switzerland AG 2024

M. Bud, *Direct Restorations*, https://doi.org/10.1007/978-3-031-55899-3_6

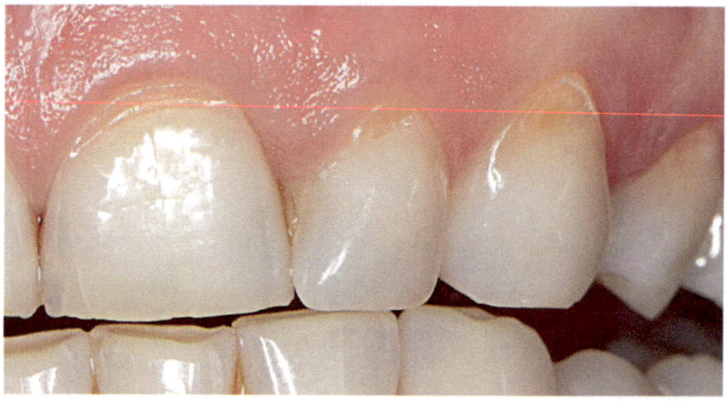

Fig. 6.1 Aspect of cervical lesions for teeth 21–23

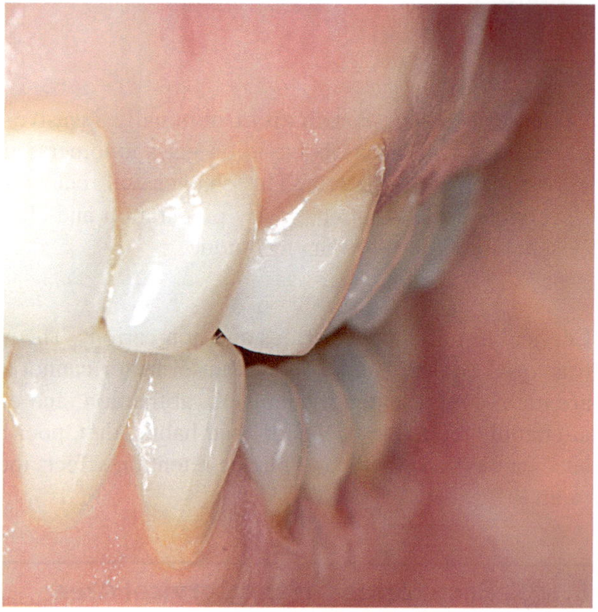

Fig. 6.2 Aspect of cervical lesions

It is possible to opt for monitoring small lesions or applying desensitizing substances, but their restoration is indicated when the lack of substance is medium or major.

The frequency of these restorations in clinical practice is high, and their restoration is not without difficulties. Most of the difficulties refer to the following aspects [7]:

- The high failure rate of these restorations through dislodging
- Frequency of excess material
- Increased incidence of secondary marginal decay

The failure of these restorations is related to several factors, among which we can mention:

- Adhesion problems caused by lack of enamel in these areas
- The different specific structure of the dentin in the cervical area that prevents adhesives from penetrating the obliterated dentinal tubules [3]
- The presence of sclerotic dentin, which decreases the quality of adhesion for both composite resins and RMGIc [8]
- Poor isolation affecting humidity control in the adhesive step of the restoration
- The mode of transmission of occlusal forces and their unfavorable distribution in the cervical area

6.2 Isolation, Cavity Preparation, and Choice of Materials

Isolation for the restoration of cervical lesions aims [9]:

- Achieving reasonable humidity control in the cavity
- Apical relocation of the gingival level to improve access and visibility and have good control of excess material and finishing

These objectives can be achieved using rubber dam and frontal, premolar (Fig. 6.3), or retraction clamps (brinkers). Apical relocation of the rubber dam sheet to improve access to the operative field can be achieved by:

- Placement of retraction cords in the sulcus prior to the application of clamps and rubber dam sheet
- Placing dental floss ligatures over the rubber dam, around the tooth
- Application of gingival retractor clamps, brinkers (type B) (Fig. 6.4)

The rubber dam sheet should be located apically so that it provides sufficient working space and the edges of the cavity do not interfere with the clamp or sheet (Fig. 6.5). Group isolation is preferred when working on a group of teeth, with the retractor clamp being moved to the tooth being treated, one at a time. Isolation of a single tooth can also be successfully achieved (Fig. 6.6). The level at which the

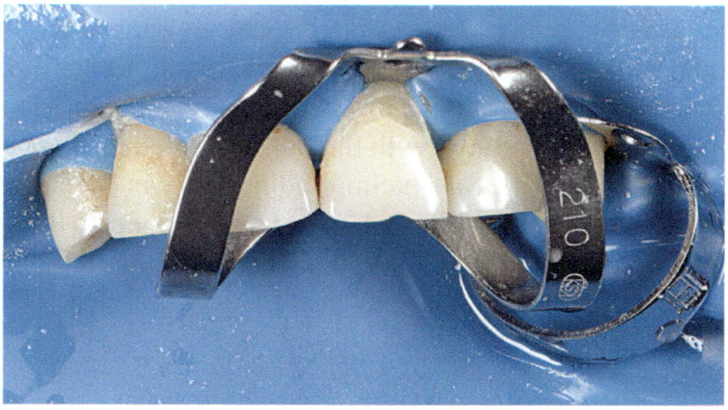

Fig. 6.3 Rubber dam isolation, clamps, and dental floss ligature

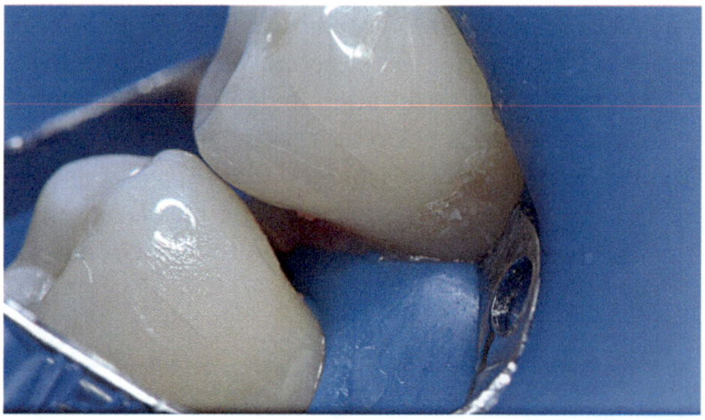

Fig. 6.4 Isolation with a rubber dam, application of gingival retractor clamp (brinker, B4)

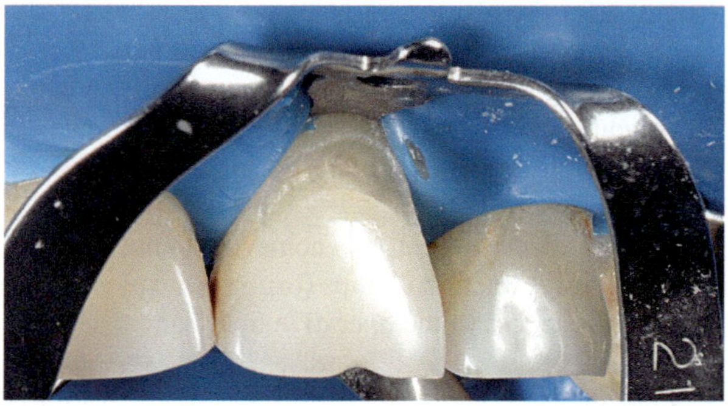

Fig. 6.5 Rubber dam sheet repositioned apically by placing a frontal rubber dam clamp

clamp is placed must allow good application and finishing of the composite and the transition zone between the tooth and composite (Fig. 6.7).

Liquid dam and Teflon tape can be used to improve rubber dam isolation. In certain situations, when the lesions extend subgingivally, it may be necessary to perform periodontal surgical interventions: gingivectomy, crown lengthening, and PET.

It is important to achieve rubber dam isolation for restoring cervical lesions, even sometimes clinicians underestimate it. The lack of it can frequently lead to the impossibility of humidity control compromising the adhesion of composite resins placed in the cavities. Clinically, this is directly related to secondary caries and partial or total dislodging of the restoration.

Cavity preparation in the cervical area must always be minimally invasive. In many cases, additional tissue removal is no longer necessary. Even in these cases, knowing that the adhesion is better on a freshly cut dentin, the cavity surface can be prepared by "wiping" with the bur. This method of preparation is supported by several studies [10]. Self-etching adhesives can be successfully used on this type of dentin. If resin-modified glass ionomer cements (RMGIc) are used, the dentin surface is treated with polyacrylic acid according to the manufacturer's instructions.

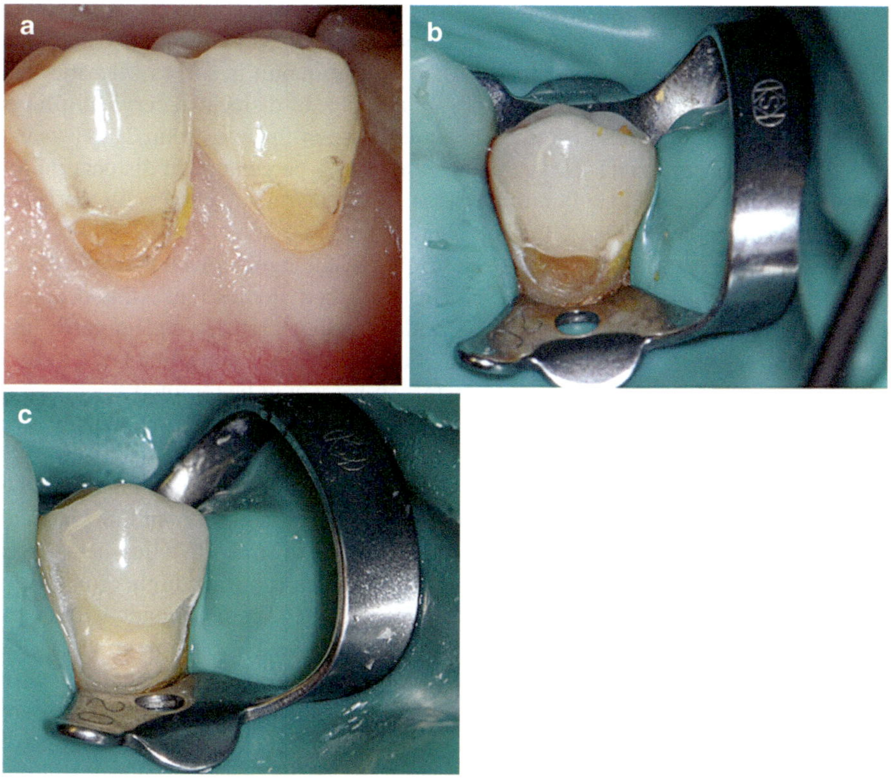

Fig. 6.6 Single tooth isolation: the aspect of the cervical caries before isolation (**a**); the aspect of the cervical cavity after single tooth isolation with the rubber dam (**b**); aspect of the class V prepared cavity (**c**)

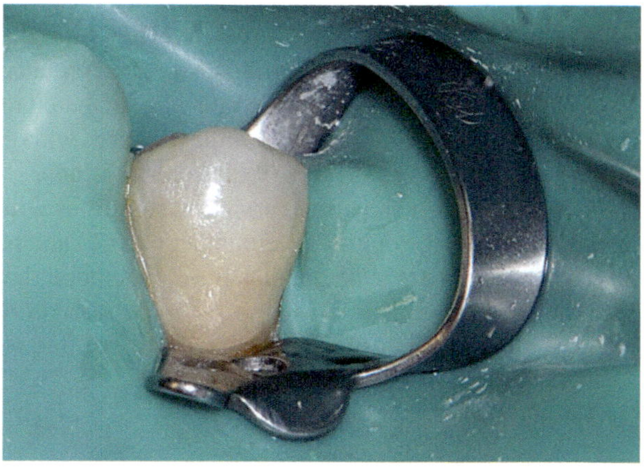

Fig. 6.7 The final aspect of a cervical cavity restoration made with resin composite

Restorations placed without prior dentin rotary preparation (cavity cleaning only) showed the highest failure rate by dislocation [10]. Moreover, the dislocation rate of these restorations increases with age as the dentin becomes sclerotic, the adhesion to it becoming weaker. Thus, the percentage of dislocated cervical fillings analyzed in a study increased from 31%, in the case of the age group 21–41 years, to 62%, in the age group 41–60 years, reaching a 71% percentage of dislocation for people over 60 years [11]. For this reason, the material of choice for geriatric patients may be conventional GIc [12].

The choice of restorative material can be quite challenging, given the wide range of composite resins and GIc available. The published studies make this decision even more difficult by the difficulty of understanding globally and unitarily the multitude of data reported by the literature. For example, we know that GIc has better adhesion to dentin than composite resins, so we would be tempted to choose it over resins. However, GIc's mechanical properties and long-term behavior are inferior to composites.

It has been stipulated that RMGIc, especially giomers, are the materials of choice for restoring lesions in the cervical area, having the best adhesion and mechanical resistance to the specific conditions in this area. In general, RMGIcs have been shown to last longer than composite resins [13]. Studies confirm a higher long-term success rate of restorations made with RMGIc (91.4%) than those made with composite resins (85.3%) [14]. In the case of evaluating the 10-year retention rate of restorations with conventional GIc, success was found in 83% of cases [15]. These results, which analyze the clinical behavior over time of different materials, are strongly influenced by the method of isolating the teeth for restoration, the age of the patients, the type of teeth analyzed, the properties of the material (generation, brand), but also the practical skills of the dentist and the lifestyle and occlusion of the patient. So, the above results must also be understood through the lens of all these aspects.

However, there are authors who, based on the superior properties of composite resins, indicate these materials as being of choice for restoring cervical lesions, associated or not with liners based on GIc/RMGIc [16]. Restoration of cervical cavities with a packable composite has been associated with a clinical success rate of only 70% [17]. The high failure rate was attributed to the stiffness of the composite used. Thus, using a flowable composite resin with greater elasticity was thought to improve the clinical success of these restorations.

A clinical study evaluating cervical restorations with a flowable composite demonstrated that all restorations were intact (100%) and had no postoperative sensitivity after 1 year [18]. Many studies have concluded that using flowable composites for non-carious cervical lesions is a good choice [19] and can be considered the materials for restoring cervical lesions [16, 20] due to their superior physical and aesthetic properties compared to GIc/RMGIc.

6.3 Working Technique

Achieving rubber dam isolation begins with applying a gingival retraction cord (Fig. 6.8) for apical relocation of the gingival level. This leads to lowering the gingival level (Fig. 6.9), providing more space to allow positioning of the rubber dam clamp at the most apical level possible without traumatizing the periodontium (Fig. 6.10). The cavity preparation is minimally invasive, without additionally removing the hard tooth structure, by slightly "wiping" the internal surface of the cavity with the bur.

The disinfection of the cavity is done with chlorhexidine applied on a cotton bullet or microbrush. Demineralization is achieved by applying 35–37% orthophosphoric acid for 15 s on dentin and 30 s on enamel (Fig. 6.11). Increasing the demineralization time from 15 to 30 s may improve adhesion to sclerotic dentin in non-carious cervical lesions, but this improvement depends on the type and brand of adhesive used [21]. The adhesive is applied by brushing for 20 s and gently dried for 5 s according to the manufacturer's instructions (Fig. 6.12). The application of the restorative material is made with as much precision as possible, without excess, so

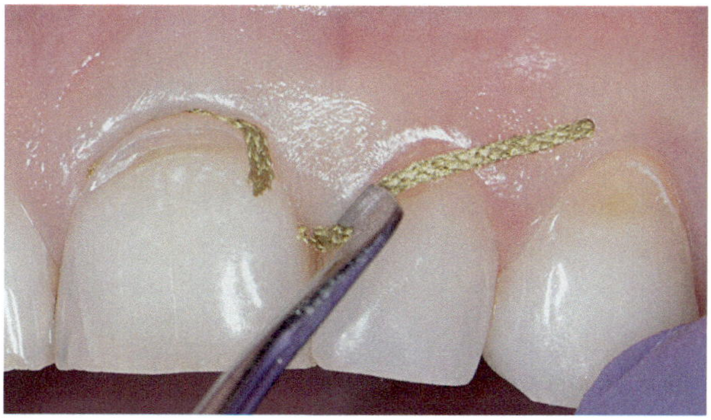

Fig. 6.8 Application of the gingival retraction cord in the sulcus for apical repositioning of the gingiva

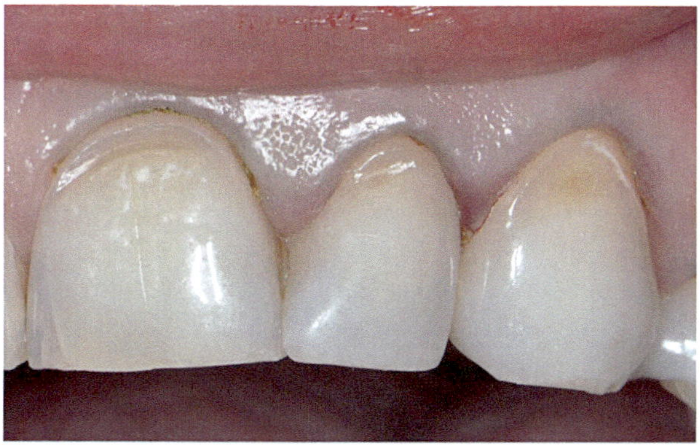

Fig. 6.9 The gingival level's aspect after applying the retraction thread in the sulcus

Fig. 6.10 Aspect of a cervical lesion on tooth 21 after application of gingival retraction cord, rubber dam sheet, and clamp to achieve group isolation

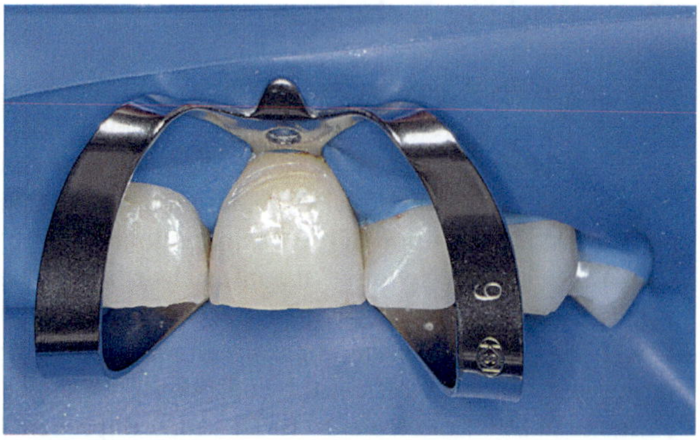

Fig. 6.11 Application of etching

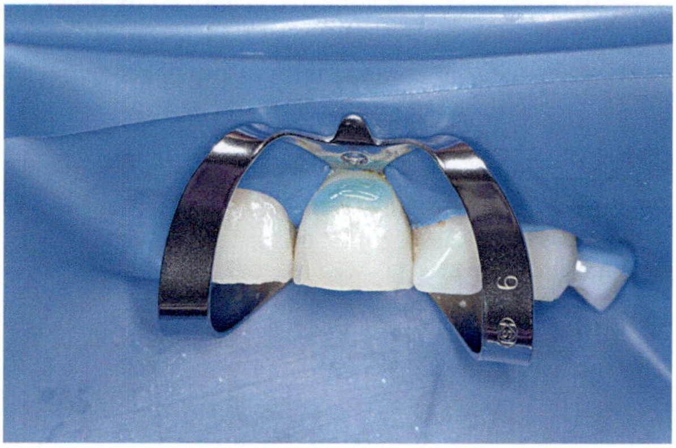

Fig. 6.12 Applying the adhesive

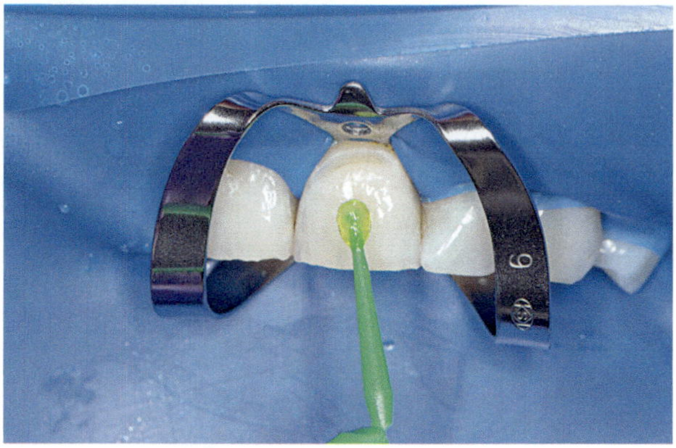

that it does not require significant interventions with rotary instruments. A modeling brush can be used to remove the excess material, improve the marginal sealing of the composite resin, and obtain a glossy surface (Fig. 6.13).

Fig. 6.13 Application of composite resin and improved marginal sealing using a brush

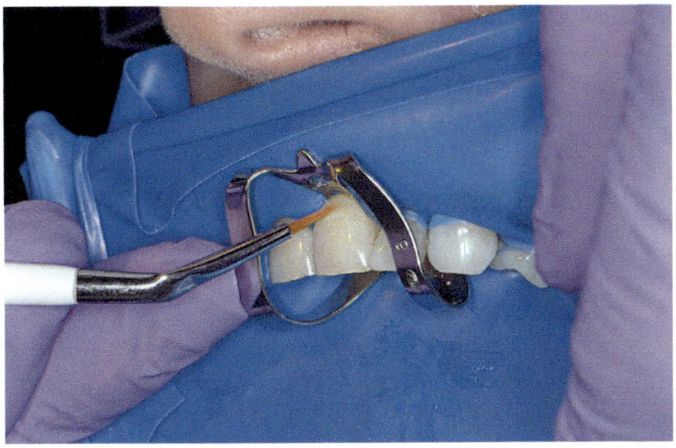

Fig. 6.14 Finishing with the yellow diamond bur

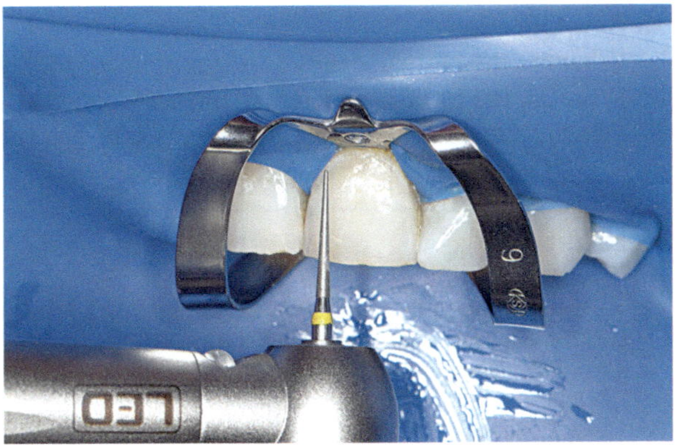

Fig. 6.15 Moving the rubber dam clamp to the next tooth to be restored [16]

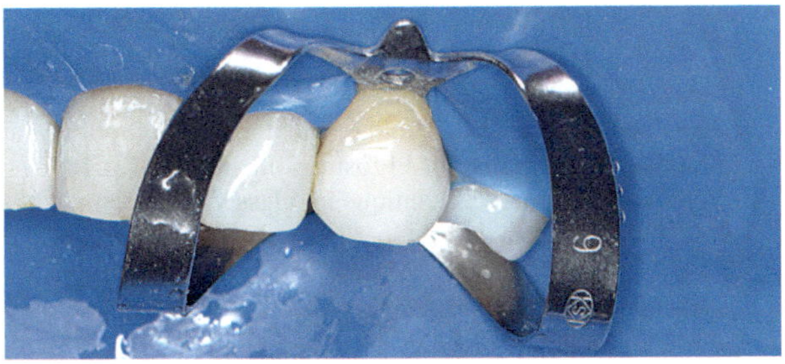

If, however, additional finishing is required, fine diamond burs (yellow or red) can be used (Fig. 6.14). The final finishing is done with rotary instruments at low speed: rubber cups, discs, spirals, and brushes with finishing pastes. Applying a surface sealant for composite resins improves marginal sealing and long-term material properties [7]. In the case presented in the image, cervical lesions at the level of several teeth were restored after rubber dam isolation. After the first was made, the clamp was moved to the next tooth, and the same steps were repeated (Fig. 6.15).

Difficulties that may arise	Possible solutions
The subgingival extension of the cavities limits visibility and access, making it impossible to fix the rubber dam sheet and achieve isolation	Gingivectomy or crown lengthening
The impossibility of good isolation with the rubber dam	Choosing materials based on GIc, less sensitive to humidity
Bleeding of the gum when inserting the retraction cord or applying the rubber dam clamps	Hemostasis with a cold water jet or specific hemostatic solutions

Conclusions

Cervical lesions benefit from a minimally invasive preparation and can be successfully restored with GIc, RMGIc, giomers, compomers, and packable or fluid composite resins. RMGIc and flowable composite resins are preferred due to their properties compatible with the specifics of the cervical area.

Review Questions

1. What are the particularities of restorations of the cervical lesions?
2. What are the recommended materials, and what advantages should they present?
3. What is the working technique for performing a cervical restoration?

References

1. Bader JD, Levitch LC, Shugars DA, Heymann HO, McClure F. How dentists classified and treated non-carious cervical lesions. J Am Dent Assoc. 1993;124(5):46–54.
2. Chan DC, Browning WD, Pohjola R, Hackman S, Myers ML. Predictors of non-carious loss of cervical tooth tissues. Oper Dent. 2006;31(1):84–8.
3. Lussi A, Hellwig E, Ganss C, Jaeggi T. Dental erosion. Oper Dent. 2009;34(3):251–62.
4. Litonjua LA, Andreana S, Cohen RE. Toothbrush abrasions and noncarious cervical lesions: evolving concepts. Compend Contin Educ Dent. 2005;26(11):767–8, 770–4, 776 passim.
5. Yoshizaki KT, Francisconi-Dos-Rios LF, Sobral MA, Aranha AC, Mendes FM, Scaramucci T. Clinical features and factors associated with non-carious cervical lesions and dentin hypersensitivity. J Oral Rehabil. 2017;44(2):112–8.
6. Hattab FN, Yassin OM. Etiology and diagnosis of tooth wear: a literature review and presentation of selected cases. Int J Prosthodont. 2000;13(2):101–7.
7. Perez CR. Alternative technique for class V resin composite restorations with minimum finishing/polishing procedures. Oper Dent. 2010;35(3):375–9.
8. Francisconi LF, Scaffa PM, de Barros VR, Coutinho M, Francisconi PA. Glass ionomer cements and their role in the restoration of non-carious cervical lesions. J Appl Oral Sci. 2009;17(5):364–9.
9. Meraner M. Soft tissue management for difficult cervical restorations. Gen Dent. 2006;54(2):117–20.
10. Lührs AK, Jacker-Guhr S, Günay H, Herrmann P. Composite restorations placed in non-carious cervical lesions-which cavity preparation is clinically reliable? Clin Exp Dent Res. 2020;6(5):558–67.
11. Bayne SC, Heymann HO, Sturdevant JR, Wilder AD, Sluder TB. Contributing co-variables in clinical trials. Am J Dent. 1991;4(5):247–50.

12. Kampanas NS, Antoniadou M. Glass ionomer cements for the restoration of non-carious cervical lesions in the geriatric patient. J Funct Biomater. 2018;9(3):42.
13. Santiago SL, Passos VF, Vieira AHM, de Navarro MFL, Lauris JRP, Franco EB. Two-year clinical evaluation of resinous restorative systems in non-carious cervical lesions. Braz Dent J. 2010;21:229–34.
14. Stewardson DA, Thornley P, Bigg T, Bromage C, Browne A, Cottam D, Dalby D, Gilmour J, Horton J, Roberts E, et al. The survival of class V restorations in general dental practice. Part 2, early failure. Br Dent J. 2011;210:E19.
15. Sidhu SK. Clinical evaluations of resin-modified glass-ionomer restorations. Dent Mater. 2010;26:7–12.
16. Perez Cdos R, Gonzalez MR, Prado NA, de Miranda MS, Macêdo Mde A, Fernandes BM. Restoration of noncarious cervical lesions: when, why, and how. Int J Dent. 2012;2012:687058.
17. McCoy RB. Clinical success of class V composite resin restorations without mechanical retention. J Am Dent Assoc. 1998;129:593–9.
18. Estafan D, Schulman A, Calamia J. Clinical effectiveness of a class V flowable composite resin system. Compend Contin Educ Dent. 1999;20:11–5.
19. Kubo S, Yokota H, Yokota H, Hayashi Y. Three-year clinical evaluation of a flowable and a hybrid resin composite in non-carious cervical lesions. J Dent. 2010;38:191–200.
20. Pecie R, Krejci I, García-Godoy F, Bortolotto T. Noncarious cervical lesions (NCCL)—a clinical concept based on the literature review. Part 2: restoration. Am J Dent. 2011;24(3):183–92.
21. Lopes GC, Baratieri CM, Baratieri LN, Monteiro S Jr, Cardoso Vieira LC. Bonding to cervical sclerotic dentin: effect of acid etching time. J Adhes Dent. 2004;6(1):19–23.

Finishing and Occlusal Fitting Techniques

7

The primary goal of this work stage is to achieve a final direct restoration without excess material, with smooth surfaces, and without surface voids or roughness. This favors increasing the restoration's longevity, reducing the probability of marginal secondary caries' occurrence, and ensuring the health of the periodontal tissues. This chapter will present how to manage the contour finishing and excess removal, working protocols for finishing the shape and occlusal adjustments, surface finishing and roughness reduction, and finishing and polishing of direct restorations of anterior teeth.

The finalization of contour, shape, and roughness after the final polymerization is the final stage of direct restoration. This finishing stage leads to obtaining the following advantages:

- Acceptable, undetectable margins of the direct restoration on probing.
- Periodontal health provided by the lack of excess and irregular surfaces.
- Occlusal (posterior) and palatal (anterior) morphology to ensure a proper occlusion.
- The glossy surface obtained retains less plaque.
- Increasing the longevity of the restoration.
- Improving the aesthetic effect.

Supplementary Information The online version contains supplementary material available at https://doi.org/10.1007/978-3-031-55899-3_7. The videos can be accessed individually by clicking the DOI link in the accompanying figure caption or by scanning this link with the SN More Media App.

© The Author(s), under exclusive license to Springer Nature Switzerland AG 2024

M. Bud, *Direct Restorations*, https://doi.org/10.1007/978-3-031-55899-3_7

Therefore, improper final morphology, the presence of excess material on the contour of the restoration, the rough surface, and marginal or surface voids increase the risks of:

- Plaque retention.
- Gingival inflammation
- Periodontal problems
- TMJ disorders
- Marginal or recurrent cavity

After the completion of the composite application stage and the completion of the final polymerization, the direct restorations are evaluated by the operator after prior drying with the air jet from the point of view of the following criteria:

- Marginal sealing. In visible and easily accessible areas, marginal sealing is assessed with the tip of a dental probe. Marginal voids or marginal excess can be detected in this way. In the area of the gingival margin, where access with the tip of the probe is impossible, the evaluation is done with dental floss or radiologically.
- Morphology, surface voids in the composite, cracks, and fractures. They can be evaluated visually or tactilely with the help of the probe. If they are large, they can require the addition of material. Adjustment of the restored occlusal relief is made by checking with articulation paper to conserve the proper static and dynamic occlusion.
- The roughness of the obtained composite surface. This is verified clinically with an explorer tip and visually by inspection.

Therefore, three categories of adjustments may be required:

(a) Contour finishes to remove excess circumferentially extruded material, partially or continuously, along the boundaries of the obturated cavity
(b) Occlusal adjustments through shape adjustments and reduction of the size giving relief to the restoration to obtain a final morphology correct and occlusally aligned with that of the opposing teeth
(c) Polishing the surface of the restoration to decrease the surface roughness

These steps are performed in the same session immediately after the final polymerization is completed and are known as the finishing, occlusal fitting, and polishing steps.

The instruments used in these steps can be hand instruments (curettes) or rotary instruments used at high or low speeds. There must be control of pulp overheating during these procedures by water cooling both in the high-speed and low-speed pieces. Rotary instruments used at high speed (in a high-speed piece) must be used with utmost care as there is a risk of accidentally removing too large amounts of the composite material or damaging the tooth in the marginal sealing area. At this stage, the use of magnification can be of considerable help.

Throughout the implementation of these stages, both the neighboring teeth and the marginal periodontium must be protected not to be damaged by touching with manual or rotary instruments.

7.1 Finishing the Contour and Removing the Excess

This step commonly begins with contour adjustments by removing excess material extruded outside the cavity's contour. Frequently, excess material is generated in the layering stage at the second-, third-, and fourth-class cavities without proper adaptation of the matrices. The excess can also be generated during the occlusal, buccal, or palatal composite superficial layer modeling.

To remove excess material, we can use the following tools:

- Diamond burs
- Metal or celluloid abrasive strips
- Rotating abrasive disks
- Curette (Fig. 7.1a)
- Scalpel blades (Fig. 7.1b)

By removing excess composite, we aim to avoid an over-contoured restoration, i.e., one that protrudes from the contour of the cavity created, in order not to produce food or plaque retention, gingival inflammation, and, last but not least, to respect the correct anatomy of the tooth. The use of magnification has been shown to reduce by 40% the risk of over-contouring fillings due to excess material [1].

Deficient adaptation of the matrix on the tooth is clinically translated into the appearance of excess material accompanied by inflammation of the interdental papilla and food retention. These can lead over time to caries on adjacent teeth (Fig. 7.2), secondary marginal caries on the restored tooth, and periodontal problems. Published studies indicate the existence of excess material in direct restorations in second-class cavities in 25–76% of cases [2]. Standard matrix systems

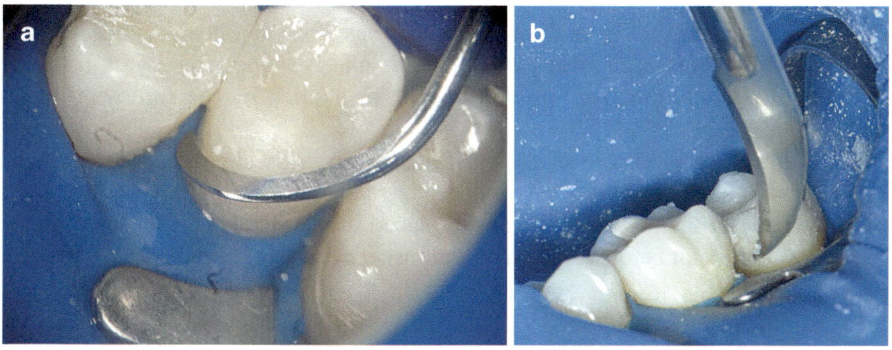

Fig. 7.1 Removal of excess composite resin generated by the lack of tight adaptation of matrices in the case of second-class cavity restorations: curette from the composite modeling kit (**a**); scalpel blade with curved tip no. 12 (**b**)

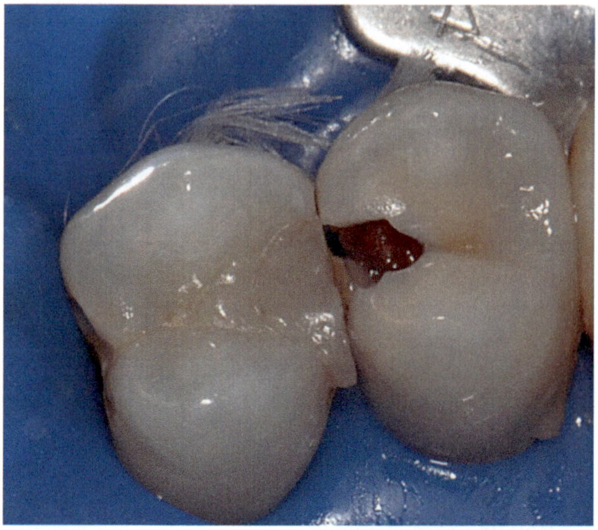

Fig. 7.2 Inadequate occlusal-distal filling on the first premolar with a major excess of material that generated food retention and, consequently, a mesial cavity on the first premolar

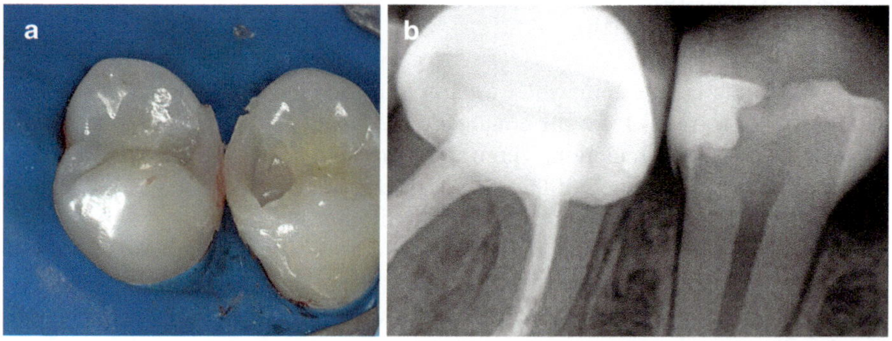

Fig. 7.3 Restoration of the proximal walls according to the centripetal technique in premolars with a consecutive generation of composite in occlusal, buccal, and oral embrasures (**a**). The excess composite resin material is visible radiologically in the gingival margin area (**b**)

cannot be adapted initially in all clinical situations, so sometimes it is necessary to supplement with auxiliary means that adapt the matrix to the anatomy of the tooth: liquid dam, Teflon tape, fixation with fingers, or fixation by pressure with instruments (e.g., mouth spatula).

Excess material in visible areas (Fig. 7.3a) can be easily identified, accessed, and removed with a curette, bur, abrasive disks, or scalpel blade (Fig. 7.4).

If the edge of the preparation was not placed in the visible (self-cleaning) area, the excess could not be observed by visual inspection but only radiographically.

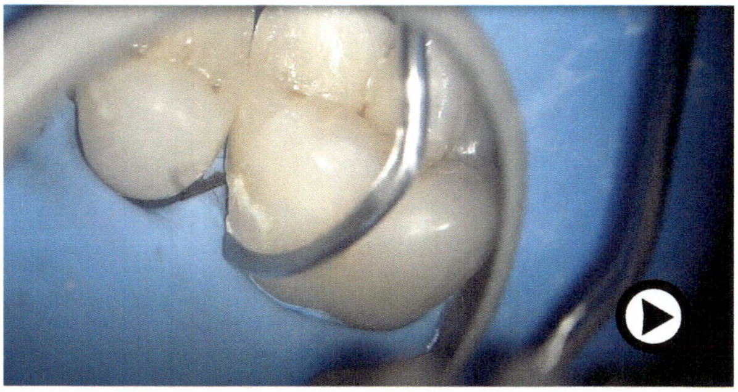

Fig. 7.4 Excess material in visible areas removed with a curette from the LM-Arte modeling kit (▶ https://doi.org/10.1007/000-bqv)

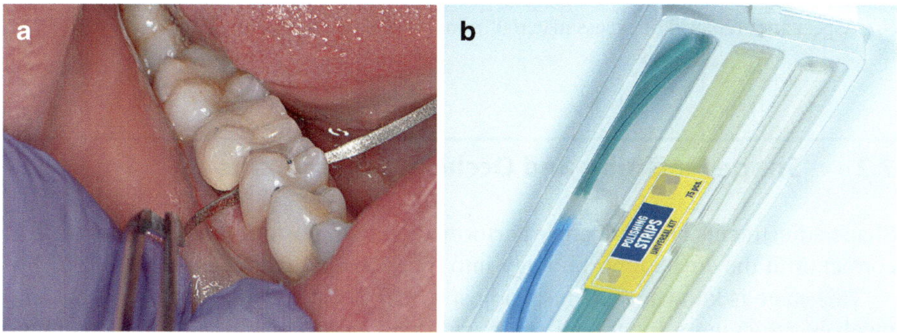

Fig. 7.5 Narrow metal abrasive strip inserted below the level of the contact point to remove excess composite resin material from the gingival margin area (**a**). Abrasive celluloid tape with an inactive zone allows interdental insertion from the occlusal side without affecting the restored contact point (**b**)

Excess material in the gingival margin area is the most difficult to identify on inspection and probing. It can be identified by flossing or radiologically (Fig. 7.3b). If this excess is detected, the most affordable way to remove it is to use a metal abrasive strip cut in half lengthwise to make it narrower. This can be inserted interdentally from the buccal or oral side directly under the contact point and, with its help, remove the excess (Fig. 7.5a). We avoid inserting the abrasive tape from the occlusal embrasure not to scrape the composite in the contact area. If the strip has an inactive, smooth, and nonabrasive zone, it can be inserted interdentally from the occlusal side without the risk of damaging the contact point (Fig. 7.5b). If excess composite at the level of the gingival margin is not detected and removed immediately after it is made, it can lead over time to bone resorption following persistent gingival inflammation (Fig. 7.6).

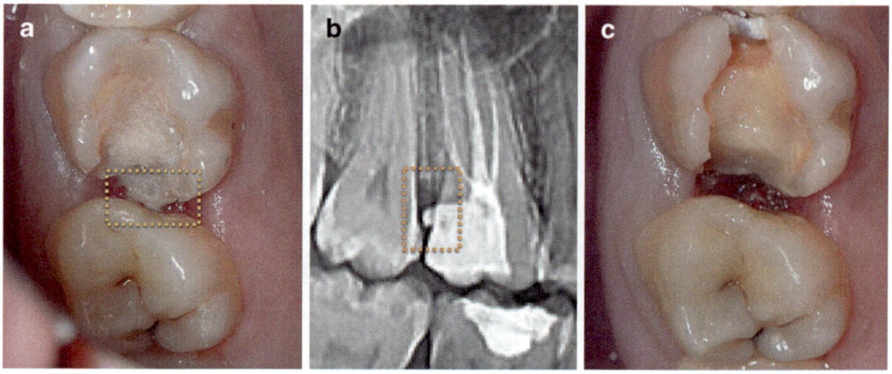

Fig. 7.6 Old obturation made of composite resin inadequate as aesthetic, morphology, marginal sealing, with excess material at the gingival margin (**a**). Excess material is visible on a radiograph (**b**). Aspect after removal of excess material from the interdental area (**c**)

7.2 Shape Finishing and Occlusal Adjustments

Shape adjustments are frequently performed on both posterior and anterior teeth to correct or fit the created morphology into function and aesthetics.

This stage is known as occlusal adjustments. Correct restoration of morphology involves achieving a functional static and dynamic occlusion with stable occlusal stops without active, passive interference or premature contacts (see Chap. 2).

Occlusal tactile sensitivity is in the case of natural teeth up to 8–10 microns [3, 4]. Thus, patients can detect dimensional differences equal to or greater than these values.

These checks are performed using conventional occlusion paper or joint films with thicknesses below 15 microns (shimstock) (Fig. 7.7a, b).

The latter are joint films made of a metallic polyester (shimstock) with a thickness of 12 μ (e.g., Arti-Fol Metallic, Bausch, Koln, Germany). They have an excellent color transfer capacity, and the film is antistatic and can be easily applied to be resistant to tearing.

Occlusion analysis can be done electronically using the T-scan system (Tekscan Inc., Boston, USA). It consists of a handpiece into which a disposable occlusal sensor is inserted. The intraoral sensor is connected to a computer via the USB port, and its software analyzes the received information. The T-scan occlusal analysis system can analyze occlusal contacts and forces transmitted to direct and indirect restorations and prosthetic work performed on vital or endodontically treated natural teeth.

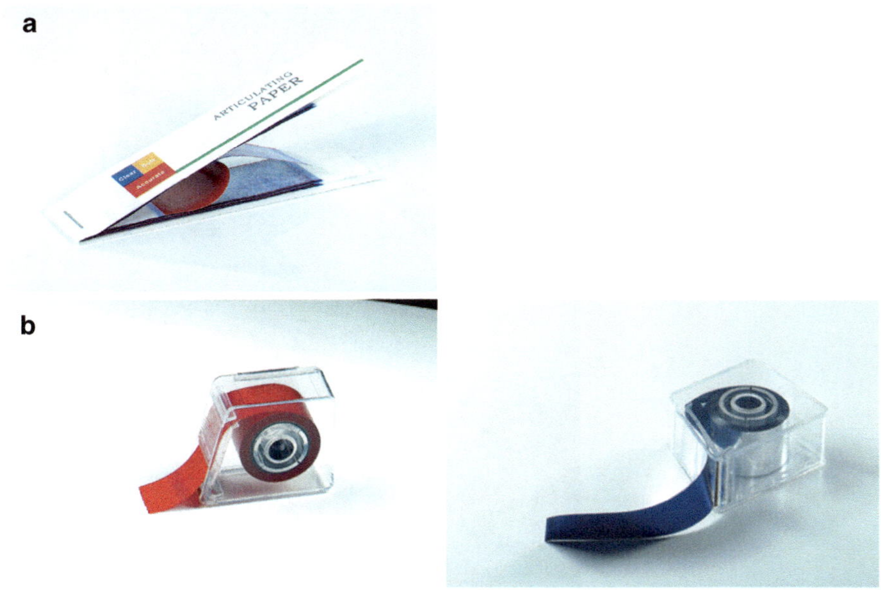

Fig. 7.7 Conventional occlusion paper (**a**) and 12-micron-thick shimstock (**b**)

7.2.1 Working Technique

The surfaces are dried, and then the patient is asked to occlude by biting on the occlusion paper (Fig. 7.8) in a centric relation, maximum intercuspation, and performing propulsive movements and left-right laterality. The occlusion is examined by analyzing the colored marks left on the teeth by the occlusion paper following these movements.

Examining the occlusion paper consists of identifying the perforations that may occur and locating the areas of contact it has produced on the tooth surfaces.

The tighter the contact, the more difficult the occlusion paper will be to remove by manual traction [5]. It has been shown that the intensity of the color left by the occlusion paper on the surface of the teeth is not proportional to the force of the contacts. Thus, in areas of closer contact, the colored marking will be imprinted on the periphery of the contact area while the said surface remains almost clean (Figs. 7.9 and 7.10).

To remove excess composite from the occlusal surface and adjust the morphology achieved by direct restoration, the following are most frequently used:

- Fine-grained (red and yellow) oval-shaped diamond high-speed piece burs (Fig. 7.11)
- Arkansas stones (Fig. 7.12)
- Multilamellar carbide burs

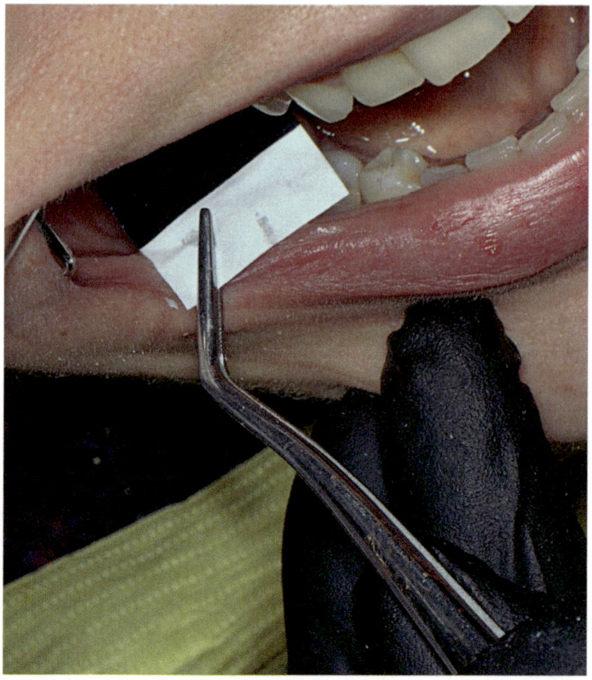

Fig. 7.8 Classic use of a conventional occlusion paper

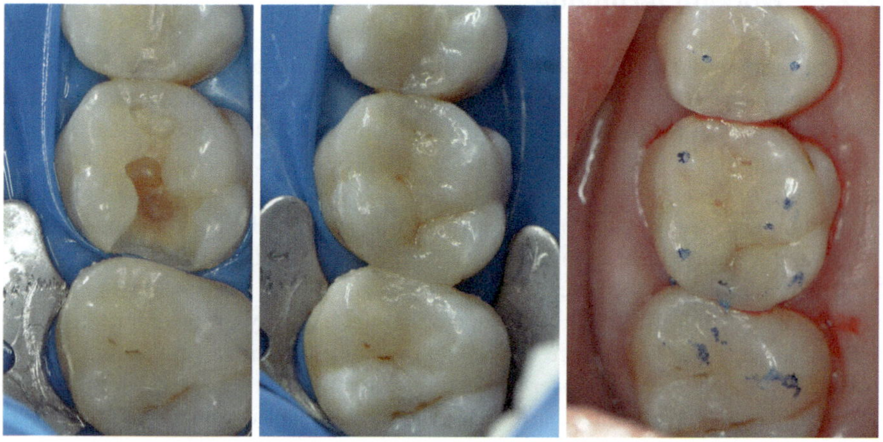

Fig. 7.9 Occlusal adjustments for a direct restoration on superior molar

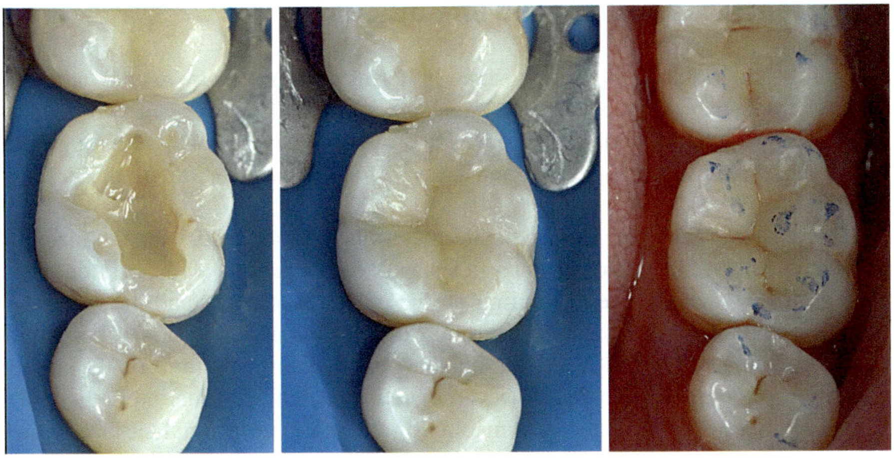

Fig. 7.10 Occlusal adjustments for a direct restoration on mandibular first molar

Fig. 7.11 Yellow diamond oval bur for occlusal adjustments

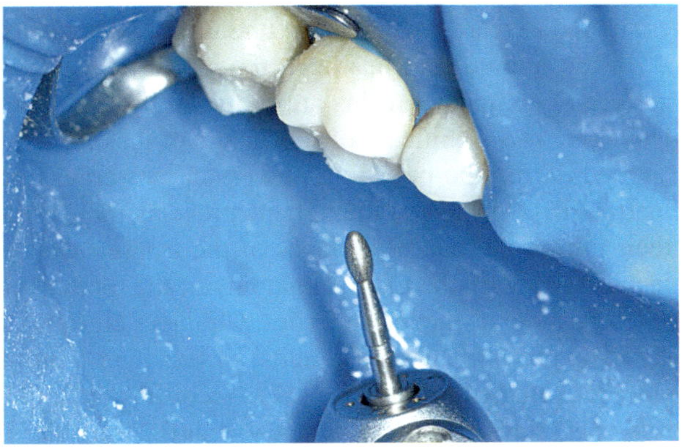

Fig. 7.12 Arkansas bur

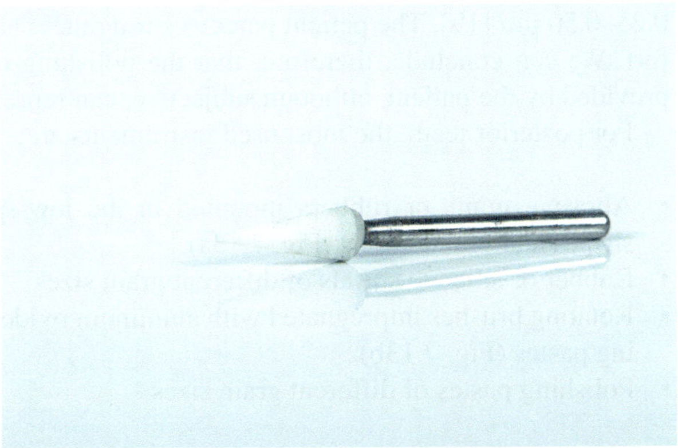

7.3 Surface Finishing and Smoothening

Finishing and polishing are important in terms of composite resins' aesthetic appearance and mechanical and physical properties [6]. Low surface roughness increases the esthetics and long-term success of composite resins, while rough surfaces cause plaque buildup, secondary caries, and discoloration of the restoration [7].

The surface roughness of composite materials is associated with the size and content of fillers, the type of filler particles, and the degree of polymerization of the material [8]. It can change depending on the polishing process and the materials' structure, flexibility, hardness, and grain. Several studies [9–11] have been published to evaluate the effectiveness of finishing and polishing systems on the surface roughness of composite resins. However, there is a lack of information in the literature [12] regarding the impact of finishing on the marginal enamel surface, which plays a vital role in the clinical outcome of the restoration. Some studies have shown that the effectiveness of the polishing system depends more on the material from which the restoration is made than on the polishing system. Composites with small, spherical particles tend to have smoother, glossier, and more wear-resistant surfaces compared to resin composites with larger or irregular particles [13].

In the literature, it has been reported that the lowest roughness values on the surface of composite resins are provided by using aluminum oxide disks [14, 15]. However, as a significant disadvantage of disks, it is stated that the frictional force applied during the polishing process causes cracks on the surface of the polymer matrix [16]. Moreover, their shape prevents their use on the occlusal surfaces, and their use on the buccal surfaces of the frontals can lead to obtaining flat surfaces inconsistent with the natural anatomy of the tooth.

Regarding aesthetic properties, Chung et al. found that a roughness value (measured by profilometry in Ra units) of less than 1 μm provided an optically smooth surface evaluated as aesthetic [17]. According to Bollen et al., the composite surface roughness threshold for plate retentive is 0.2 μm [18]. The ultimate criterion remains patient feedback. The study by Jones et al. shows that the patient can detect with their tongue roughness whose average values are greater than or equal to 0.25–0.50 μm [19]. The patient perceives roughness above these values as discomfort. We can conclude, therefore, that the polishing correlated with the feedback provided by the patient, although subjective, can represent a practical criterion.

For posterior teeth, the most used instruments are:

- Abrasive gums or rubbers mounted in the low-speed handpiece of different shapes and granulations (Fig. 7.13a)
- Rubber or silicone spirals of different grain sizes
- Rotating brushes impregnated with aluminum oxide used with or without polishing pastes (Fig. 7.13b)
- Polishing pastes of different grain sizes

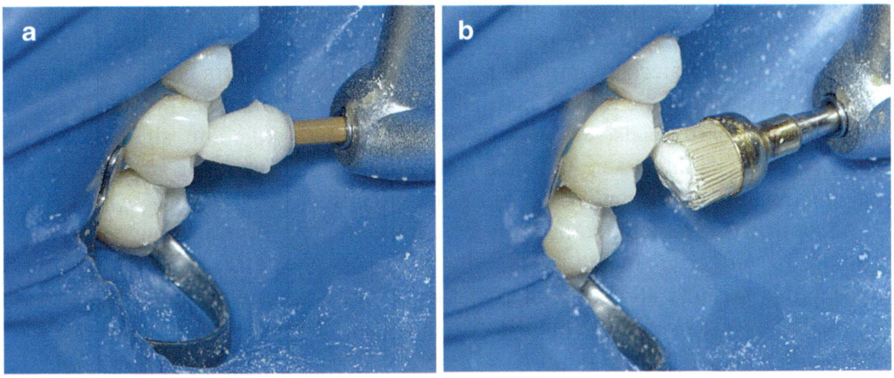

Fig. 7.13 Abrasive rubbers for the low-speed handpiece (**a**). Rotary brush for composite finishing used at low speed in the low-speed handpiece with finishing paste (**b**)

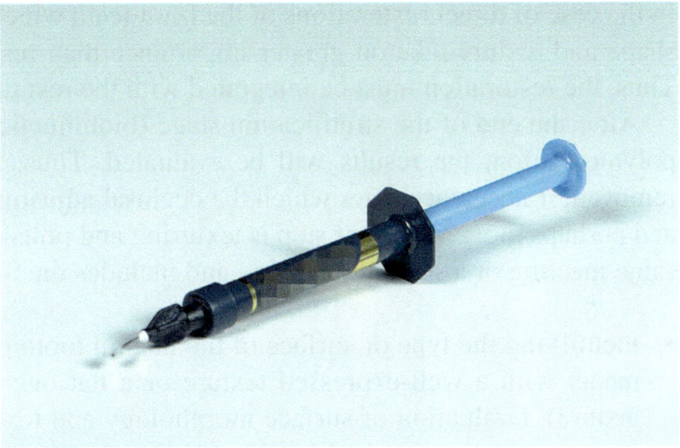

Fig. 7.14 Surface sealant for composite resins

Their use is always done from large grain to smaller grain, i.e., from dark to light colors. Multi-grit paste systems should be used similarly, in the order indicated by the manufacturer, from coarse to fine grit.

7.3.1 Composite Surface Sealants

Glazing materials or "surface sealants" modify the surface characteristics of restorative materials (Fig. 7.14).

These surface sealants are low-viscosity resins that polymerize on the surface of the composite resin restoration to penetrate microstructural defects and smooth the surfaces. On the other hand, it has been shown that bacterial adhesion significantly decreases on sealed surfaces [20]. These materials are known to maintain ideal surface properties, provide adequate marginal sealing, and improve the surface quality of the composite restoration [21]. These agents aim to reduce the water absorption of the material, minimizing discoloration of the resin composite by protecting the surface of the restoration with a thin film of sealant [22].

Surface sealants are also effective on the color stability of composites, depending on the type of sealant and composite material used. However, using surface sealants may not always bring benefits regarding color stability [23].

According to the manufacturer's instructions, after the finishing stage of the restoration, its surface is treated by applying orthophosphoric acid for 20 s, followed by generous washing and drying. Apply the sealant by brushing with a microbrush, remove the excess by gently blowing with an air jet, and polymerize for 20 s, preferably under a layer of glycerin (as an oxygen barrier).

7.4 Finishing Direct Restorations on Frontal Teeth

In the case of direct restorations of the front teeth which involve the buccal surface, shape and texture take on greater importance than restorations in the lateral area. Thus, the restoration must be integrated with the rest of the natural tooth crown.

After the end of the stratification stage (biomimetic or simplified) and the final polymerization, the results will be evaluated. Thus, the excess material will be removed, if necessary, after which the occlusal adjustments will be made. The final and perhaps most important step is texturing and polishing. This can be done in the same meeting or a separate meeting and includes the following:

- Identifying the type of surface of the natural tooth on which the restoration was made: with a well-expressed texture or a flat one (with erased or nonexistent texture). Evaluation of surface morphology and texture is done after drying the crown with air spray, by visual inspection, and by changing the angles and light in which the evaluator looks at the tooth. For a more accurate evaluation of the texture, an articulation paper can be used that slides under pressure on the buccal surface. The raised or prominent areas will be colored, and the grooves will remain unimpregnated.
- The continuation at the level of the restoration's buccal surface, shape, and texture existing on the natural crown. This is done with manual or rotary tools at high and low speeds.
- Polishing the obtained surface with rotary instruments at low speed.

7.4.1 Working Technique

In order to exemplify a possible working technique, we will present the following case of an incisal fracture at the level of tooth 2.1 without involving the pulp chamber and the mesial extension below the level of the contact point. The fragment was not recovered, the therapeutic decision being to make a direct restoration from composite resins.

After the installation of anesthesia, the rubber dam isolation of the entire frontal group and the choice of color before the appearance of dehydration of the teeth are performed (Fig. 7.15a, b). We select the shade of dentin in the cervical area and the shade of enamel in the incisal third by placing portions of the two composites and polymerizing them (Fig. 7.15c).

The palatal silicone key was created with the direct technique by placing the palatal silicone (Fig. 7.16a). After setting the material, the excess silicone was trimmed from the fractured area with a scalpel, and the final shape of the key was achieved by removal with a fine cylindrical bur with a rounded tip (mounted in the high-speed piece) (Fig. 7.16a, b). Thus, a suitable conformation of the silicone key was obtained to support the application of the first layer of palatal composite. We applied a biomimetic layering technique using palatal and proximal enamel and two shades of dentin.

The application of the enamel composite on the silicone key was made extraoral after marking the cavity limit on the key (Fig. 7.17a–c). Removing the silicone key from the teeth provides more working space and increased control for applying the first layer of palatal composite. When the silicone key is reattached to the teeth, the marginal palatal sealing of the composite applied to the key is checked. This can be improved by packing with a microbrush or brush or adding a fluid composite. After

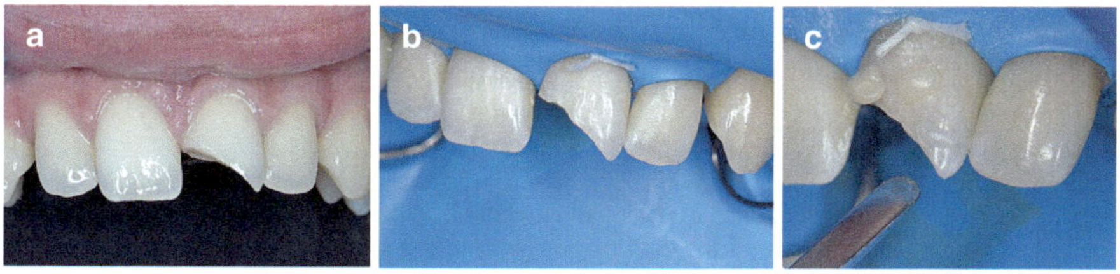

Fig. 7.15 Incisal fracture involving the mesial angle, without involving the pulp chamber for tooth 21 (**a**); isolated with rubber dam for a direct restoration (**b**); determination of dentin and enamel shades before the start of the procedure to prevent its change induced by dehydration (**c**)

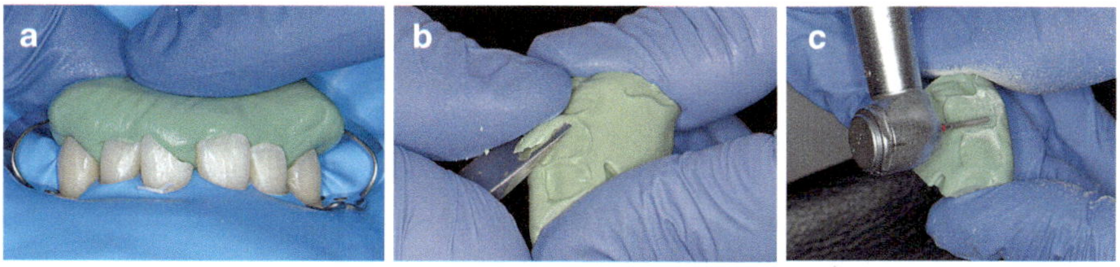

Fig. 7.16 Putty silicone impression of the initial situation (**a**); cutting with a scalpel the excess silicone that penetrated the fractured area (**b**); finishing the shape with a high-speed piece bur (**c**)

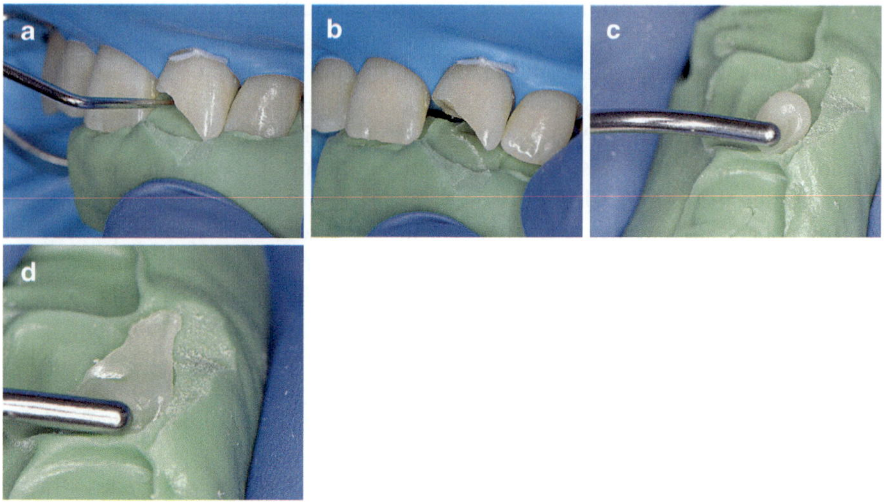

Fig. 7.17 Marking the palatal border of the cavity on the silicone key by gently scratching with the probe or sharp instrument (**a**); removing the silicone key (**b**) for easier extraoral manipulation of the composite applied to the key for the restoration of the palatal wall (**c**, **d**)

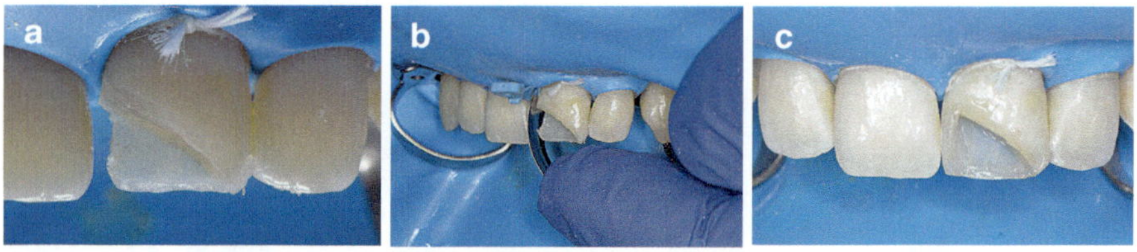

Fig. 7.18 Aspect of the enamel composite palatal wall obtained with the silicone key (**a**). Fixing the Palodent sectional matrix in a vertical position (**b**) in order to restore the mesial wall (**c**)

the polymerization of the composite, the palatal key can be removed (Fig. 7.18a). Later, the proximal wall was restored using a metallic sector matrix (Palodent classic) fixed cervically with an interdental wedge and incisally with a finger (Fig. 7.18b). We obtain a delimited area open only to the buccal, where two shades of dentin will be layered (Fig. 7.18c).

7.4.2 Finishing, Shaping, and Polishing

7.4.2.1 The Shape, Volume, and Contour of the Restoration

(A) Excess material and buccal profile

Checking for excess cervical material can be done with a curette (Fig. 7.19), scalpel blade, or burs. Proximal finishing can also be done with abrasive strips without damaging the contact point. They must be inserted interdentally in

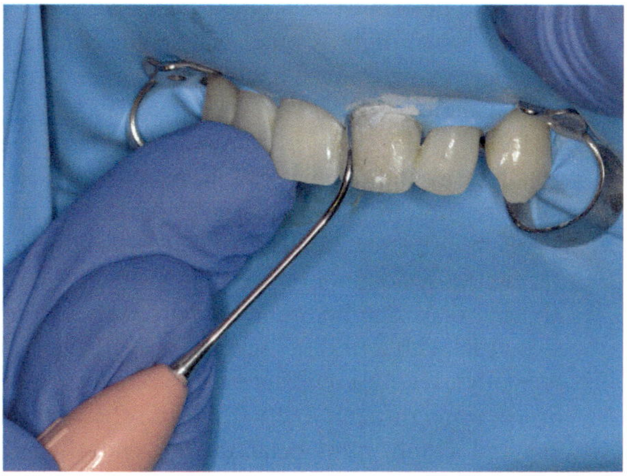

Fig. 7.19 Removal of interdental excess material from the gingival area with the curette

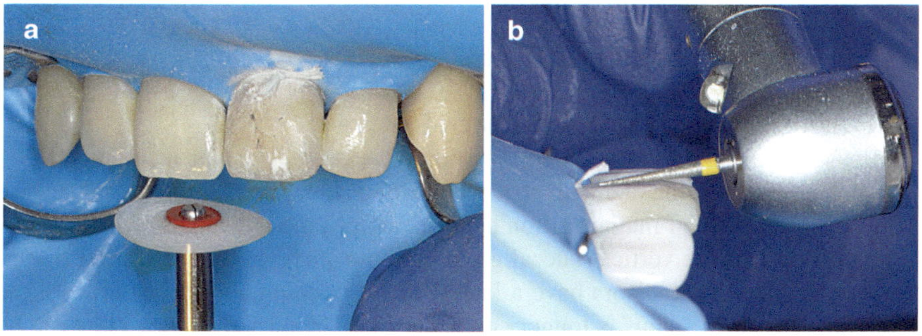

Fig. 7.20 Finishing with flexible abrasive disks of several grits (**a**) and fine high-speed piece diamond burs (**b**)

their nonabrasive area or directly from the buccal side below the level of the contact point. In the buccal and incisal areas, excess composite can be removed with abrasive disks or diamond burs (Fig. 7.20a). Then follow the profile shape of the buccal surface and the angulation between its three portions: cervical, middle, and incisal (Fig. 7.20b).

(B) Transition lines

Correcting the shape aims at obtaining a symmetry of shape and proportionality with the neighboring and contralateral teeth. The evaluation of the crown shape is done by analyzing the buccal surface, which is relatively flat, and the transition lines between it and the proximal surfaces, which are roughly convex. Light reflects on the right buccal area, making it easily perceptible compared to the proximal surfaces outside it. Thus, the buccal embrasures remain in a shadow area. The distance between these buccal edges, mesial and distal, is directly correlated with the perception of the shape of the buccal surface of the crown as a whole. In order to visually perceive a crown as narrow, the transition lines must be brought closer, thereby reducing the planar buccal surface on which light is reflected. On the contrary, moving the transition lines apart and increasing the flat buccal area creates the illusion of a wider crown.

(C) Incisal angles

Defining the shape of the incisal angles is an essential step that leads to obtaining a good symmetry of the restored tooth with its counterpart. In women, they are more rounded, and in men, they are straighter. The mesial angle is frequently sharper, and the distal angle is more rounded.

The most commonly used tools for making shape corrections are rotary abrasive disks and fine diamond burs. Although most companies produce abrasive disks with four different types of grits, only the two intermediate grits are typically used for composite removal and reshaping. The hardest ones are too invasive and difficult to control precisely, with the risk of removing too much material. On the other hand, the fine ones do not remove the composite. They can only produce a polishing effect on the material.

7.4.3 Macro- and Microtexture

7.4.3.1 Vertical and Horizontal Macrotexture

For reasonable control of the execution of this procedure, it can be recommended to use a pencil to trace the elements that will have to be created on the buccal surface (Fig. 7.21). The use of magnification helps to achieve these elements of finesse.

In most cases, the vertical buccal grooves in the shape of "V" or "Eiffel tower" on the upper central incisors have a larger incisal opening and narrow toward the cervical. The distal sulcus is longer cervically than the mesial sulcus. They can be made with fine diamond burs (cylindrical, finishing, flame) used at low speed for better control. Another way of making the grooves is by using spherical low-speed burs. The edges of the grooves are finished with fine diamond burs. The use of magnification helps to achieve these elements of finesse. They can be made with fine round diamond burs used at low speed for better control.

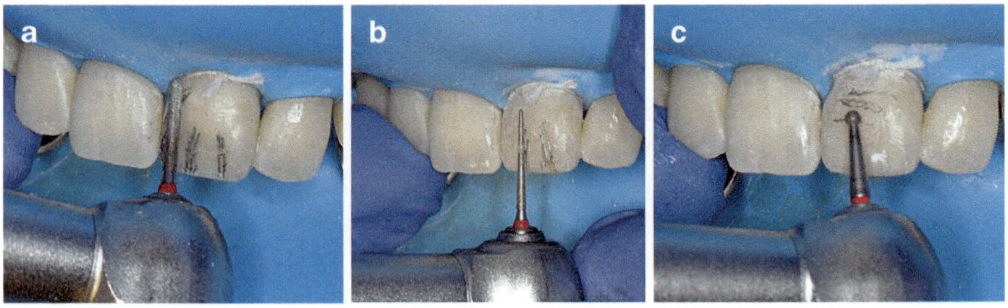

Fig. 7.21 Drawing with a pencil the transition lines and buccal grooves (**a**), making them with fine yellow or red diamond burs (**b**), making the horizontal striations in the cervical area (**c**)

The horizontal macrotexture is represented by two to three parallel grooves located in the cervical third to a maximum in the middle buccal third. They lie between the transition lines.

After their realization, these macrostructure elements are polished with rubbers at low speed (Fig. 7.22a, b). For rubber systems that offer multiple grits, it is necessary to use the complete set, starting from the largest to the smallest grit. With these rubbers, the previously created grooves are entered to obtain a surface and a smooth transition between the grooves and the buccal surface (Fig. 7.23).

7.4.4 Vertical and Horizontal Microtexture

Vertical microtexture elements are usually represented by small vertical grooves located in the middle third of the V-shaped grooves, the previously created macrotexture. The horizontal microtextural elements are represented by fine grooves from the cervical third to the incisal third and extending between the transition lines

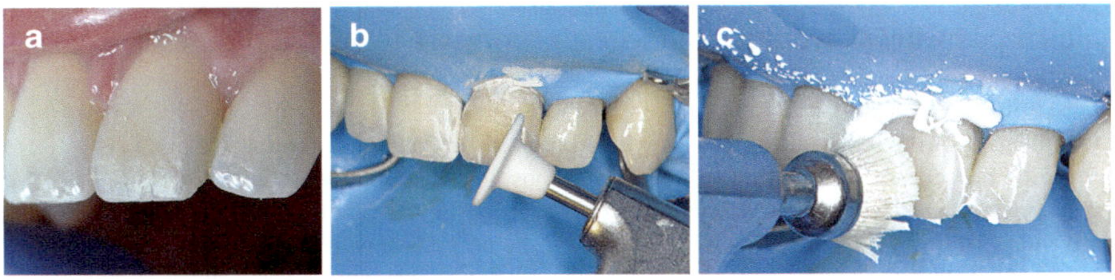

Fig. 7.22 Aspect of the restoration before finishing (**a**). Finishing with different rubber grits (**b**) and polishing with brushes and abrasive pastes (**c**)

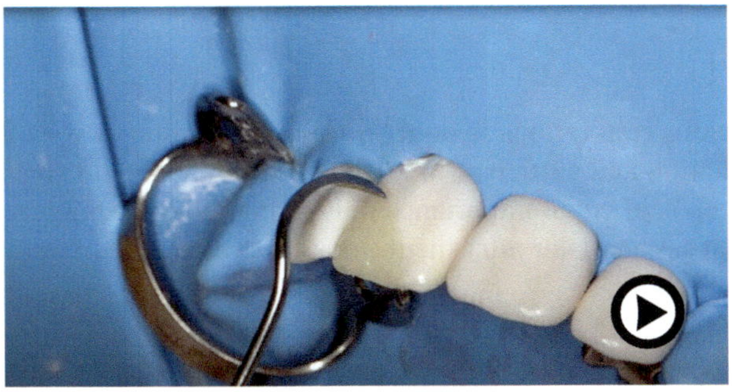

Fig. 7.23 Finishing the buccal surface of direct frontal restorations (▶ https://doi.org/10.1007/000-bqt)

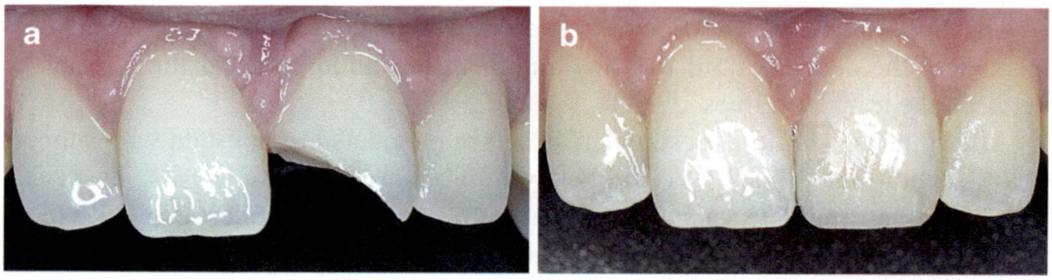

Fig. 7.24 The initial aspect (**a**) compared to the final aspect after restoration, immediately after the removal of the rubber dam sheet (**b**)

(called perikymata). They are extremely thin and close together. They can be made with fine diamond burs with a sharp tip at low speed and used at a 45° angle by continuously moving the bur in the same direction (either from mesial to distal or in the opposite direction). These elements can be polished with soft, fine rubbers or silicone spirals. For a natural glossy appearance, a fine polishing paste based on aluminum oxide or diamond paste with particles below 0.5 microns can be applied with soft brushes at low rotation so as not to scratch the surface (Fig. 7.22c).

The final result evaluated immediately after removing the rubber dam foil can be influenced by the dehydration of the teeth during the treatment (Fig. 7.24).

Difficulties that may arise	Possible solutions
Overheating of the tooth during finishing procedures. Although working without water has the advantage of observing the surface better and keeping the polishing paste longer, it leads to sensitivity	Finishing can be done intermittently using a continuous or intermittent water jet to avoid irreversible pulpal damage caused by overheating the tooth. If the procedure were performed under anesthesia, the patient would be unable to signal the sensitivity or pain caused by overheating to the doctor
Unwanted excessive removal of the composite due to the use of high-speed piece (high-speed piece) diamond burs	Redoing of the composite additive procedure

Conclusion

Finishing previous restorations is done in well-defined stages with specific laborious instrumentation and sufficient time allocated by the doctor to achieve optimal results. This step is of equal importance to layering. The finishing step can be done as an individual session later after the restoration is completed.

Did You Get It?

1. What are the advantages of the finishing stage?
2. What risks can be created by not completing the finishing stage of the restorations?
3. How can contour finishing be performed to remove excess extruded material?
4. How can occlusal adjustments be achieved through shape adjustments and reduction of relief size of the restoration?

5. How can restoration surface polishing be performed to decrease surface roughness?
6. What is the working technique for finishing restorations in the frontal area?

References

1. Frankenberger R, Kramer N, Pelka M, Petschelt A. Internal adaptation and overhang formation of direct class II resin composite restorations. Clin Oral Investig. 1999;3(4):208–15.
2. Brunsvold MA, Lane JJ. The prevalence of overhanging dental restorations and their relationship to periodontal disease. J Clin Periodontol. 1990;17(2):67–72.
3. Tryde G, Frydenberg O, Brill N. An assessment of the tactile sensibility in human teeth. An evaluation of a quantitative method. Acta Odontol Scand. 1962;20:233–56.
4. Siirila HS, Laine P. The tactile sensibility of the parodontium to slight axial loadings of the teeth. Acta Odontol Scand. 1963;20:415–29.
5. Harper KA, Setchell DJ. The use of shimstock to assess occlusal contacts: a laboratory study. Int J Prosthodont. 2002;15(4):347–52.
6. Lopes IAD, Monteiro PJVC, Mendes JJB, Gonçalves JMR, Caldeira FJF. The effect of different finishing and polishing techniques on surface roughness and gloss of two nanocomposites. Saudi Dent J. 2018;30:197–207.
7. Lopes GC, Vieira LC, Araujo E. Direct composite resin restorations: a review of some clinical procedures to achieve predictable results in posterior teeth. J Esthet Restor Dent. 2004;16:19–32.
8. Nagem FH, D'azevedo MT, Nagem HD, Marsola FP. Surface roughness of composite resins after finishing and polishing. Braz Dent J. 2013;14:37–41.
9. Yap AU, Yap SH, Teo CK, Ng JJ. Finishing/polishing of composite and compomer restoratives: effectiveness of one-step systems. Oper Dent. 2004;29:275–9.
10. Uppal M, Ganesh A, Balagopal S, Kaur G. Profilometric analysis of two composite resins' surface repolished after tooth brush abrasion with three polishing systems. J Conserv Dent. 2013;16:309–13.
11. Barbosa SH, Zanata RL, Navarro MF, Nunes OB. Effect of different finishing and polishing techniques on the surface roughness of microfilled, hybrid and packable composite resins. Braz Dent J. 2005;16:39–44.
12. Sumali C, Hidayat A, Kusnoto J, Sudhana W. Effect of one-step and multi-steps polishing system on enamel roughness. J Dent Indon. 2012;19:65–9.
13. Amaya-Pajares SP, Koi K, Watanabe H, da Costa JB, Ferracane JL. Development and maintenance of surface gloss of dental composites after polishing and brushing: review of the literature. J Esthet Restor Dent. 2022;34(1):15–41.
14. Aytac F, Karaarslan EŞ, Agaccioglu M, Tastan E, Buldur M, Kuyucu E. Effects of novel finishing and polishing systems on surface roughness and morphology of nanocomposites. J Esthet Restor Dent. 2016;28:247–61.
15. Babina K, Polyakova M, Sokhova I, Doroshina V, Arakelyan M, Novozhilova N. The effect of finishing and polishing sequences on the surface roughness of three different nanocomposites and composite/enamel and composite/cementum interfaces. Nanomaterials (Basel). 2020;10(7):1339.
16. Yadav RD, Raisingani D, Jindal D, Mathur R. A comparative analysis of different finishing and polishing devices on nanofilled, microfilled, and hybrid composite: a scanning electron microscopy and profilometric study. Int J Clin Pediatr Dent. 2016;9:201–8.
17. Chung K-H. Effects of finishing and polishing procedures on the surface texture of resin composites. Dent Mater. 1994;10:325–30.

18. Bollen CM, Lambrechts P, Quirynen M. Comparison of surface roughness of oral hard materials to the threshold surface roughness for bacterial plaque retention: a review of the literature. Dent Mater. 1997;13(4):258–69.
19. Jones CS, Billington RW, Pearson GJ. The in vivo perception of roughness of restorations. Br Dent J. 2004;196:42–5.
20. Kim DH, Kwon TY. In vitro study of Streptococcus mutans adhesion on composite resin coated with three surface sealants. Restor Dent Endod. 2017;42(1):39–47.
21. dos Santos PH, Pavan S, Suzuki TYU, et al. Effect of fluid resins on the surface roughness and topography of resin composite restorations analyzed by atomic force microscope. J Mech Behav Biomed Mater. 2011;4(3):433–9.
22. Hepdeniz OK, Temel UB, Ugurlu M, Koskan O. The effect of surface sealants with different filler content on microleakage of class V resin composite restorations. Eur J Dent. 2016;10:163–9.
23. Korkut B, Bud M, Kukey P, Sancakli HS. Effect of surface sealants on color stability of different resin composites. Med Pharm Rep. 2022;95(1):71–9.

Part III

Direct Additive Restorations and Indirect Restorations (Onlays)

Injection Molding: For Incisal Edges and Direct Onlays

8

Complex oral rehabilitation aims at both aesthetic and functional restoration. Contemporary dental materials, clinical digital planning techniques, and mock-ups allow the dentist and the patient to evaluate the proposed treatment plan visually and clinically. However, making final restorations, direct or indirect, is still very difficult and time-consuming, requiring specific skills and attention to detail. This chapter will present the i**njection molding technique for incisal edges and direct onlays:** indications; materials used; working protocol; special features for anterior teeth, palatal veneers, and incisal edges; special features for posterior teeth (direct onlays); and Vailati three-step technique for complex rehabilitation.

When changing the smile requires interventions on several anterior teeth, indirect restorations are preferable to direct ones. This happens for efficiency and predictability of the result and for reasons related to the materials' properties. The choice of a direct composite resin restoration technique should be based on survivability relative to the esthetic properties and ease of use of composite resins. The realization of direct restorations is a time-consuming and often unpredictable process, with the dentist having great freedom to choose the shape and dimensions of the restorations. As a rule, they do not use predefined shapes or contours of the tooth.

8.1 Indications and Materials

The indications for the injection molding technique with the stent are both for provisional test restorations and permanent direct additive restorations. However, this last category of indications is debatable, depending on the type of composite used and the manufacturers' indications.

Supplementary Information The online version contains supplementary material available at https://doi.org/10.1007/978-3-031-55899-3_8. The videos can be accessed individually by clicking the DOI link in the accompanying figure caption or by scanning this link with the SN More Media App.

© The Author(s), under exclusive license to Springer Nature Switzerland AG 2024

M. Bud, *Direct Restorations*, https://doi.org/10.1007/978-3-031-55899-3_8

For clinical cases where the VDO is reduced due to generalized abrasions or erosions (Figs. 8.1, 8.2, and 8.3), it can be decided to raise the occlusion with the increase of the VDO. For this purpose, as a rule, patients are proposed to test the new VDO for a predetermined period. This can be achieved with the help of a removable splint or direct additive restorations maintained for 1–3 months. Thus, in these cases, several teeth are involved. The injection technique is highly advantageous for several reasons, among which we can mention:

- It is a fast treatment.
- The results are predictable.
- The working technique is easy.
- The stent can be made exclusively in the office without the involvement of the laboratory.

With the improvement of the properties of the flowable composite materials, long-lasting restorations can also be performed, depending on the manufacturer's indications of each material.

8.1.1 Materials

Increasing the filler loading of composite resins improves functional wear resistance and physical properties. Also, composite resins with smaller particles are easier to polish, keep their gloss for extended periods, and are more wear resistant.

The flowable composite resins with a lower viscosity also have a good adaptation on the walls of the cavities, being for this reason indicated to be injected into stents that can restore the morphology of the teeth [1, 2]. Given that these restorations will be subjected to occlusal forces, it is recommended to use high-load composites that resist wearing without being covered by packable composites. There are such specially designed materials (G-aenial Injectable, G—filler 69% wt) (Fig. 8.4a) as part of a kit for the injection molding technique (e.g., injection molding kit, GC), but other materials with similar properties can be successfully used for this procedure (e.g., SDR, Dentsply Sirona—filler 71.5% wt).

The materials used to make the stent must be transparent to have good visual control of the injection and to allow the proper polymerization of the composite resin after its injection (e.g., Exaclear, GC) (Fig. 8.4b). Among the advantages of a transparent stent (Fig. 8.5) compared to a partially transparent or even opaque stent we can mention:

- Visual control of the amount of flowable composite injected and the distribution of the material
- Control of excess composite that can be extruded from the stent
- Procedure precision
- Good final results

Review Questions

1. What are the advantages of using injection molding?
2. What composite resin materials can be used for injection molding and why?
3. What materials can be used to make the stent for the injection molding technique and why?

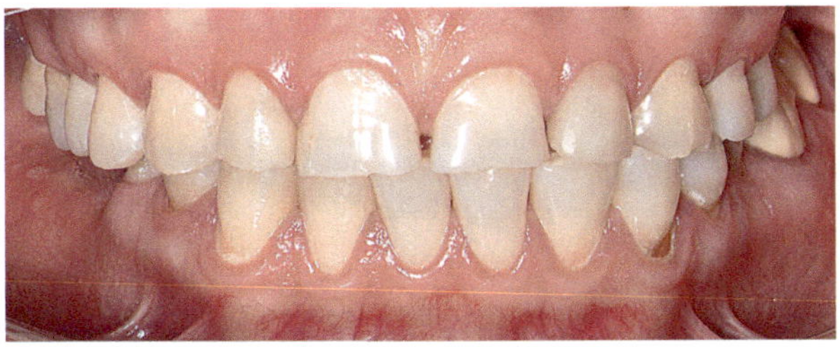

Fig. 8.1 The initial aspect from the frontal view in occlusion

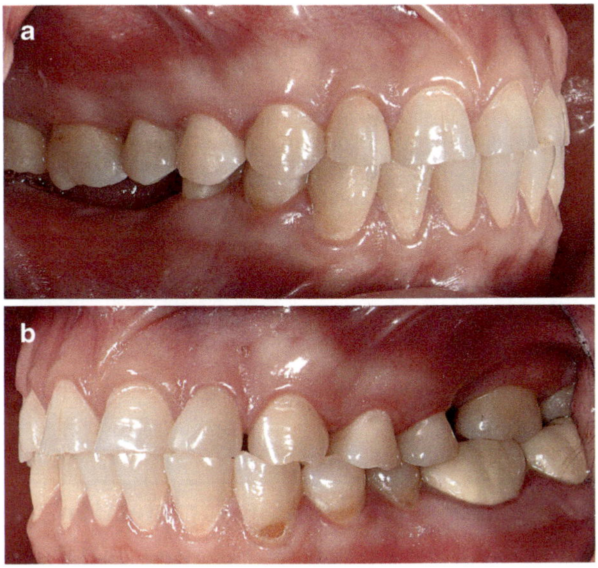

Fig. 8.2 Initial aspect in occlusion, buccal view quadrants 1 and 4 (**a**) and quadrants 2 and 3 (**b**)

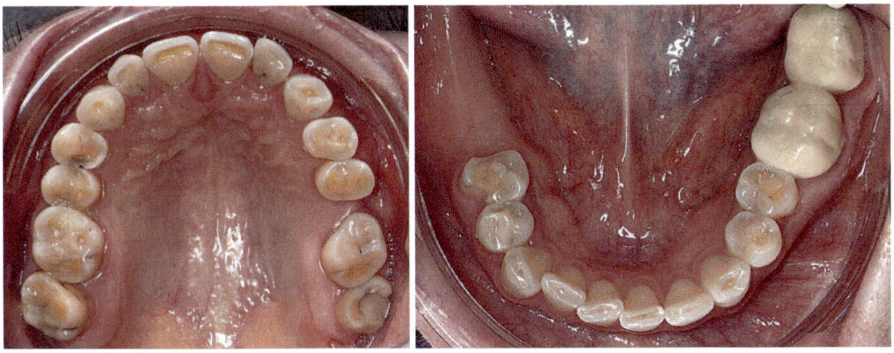

Fig. 8.3 Initial aspect, occlusal photographs

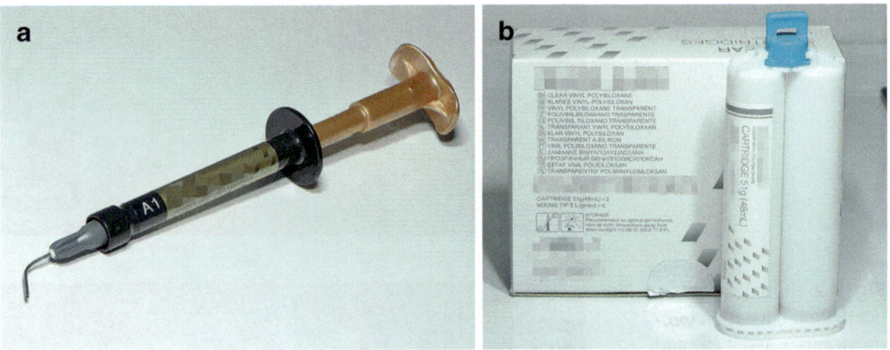

Fig. 8.4 The flowable composite resin for the injection technique G-aenial Injectable (**a**) and transparent silicone for fabricating the stent (**b**)

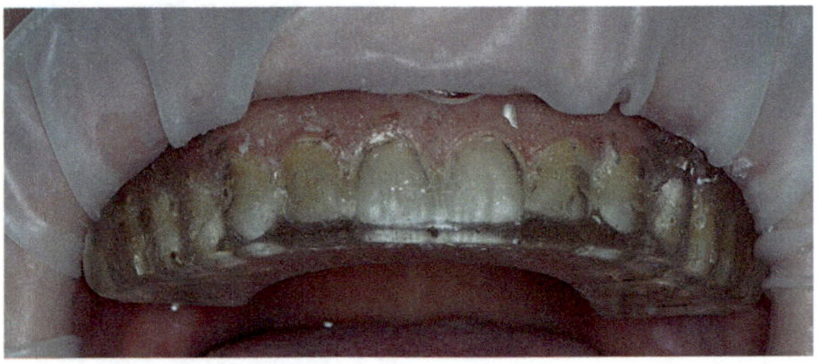

Fig. 8.5 Transparent stent for injection molding

8.2 Working Technique for Injection

The main idea: The technique requires a wax-up (or digital equivalent), a transparent stent that will serve as a conformer for the injection of composite. The result proposed in the case design will thus be obtained.

8.2.1 Planning

An impression of the initial intraoral situation will be taken conventionally or digitally. The planning is done according to the impression, either conventionally with wax on the model (Fig. 8.6a) or digitally using Digital Smile Design software (Fig. 8.6b). For a digital workflow, the mock-up can be 3D printed or milled. Also, the mock-up can be made conventionally using an impression of the printed model of the proposed final design.

8.2.2 The Fabrication and Preparation of the Stent

In order to make the transparent silicone stent, the model/cast with the wax-up representing the proposed situation is immersed in water for 5 min before the impression (Fig. 8.7a). Lubrication or wetting can help prevent the impression of silicone from sticking to the model/cast.

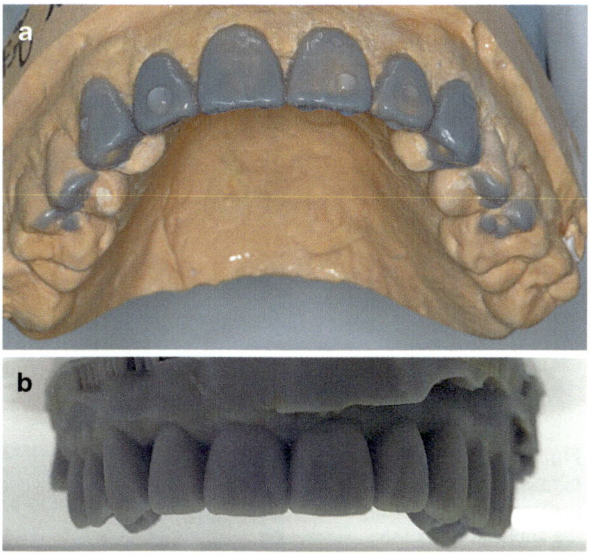

Fig. 8.6 Wax-up design (**a**) or a 3D printed model (**b**)

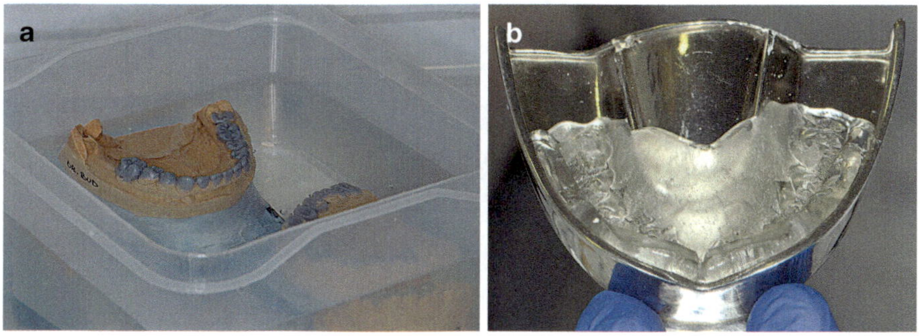

Fig. 8.7 Immersion of the model/cast with the wax-up in water for 5 min prior to impression using transparent silicone for the stent (**a**). Applying silicone in a non-retentive impression tray allows easy removal of the stent obtained after the setting time (**b**)

The impression is made with transparent silicone (e.g., Exaclear, GC) in the impression tray without retentions (Fig. 8.7b). This allows for the easy removal of the resulting stent from the tray and its preparation for injection. Both technician and dentist can fabricate the stent. If it is decided to fabricate the stent in the dental laboratory, the technician can decide to "reinforce" it with a rigid transparent plastic. This gives it more resistance to handling and stiffness for easier adaptation in the field.

The preparation of the silicone stent consists of the following:

- Removal of excess material.
- Verification of easy insertion and disinsertion in the oral cavity in the correct position.
- Creating centered occlusal perforations for each tooth (Fig. 8.8) through which the injection of the flowable composite will be performed. They can be made by piercing with a needle or with a bur. Making them from the inside of the stent allows a more precise centering of the perforation in the middle of the occlusal surface.

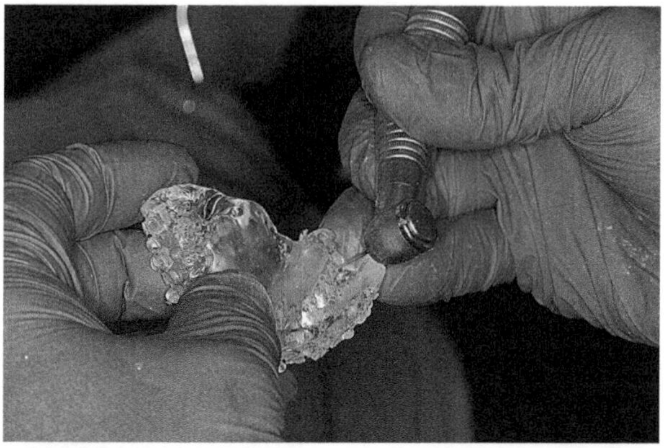

Fig. 8.8 Making perforations with a bur in the middle of the occlusal surface of each tooth

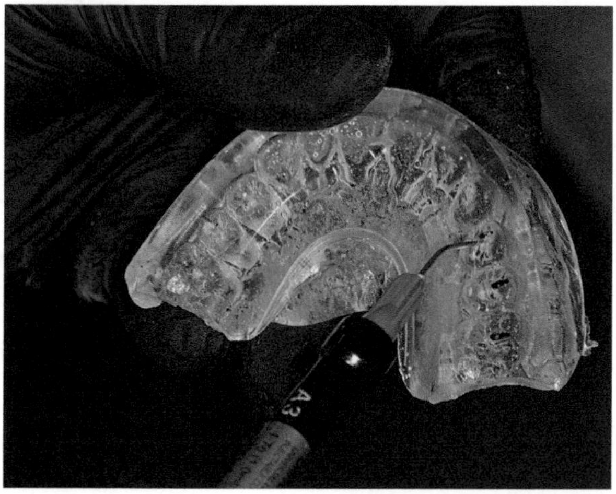

Fig. 8.9 Checking the permeability of the perforations by inserting the applicator tip of the flowable composite syringe

- Cleaning and removing any debris of silicon produced during perforation.
- Checking permeability by inserting the applicator tip of the flowable composite syringe to be used (Fig. 8.9).
- Lack of gingival inflammation that can produce slight bleeding that affects adhesion.

8.2.3 The Isolation of the Operating Field

Although this adhesive technique indicates a good isolation, using a rubber dam sheet can make it difficult or even impossible to apply the stent over the teeth. For this reason, a classic lip retractor (or OptraGate) can be a much more practical method of retracting soft tissues and improving visibility and access. Since most restorations are on the incisal and occlusal areas, moisture control is relatively easy to maintain. These direct injection onlays are usually temporary, so perfect isolation is unnecessary. If they are carried out for longer, try to isolate as effectively as possible.

8.2.4 Preparation of Teeth for Adhesion

The teeth are cleaned of pigmentation or plaque (ultrasound, airflow, professional brushing). With the soft tissue retractor in place (e.g., OptraGate, Ivoclar Vivadent), the teeth will be prepared one by one for adhesion, similar to cementing indirect restorations.

Thus, the adjacent teeth will be isolated by covering the proximal surfaces with thin Teflon tape. Clear celluloid strips can also be used for separation, but the silicone key must be sectioned for each tooth in this case. The surfaces to be prepared for adhesion will be etched with orthophosphoric acid (35–37%) 15 s on dentin and 30 s on enamel and then washed with water and air-dried. The adhesive is applied for 20 s and then air-dried for 5 s.

8.2.5 Injection of Flowable Composite

After applying the adhesive system to the tooth, the stent is applied. This is pressed firmly with the fingers to be placed in the correct position, fixed, and adapted to the operating field to prevent the material extrusion during the injection (Fig. 8.10). The injection is done by inserting the tip of the applicator through the previously made perforation until it meets the tooth. Touching the tooth is a check of the permeability of the perforation that allows the injection. At the time of injection, the applicator tip can be slightly withdrawn to facilitate the flow of material to reach the entire volume that must be filled. The injection is done slowly to allow the flowable composite resin to fill tight all areas. The transparent stent allows visual control of the injection. When the volume fills, and the composite begins to flow back, the injection can be stopped, and the applicator tip removed. The composite is polymerized for 10–20 s on each surface, according to the manufacturer's instructions of the material used, after which the stent is removed, and the result is evaluated (Fig. 8.11a, b).

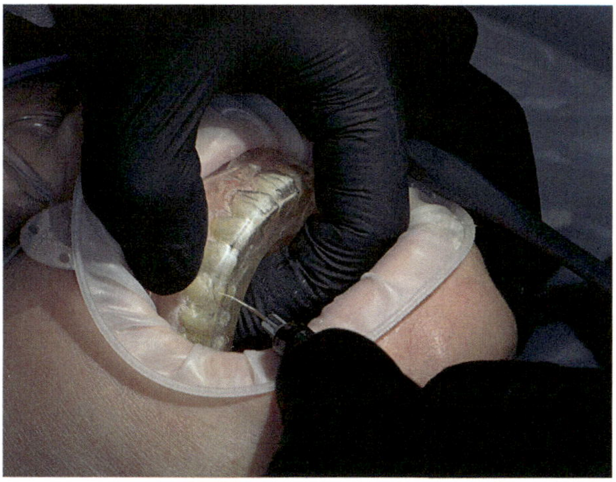

Fig. 8.10 Placing the stent on the arch in order to inject the flowable composite

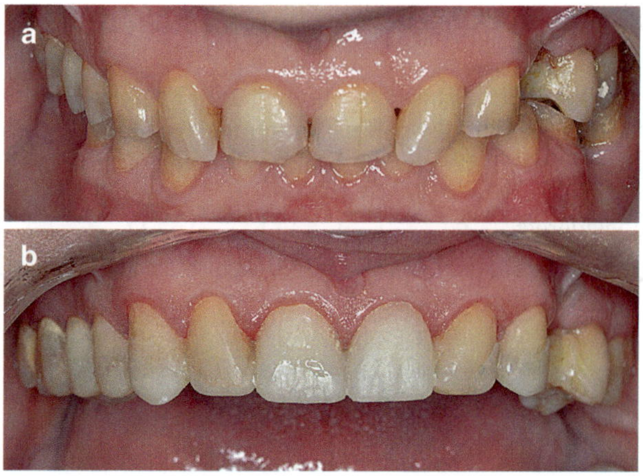

Fig. 8.11 Aspect before (**a**) and after adhesive addition of flowable composite by injection on the upper anterior teeth (**b**)

8.2.6 Cleaning Up Excess and Finishing

This step is crucial for maintaining periodontal health. Additive adhesive restorations must be finished and polished after the removal of excess to achieve a glossy and smooth composite surface.

Difficulties that may arise	Possible solutions
Proximal of cervical reflow of flowable composite	Checking the cervical adaptation of the stent, isolating the adjacent teeth with Teflon tape
Traumatizing the periodontium by removing excess composite	Realization of a more precise stent from a transparent material (e.g., Exaclear, GC)
Bleeding of the gum at the time of stent application indicates an inflamed periodontium and prevents the necessary isolation for an adhesive procedure	The cause of the inflammation should be removed, and the injection procedure should be postponed until the gingival inflammation disappears

Review Questions

1. What are the steps in making additive direct restorations by injection molding using a stent?

8.3 Particularities of Anterior Teeth: Palatal Veneers and Incisal Edges

Main idea: The injection molding technique can be used for frontal teeth as part of a larger treatment plan. The obtained restorations can be temporary or permanent, for one or more teeth.

8.3.1 Working Technique

The working steps are the same as described in the previous section (Sect. 8.2), with some particularities imposed by the specific morphology of the frontal teeth (Fig. 8.12).

For injection molding of the frontal teeth, the following recommendations can be considered:

- The perforation for the injection can be made in the stent in the middle of the incisal edge or toward the incisal angles (Fig. 8.13a). In the area of the

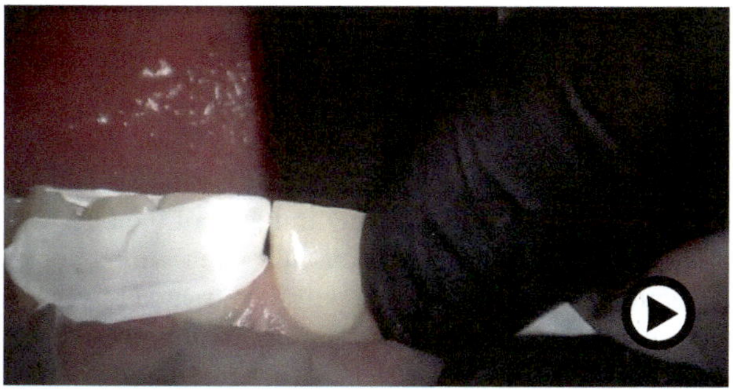

Fig. 8.12 Palatal veneers by flowable composite resins using injection molding technique (▶ https://doi.org/10.1007/000-bqw)

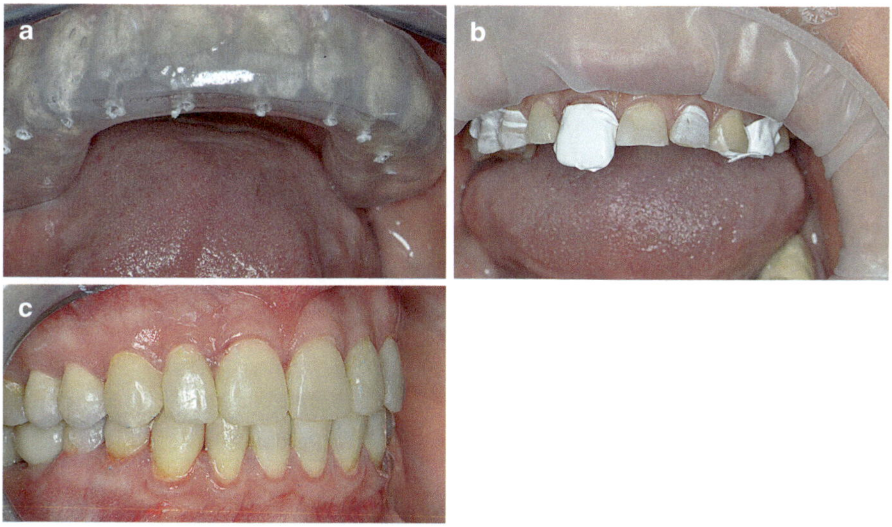

Fig. 8.13 Adhesive addition of composite by injection molding to restore the coronal shape of the frontal group: preparation of a transparent stent based on a wax-up (**a**); successive injection after isolation of adjacent teeth (**b**); final aspect (**c**)

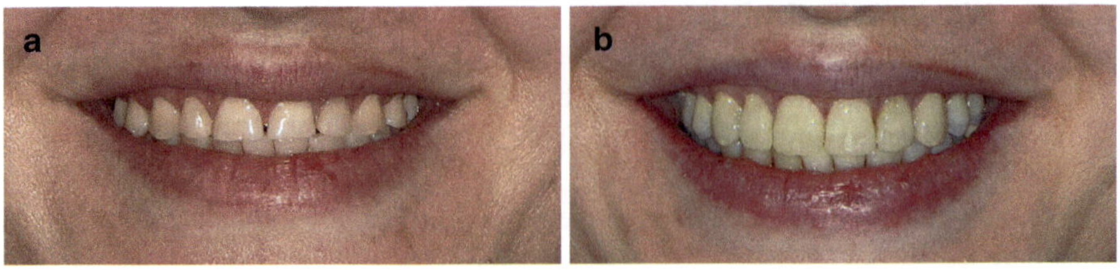

Fig. 8.14 Initial (**a**) and final (**b**) aspect after additive adhesive restoration by injection with flowable composite for the upper anterior teeth

perforation, there will always be an excess of material that will have to be removed and finished after light curing.

- The adjacent teeth are isolated with Teflon tape, and the injection is made to each tooth separately (Fig. 8.13b) until all teeth are completed (Fig. 8.13c).
- They are made individually for better aesthetics, hygiene, and periodontal health.
- Inserting the applicator tip of the flowable composite syringe through the stent can be done until it reaches below the central area of the buccal surface. Thus, a more straightforward injection in the cervical area will be ensured, following that, as the injection progresses, the tip will be retracted toward the incisal.
- Finishing and polishing should follow the same steps as in anterior direct restorations. This ensures good aesthetics even if the restoration is made provisionally (Fig. 8.14).
- The patient should receive recommendations regarding mechanical care, hygiene, and monitoring of the restorations.

Difficulties that may arise	Possible solutions
Obtaining a chromatic difference that affects aesthetics. This can happen because some of the flowable injectable composite may not have the same opacity as a dentin composite	If the restoration is provisional, having a major functional purpose, the patient must temporarily accept certain aesthetic limits. The restoration can be improved by adding additional composite in certain areas for aesthetic correction
Maintaining the integrity of the restoration during the provisional period (1–3 months), considering the mechanical vulnerability to fracture of the composite incisal angles	If fractures occur (albeit rare), they are repaired with a composite resin. The patient is advised to pay extra attention during this period
Correct stent placement is impossible due to too thick Teflon tape that prevents a tight fit. Thus, excess material or oversized occlusal restorations may occur	Use thinner Teflon tape or section off the silicone key and use clear celluloid tape

8.4 Particularities for Posterior Teeth: Direct Onlay

Main idea: The injection molding technique can be used for lateral teeth as part of a larger treatment plan, as a temporary step, or as a minor treatment for one or more teeth.

8.4.1 Working Technique

The working steps are the same as described in the previous section (Sect. 8.2) with some differences. It differs according to their purpose, thus:

- Direct posterior onlays can be splinted, on the first three posterior teeth (PM1, PM2, and M1) when the onlays are made provisionally as part of a complex restoration with VDO elevation
- Individually (single units) with the isolation of the adjacent teeth when they are performed both provisionally and for long term

Thus, for injection molding on the lateral teeth, the following recommendations can be considered:

- The perforation for the injection can be made in the stent in the middle of the occlusal surface to facilitate good access for the injected material in all areas.
- In the case of permanent restorations, the adjacent teeth are isolated with Teflon tape, and the injection is made to each tooth separately until all teeth are completed (single units onlays).
- Inserting the applicator tip of the flowable composite syringe through the stent as deeply as possible to ensure the most efficient injection.
- Finishing and polishing must follow the steps specific to direct restorations.
- The patient should receive recommendations regarding mechanical care, hygiene, and monitoring of the restorations.

Difficulties that may arise	Possible solutions
The silicone is not thick enough and can deform, affecting the morphology of the restoration	The key must be redone, ensuring a greater thickness of silicone
The occlusal perforation made with the bur or needle may not be perfectly cleaned. There is a risk that silicone debris will be included in the composite restoration	Carefully inspect the stent, cleaning with an air jet or microbrush
Interdental or cervical extrusion of the flowable composite	Checking the cervical adaptation of the stent, isolating the adjacent teeth with Teflon tape
Traumatizing the periodontium by removing excess composite	Realization of a more precise stent from a transparent material (e.g., Exaclear, GC)

8.5 Vailati Three-Step Complex Rehabilitation Technique with Increasing of VDO

Main idea: The indication for increasing the VDO involves careful planning and a trial period that can also be achieved with additive restorations made most effectively by injection molding.

This technique has been described as one of the minimally invasive conservative techniques which the dentist completes by adding composite resins without preparations that may be necessary in the case of other restorations (onlays, crowns, etc.).

This is how the authors Francesca Vailati and Cristoph Belsel [3] summarized this technique:

"Traditionally, patients with severe generalized erosions benefit from complex rehabilitation, crowns being frequently recommended to patients. An innovative concept was developed to facilitate the clinician's task during the planning and execution of adhesive restorations: the three-step technique. Three laboratory stages are alternated with three clinical stages, allowing the clinician and laboratory technician to work together to achieve a predictable esthetic and functional outcome. During the first stage, an aesthetic assessment, establishment of the VDO, and the occlusion plan are performed. The patient's posterior quadrants are restored to an increased vertical dimension in the second stage. Finally, in the third step, the previous guidance is restored. Using the three-step technique, the clinician can transform a complete rehabilitation into an individual rehabilitation of each quadrant."

This three-step technique aims to achieve an additive adhesive restoration using direct posterior provisional restorations at a new VDO established by the dentist. Therefore, direct injection onlays will be made for the posterior area and palatal, or sometimes buccal veneers will be made similarly, to restore the anterior guidance, if necessary.

Steps	Laboratory	Cabinet	The purpose of this step
Step 1: Aesthetics	Upper anterior wax-up	Direct mock-up in the anterior area	Aesthetic validation of occlusion plan and VDO
Step 2: Posterior support	Posterior wax-up	Direct onlays in the posterior area	Achieving a stable occlusion
Step 3: Anterior guidance	Palatal veneers	Palatal veneers obtained by injection or in the laboratory	Restoration of anterior guidance

8.5.1 Step 1

This first step begins with case documentation with standard photographs and impressions for study models. Intermaxillary relations are determined using a face-bow, and this information is sent to the laboratory. Following the case analysis by the medical team, together with the technician and patient, a proposal for aesthetic modification of the upper arch is agreed upon. This is prefigured as a wax-up (Fig. 8.15a, b) or digitally using DSD software. Based on this, the patient will receive the transfer to the oral cavity of the proposal in the form of a maxillary mock-up directly on the buccal surfaces of the frontal teeth and possibly the premolars (Fig. 8.16a, b).

8.5.2 Step 2

Establish lateral occlusal support by making direct onlays on the first three posterior teeth (PM1, PM2, M1) (Fig. 8.17). The second molar will not be included for several reasons:

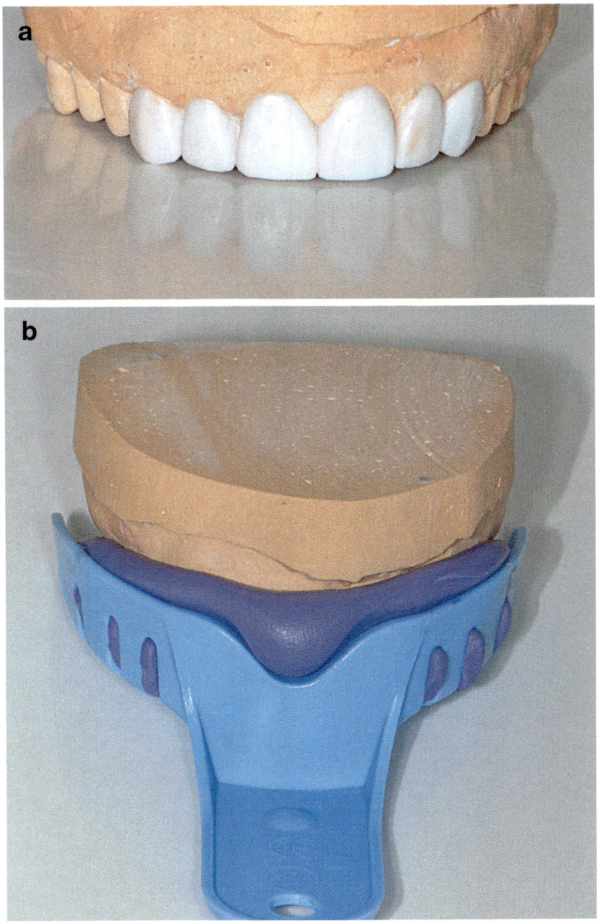

Fig. 8.15 Step 1: Wax-up (**a**) impression with putty silicone (**b**) in order to make the mock-up

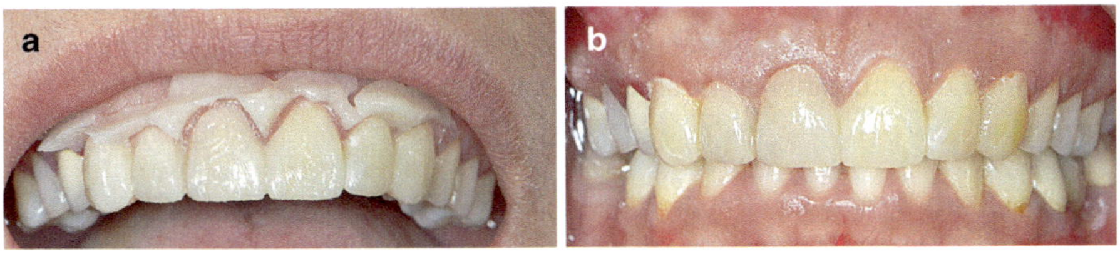

Fig. 8.16 Step 1: Mock-up of the anterior teeth (**a, b**)

- It is a reference for the VDO increase.
- It helps to fix the stent during the injection.
- It brings not benefit for the occlusal stability, three lateral teeth being enough to achieve a stable occlusion.

There is no consensus on the optimal period of provisional restorations at the new VDO size. Most often, practitioners propose their patients 1 month, after which,

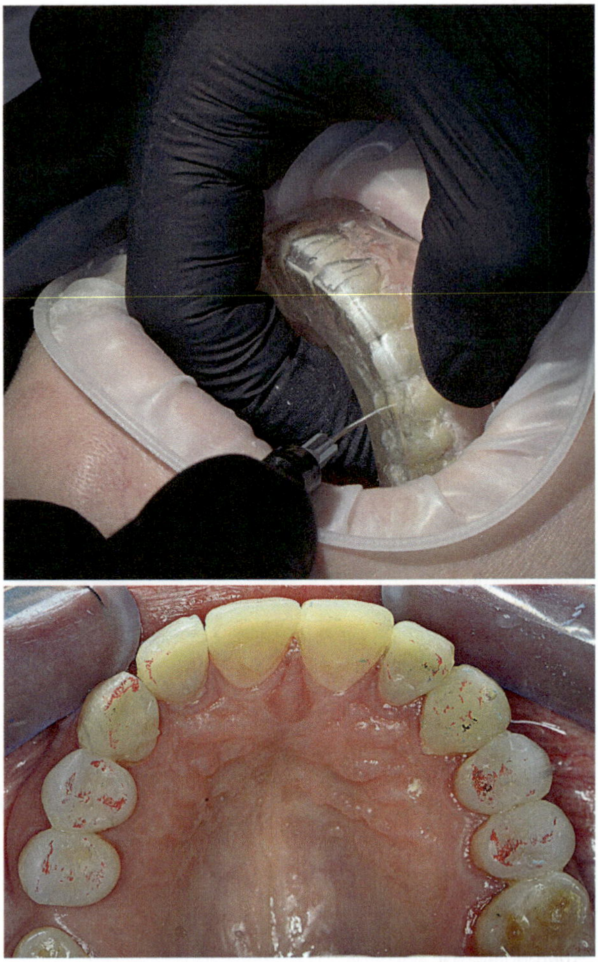

Fig. 8.17 Step 2: Restoring the posterior support through direct onlays made by injection molding

in the absence of TMJ and muscle symptoms, the new VDO is validated and maintained for the continuation of treatment through definitive prosthetics.

8.5.3 Step 3

The restoration of the anterior guidance can be achieved by palatal veneers made by injection (Fig. 8.18) or composite or ceramic veneers made in the laboratory can be bonded. In the case of ceramic palatal veneers, the hardness characteristics of the ceramics must be analyzed, and the impact they can have on the lower antagonists in terms of the abrasion produced must be evaluated.

For making palatal veneers by injection, the teeth must be perfectly cleaned so that the palatal surface can be prepared for adhesion (Fig. 8.19). A transparent silicone stent is made in the office or laboratory, perforations are made in the middle of the palatal surfaces, and their permeability is checked (Fig. 8.20).

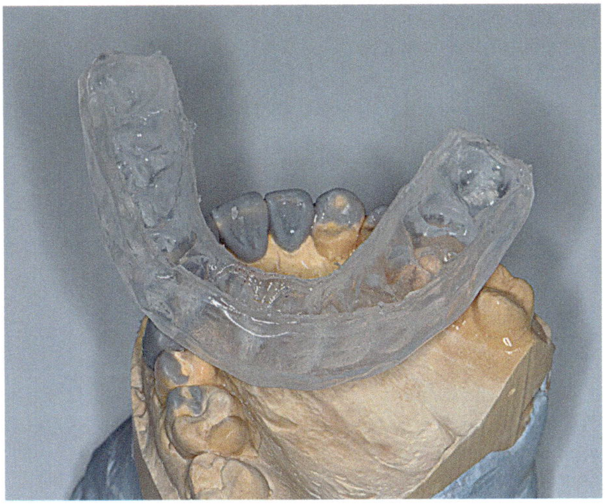

Fig. 8.18 Step 3: Restoring the anterior guidance: wax-up of the palatal veneers and the stent

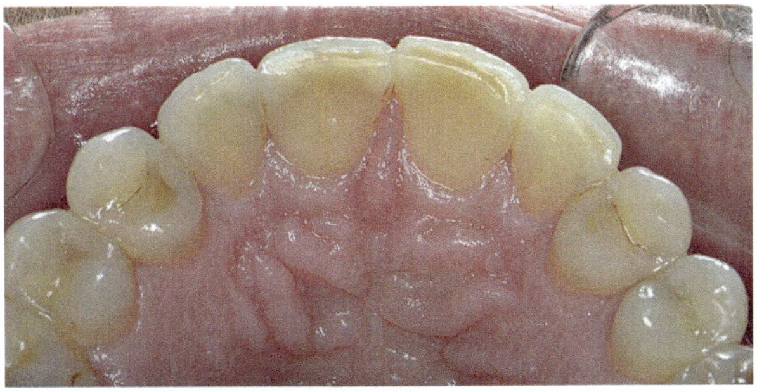

Fig. 8.19 Step 4: Preparation of the palatal surfaces for adhesion

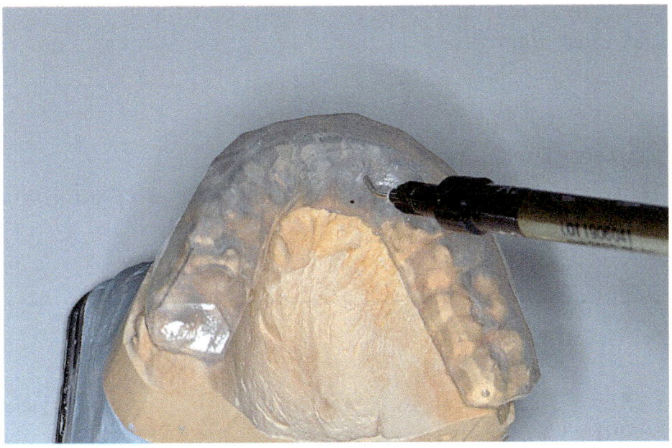

Fig. 8.20 Step 5: Preparing the injection mold and creating and checking the perforations

The veneers are made one at a time by isolating the adjacent teeth with Teflon (Fig. 8.21) to provide good aesthetics, the possibility of proper hygiene, and the maintenance of healthy gingiva. Occlusal adjustments, finishing, and polishing are performed (Fig. 8.22).

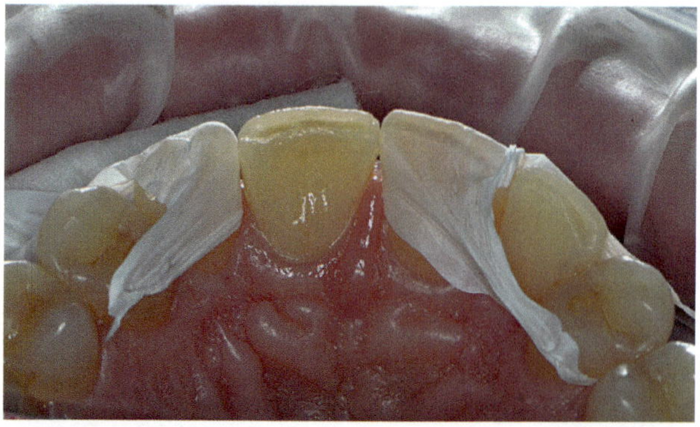

Fig. 8.21 Step 6: Preparation of adjacent teeth with Teflon tape

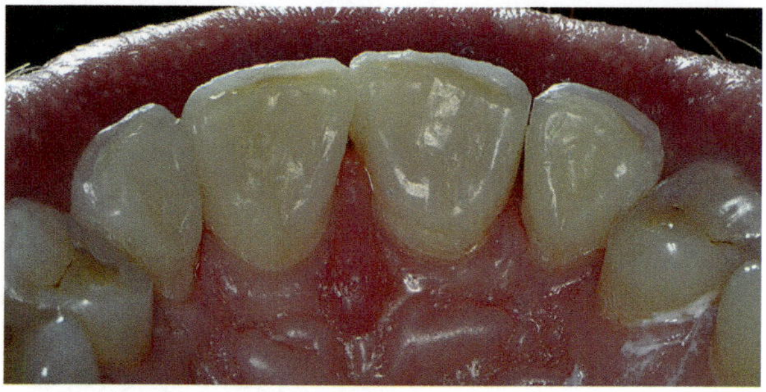

Fig. 8.22 Step 7: Final aspect of palatal veneers after injection of flowable composite

Difficulties that may arise	Possible solutions
The patient is not compliant and does not go through all the steps of treatment	This type of treatment should only be proposed to compliant patients because its partial implementation cancels the intended results
Splinting the posterior onlays can create hygiene maintenance problems and cause gingivitis	Separate injection to obtain single unit restorations on each tooth

Review Questions

1. What are the stages of the Vailati three-step additive technique, and what do they consist of?

References

1. Terry DA, Powers JM. A predictable resin composite injection technique, part I. Dent Today. 2014;33(4):96–101.
2. Terry DA, Powers JM, Mehta D, Babu V. A predictable resin composite injection technique, part 2. Dent Today. 2014;33(8):12.
3. Vailati F, Belser UC. Full-mouth adhesive rehabilitation of a severely eroded dentition: the three-step technique. Part 1. Eur J Esthet Dent. 2008;3(1):30–44.

Indirect Restorations

9

Dental structural defects can be the consequence of multiple factors, and cavities are the predominant cause, with an estimated prevalence of over 90% in the general population worldwide [1]. Other factors such as erosion, abrasion, attrition, fracture, and combinations may contribute to hard tooth tissue loss. These situations can give rise to sensitivity, pain, pulp tissue involvement, secondary caries, and periodontal and occlusal problems (antagonistic extrusions, interferences, etc.).

All this generates the need for tooth restoration [2], with indirect partial restorations being a minimally invasive alternative to conventional crowns. They have good aesthetic results, color stability, biocompatibility, and high long-term survival rates [3]. This chapter will present how to make tooth preparation for indirect restorations, working protocols for immediate dentin sealing (IDS), cavity optimization, re-preparation, impression and provisional restoration, and cementation.

Partial restorations are classified according to the restored area. There are several types of indirect restorations, some of the most commonly performed by dentists being:

- Inlays—do not cover the cusps but only address the negative occlusal relief
- Onlays—extend on both the negative and the positive relief of the occlusal surface covering at least one cusp [3]
- Overlays—cover the entire occlusal surface [4]
- Endocrowns—can be made on endodontically treated teeth where they cover the entire occlusal surface extending to the entrance to the root canals

---

Supplementary Information The online version contains supplementary material available at https://doi.org/10.1007/978-3-031-55899-3_9. The videos can be accessed individually by clicking the DOI link in the accompanying figure caption or by scanning this link with the SN More Media App.

© The Author(s), under exclusive license to Springer Nature Switzerland AG 2024

M. Bud, *Direct Restorations*, https://doi.org/10.1007/978-3-031-55899-3_9

9.1 Tooth Preparation

Main idea: The preparation of teeth for an indirect restoration should lead to obtaining a geometry as simple as possible, with rounded angles, non-retentive, without thin enamel walls, which ensures a sufficient thickness of the prosthetic restoration to be resistant under the action of occlusal forces.

Before starting the tooth preparation for an indirect restoration, there is an evaluation stage by visual inspection, the use of an explorer, and complementary examinations (vitality tests, radiographs).

When evaluating the tooth to be prepared for an indirect restoration, we assess the following aspects:

- The initial contour of the cavity and plan the future shape that will result after the preparation of the cavity. The final margins of the preparation for indirect restorations must be placed supragingivally. Proximally, avoid placing the limit of the preparation at the level of contact points for hygiene and long-term prophylaxis reasons.
- The thickness of the remaining walls. Remaining vertical walls less than 1.5 mm thick do not provide strength and must be removed to achieve cusp protection.
- The occlusal contacts with the antagonists. They must be identified with the occlusion paper to avoid opposing tooth contact with composite-tooth transition line (Fig. 9.1).
- The proximal contact with the adjacent tooth should be removed (Fig. 9.2).

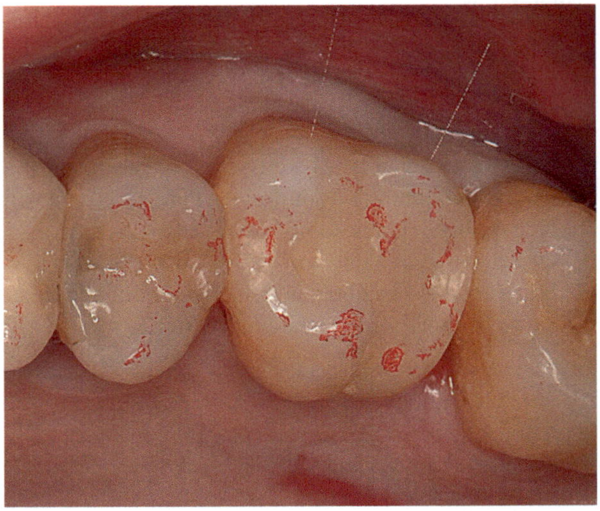

Fig. 9.1 Checking occlusal contacts using articulating paper

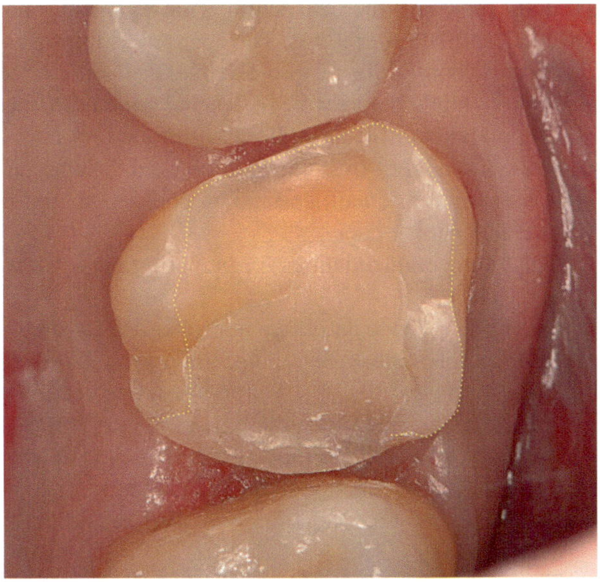

Fig. 9.2 Tooth preparation for overlay, proximal separation, and deep margin elevation with composite resins

9.1.1 Pre-prosthetic Treatment: The Supragingival Margin Elevation

This procedure aims to reposition the cavity margins supragingivally. The aspects improved by the supragingival localization of the margins of preparations for indirect restorations are:

- Impression
- Marginal fitting of the prosthetic restoration
- Isolation with a rubber dam for adhesive cementing
- Cementation
- Cleaning excess luting material
- Finishing after cementing and final quality control

In the area where the margins have been relocated supragingivally with composite, the circumferential sealing of the onlay will not be done on the enamel but the composite. For a good long-term prognosis in such cases, the ratio between enamel and composite areas must be carefully evaluated (Fig. 9.2).

Preparing a tooth for indirect restorations requires more extensive preparation than direct restorations [5, 6].

The concept of "biomimetic dentistry," used more often in recent years, aims to obtain dental restorations that reproduce the biomechanics and aesthetics of natural teeth as closely as possible, replicating what nature has created [7]. The biomimetic approach aims to increase the longevity of the remaining dental tissues [8] by partially replacing the lost dentin with composite materials and the enamel with indirect ceramic restorations. The continuous improvement of the various materials (adhesives, composite resins, ceramics) allows for obtaining dental restorations resistant to high compressive forces and good aesthetics.

The preparation is carried out with diamond burs at high speed. Thus, round-tipped cylindrical or oval burs can be used. The recommended granulation for the burs is medium or small, and the preparation should be finished with a low speed using rotary rubber cups.

General recommendations for preparing posterior teeth for indirect restorations:

- Diverging walls to achieve a non-retentive cavity.
- Rounded internal angles, the geometry of the preparation as simple as possible.
- The thickness of the restoration should be relatively constant at approximately 1.5–2 mm, depending on the type of material used (Fig. 9.3).
- Preparation of 90° (Fig. 9.4) or beveled enamel edges.
- Chamfer on the functional cusps and a butt finish on the nonfunctional cusps.
- The edges of the preparation placed outside the areas of contact with the antagonists.
- The edges of the preparation should be in enamel around the entire preparation circumference in order to obtain maximum adhesion.
- Elimination of retentive areas and cusps not supported by dentin by lining the undercut area.
- The edges of the preparation must be supragingival to allow rubber dam isolation for the cementation step.
- Removing other inadequate old fillings on the tooth and extending the preparation in these areas.

9.1.2 Preparing the Cusps and Making the Isthmuses

The occlusal reduction must ensure a uniform and sufficient thickness to allow the inlay to have the thickness required for resistance according to the technical recommendations of the material. Cusps supported by thin vertical walls, less than 1.5 mm

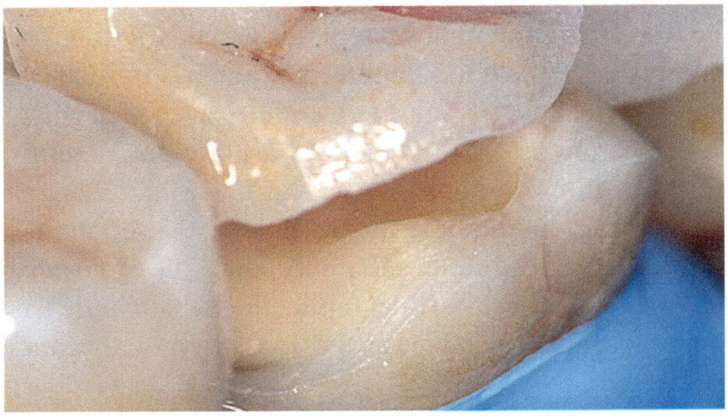

Fig. 9.3 Ceramic onlay—try in step

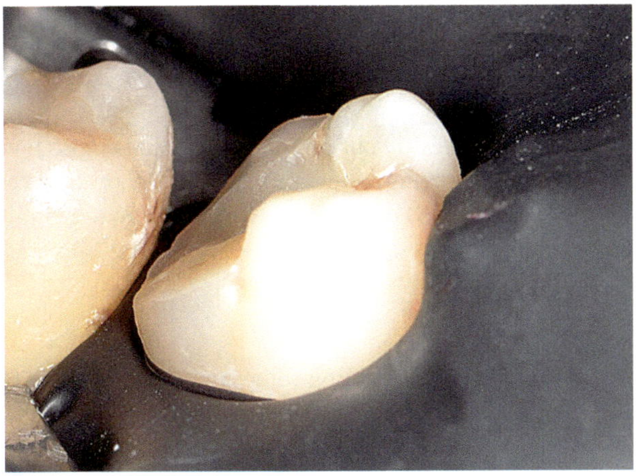

Fig. 9.4 Onlay preparation on the lower molar with the edges prepared at 90°

thick, can fracture easily. Thus, the height of these walls can be reduced [9] so that the inlay extends over them to cover them. This procedure is called cusp protection. Reducing the height of the cusps must provide space for sufficient material thickness to withstand occlusal forces [10].

Guidelines for reducing the height of the cusps:

- Approximately 1.5–2 mm evenly on occlusal surfaces and functional cusps.
- The width of the isthmus must be at least 2 mm.
- The proximal edges of the preparation must be at least 0.5 mm from the adjacent teeth.
- For vital teeth, the necessary cusp protection is about 2 mm.
- For endodontically treated teeth, the required cusp protection is approximately 3 mm.

Difficulties that may arise	Possible solutions
Keeping vertical walls too thin out of a desire to be minimally invasive	This will adversely affect the long-term prognosis, so cusp protection is indicated
Preparation of the proximal areas located below the level of the contact points	In these areas with more difficult access, using oval burs can help obtain edges with 90°

Review Questions

1. What are the main indirect restorations frequently performed by dentists?
2. What aspects do we look for when evaluating a tooth to be prepared for an indirect restoration?
3. What aspects are improved by the supragingival localization of the margins of preparations for indirect restorations?
4. What are the general recommendations for preparing posterior teeth for indirect restorations?

9.2 Immediate Dentin Sealing (IDS) and Cavity Design Optimization

Main idea: Freshly cut (prepared) dentin is more favorable for adhesion, so an immediate coating is recommended. The procedure is called immediate dentin sealing (IDS) and can be performed by the single application of an all-in-one adhesive system or by the combined application of both the adhesive system and a flowable composite.

Immediate dentin sealing after cavity preparation for direct restorations is indicated in all cases [11] following Bertschinger's initial studies [12] in 1996 and aims to:

- Limit excessive preparation
- Protect the pulp and dentine and decrease sensitivity in the period between appointments
- Improve the dentin adhesion of the definitive restoration

Contamination of these dentin surfaces by placing temporary fillings (without being previously sealed with an adhesive material) can reduce the adhesion of definitive restorations to the dentin area [13]. The quality of the bond will increase if immediate dentin sealing is achieved, regardless of the adhesive system used. Furthermore, using a three-step etch-and-rinse adhesive system or combining an adhesive system with a flowable composite layer improves long-term bond strength [14] significantly.

The decrease in postoperative sensitivity following immediate dentin sealing is the subject of much research, with inconclusive results [15].

Initially, the procedure only involved applying a layer of adhesive over the dentin. The steps for immediate dentin sealing with adhesives are as follows [16]:

1. Identification of exposed dentin areas
2. Demineralization with orthophosphoric acid 37% for 5–15 s
3. Washing and drying
4. Applying and drying the adhesive to obtain an even layer without excess
5. Preliminary polymerization for 20 s
6. Application of an oxygen inhibitor gel (glycerin) and final polymerization for another 10 s

Any light-curing liner can be applied for immediate dentin sealing (Fig. 9.5). Moreover, this stage can be combined with the next one, that of cavity design optimization. The liner applied to the entire dentinal surface also helps to eliminate retentive areas. You can use flowable composites (classic or bulk), GIc modified with resins, or their variants: giomers, compomers, etc.

Difficulties that may arise	Possible solutions
If the preparation was done without rubber dam isolation, difficulties might arise concerning isolation	Isolation with a rubber dam for the preparation step and sealing of the dentin
Precise application of sealant	It is applied in very thin layers and only on the dentine area

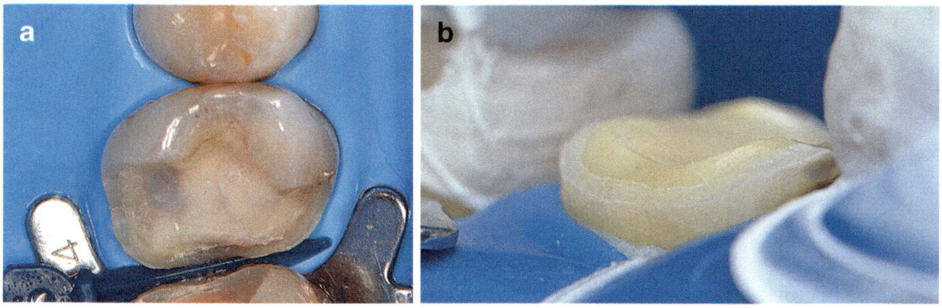

Fig. 9.5 Tooth preparations for indirect restorations where the dentin surfaces were sealed with RMGIc (**a**) and flowable composite (**b**)

Review Questions
1. What is immediate dentin sealing, and what is its purpose?
2. With what materials and how can immediate dentin sealing be achieved?

9.2.1 Optimizing the Design of the Prepared Cavity

The main idea: Optimizing the design of the preparation for indirect restorations is aimed at eliminating retentive areas, relocating certain margins of the cavity, and cleaning the enamel contour from possible restorative materials unintentionally placed on the circumferential limits of the preparations.

Immediate dentin sealing with adhesive is, in many cases, followed by applying a flowable composite [17] to the dentin area to optimize the cavity shape by lining the retentive areas (Fig. 9.6). If the clinical situation requires it, in this phase, the gingival margins can be occlusally relocated by adding flowable or packable composite material. When using composite resins, after an initial polymerization of 5 s of the final layer, it is recommended to apply an oxygen barrier (e.g., glycerin) prior to the final polymerization [9].

Sasse et al. (2015) showed in their studies that the use of composite materials to optimize the shape of the cavity has a minor influence on the fracture resistance of ceramic restorations [18]. During this step, it is constantly checked that the enamel area remains clean without leakage of materials that prevent good adhesion of the indirect restoration to the enamel (Fig. 9.7). This step is completed by finishing using a fine diamond bur.

Difficulties that may arise	Possible solutions
Incorrect assessment of the shape of the preparation obtained may present retentive areas	Evaluation using a mirror from several angles
Material extrusion outside the dentine area	It must be removed with a bur if it has also been placed on the enamel area

Review Questions
1. What is the purpose of the cavity design optimization for indirect restorations?
2. How cavity design optimization for indirect restorations can be done?

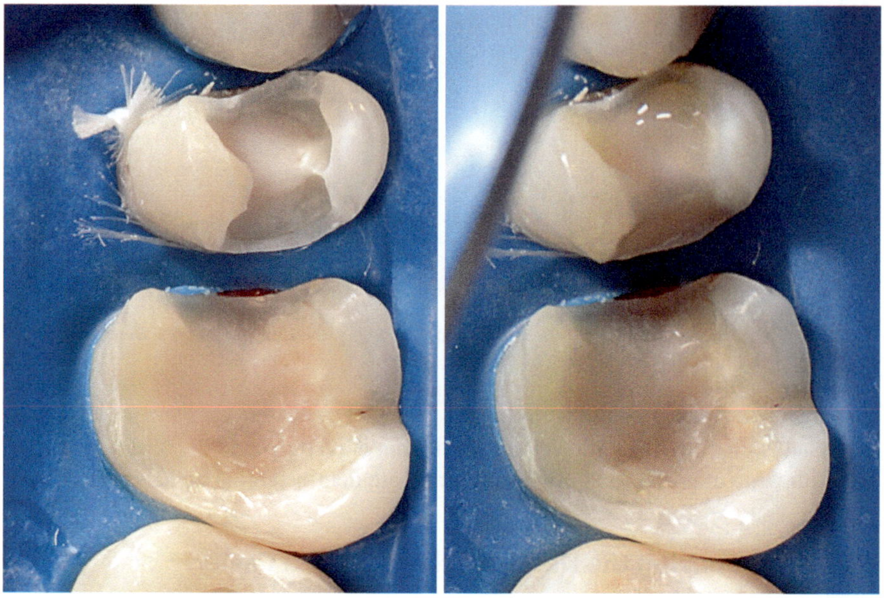

Fig. 9.6 Cavity design optimization by lining the retentive areas

Fig. 9.7 Cleaning the enamel margins of restorative materials involuntarily placed on the enamel

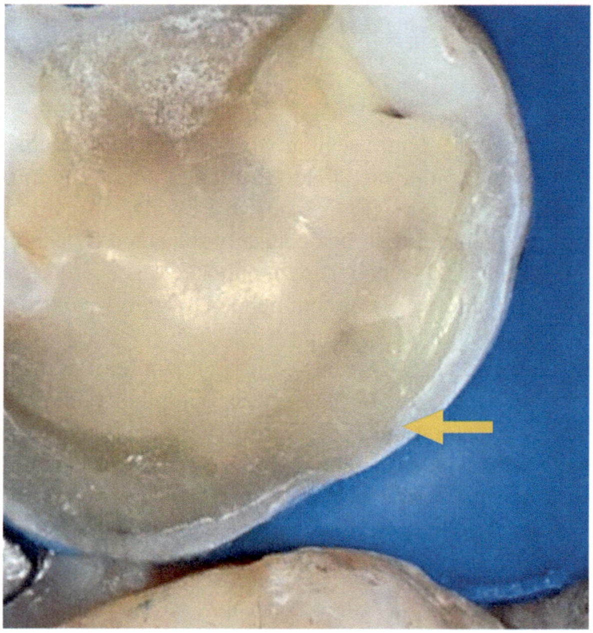

9.3 Re-preparation, Finishing Edge Preparation, and Stress Relocation for Onlays

Main idea: Modifying the shape of the edges of prepared cavities aims to increase adhesion and esthetics while also bringing mechanical benefits.

The 90° angle preparation of the cavo-superficial angle of the cavities for onlays/overlays is used for several reasons, such as ease of preparation, impression, and inlay fabrication.

It has been shown that the most common problems encountered with indirect restorations are their fracturing and debonding. Therefore, working techniques have been developed to remedy these problems.

The option of preparing the enamel edges of the cavity by making an extended bevel produces the relocation of stress to the tooth's interior, thus increasing the mechanical resistance to fracture and decimation [19]. Such a design, in which all the outer edges of the preparation are relocated cervically (Fig. 9.8), ensures a homogeneous centripetal distribution of stress toward the center of the tooth. So, it

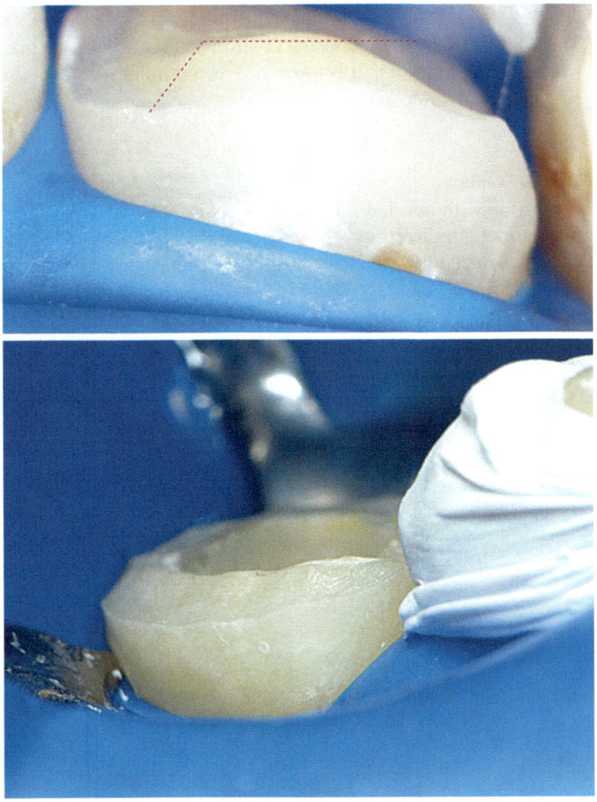

Fig. 9.8 Chamfer preparation of cavity edges to redirect centripetal stress toward the tooth's center

decreases the cyclic fatigue of the adhesive interface. This type of preparation, somewhat flattened, with simple geometry, ensures the retention of the restoration because of adhesion, not because of the cavity geometry.

The clinical advantages of relocating the edges of the preparation (Fig. 9.9) are the following [20]:

1. Improving adhesion by increasing the enamel surface available for adhesion and the perpendicular sectioning of enamel prisms (enamel rods) compared to the sharp preparation of the edges when the prisms are sectioned parallel to their axis.
2. Aesthetic improvement by achieving a gradual transition between the tooth and the indirect restoration.
3. The apical relocation of the contour of the preparation reduces the difference in level between the tips of the cusps that will be covered and the base of the preparation, simplifying the geometry of the preparation.
4. Increasing the fracture resistance of the tooth [19].

Difficulties that may arise	Possible solutions
Creating bevels in hard-to-reach (proximal) areas	The use of oval burs or skip the beveling in this area. The buccal and oral bevel may be sufficient
The impossibility of good visual control, so that when making a bevel that is too concave, too much enamel can be removed	Using magnification can help to better control this step

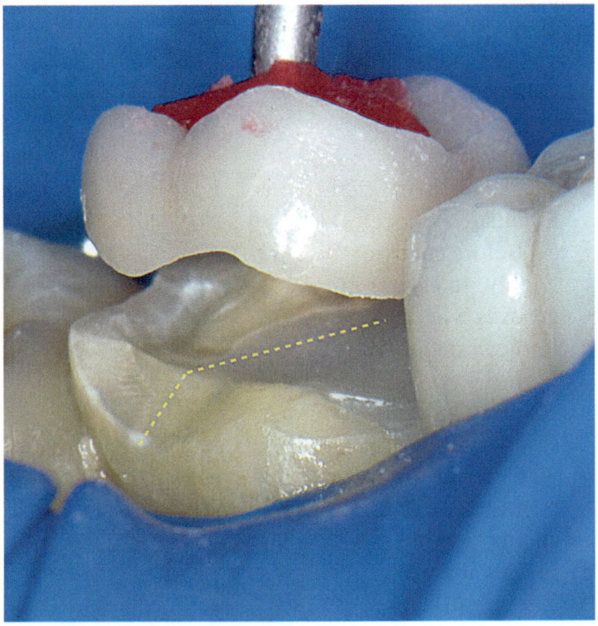

Fig. 9.9 Onlay preparation with beveled for centripetal redirection of stress induced by occlusal forces

Review Questions

1. What is and for what purpose can the re-preparation of the edges of an onlay cavity be performed?
2. What are the clinical advantages of relocating the edges of the inclined preparation "in the roof"?

9.4 Impression and Provisional Restoration

Main idea: The classical or digital optical impression is performed similarly to any prosthetic preparation. Quadrant or full arch trays are used for the silicone impression, and an intraoral optical scanner is used for the digital impression.

9.4.1 Working Technique

Two different viscosities of silicones are used, and the dentist can decide for the impression in one or two steps, double impression, or technique of simultaneous imprinting with two viscosities. Two-step impressions can lead to better results.

Putty silicone is first used and then elimination of retentive areas in the impression. Fluid consistency silicone is applied over the preparation and interdental, and a light air jet is applied to favor the penetration and distribution of the fluid in all areas (interdental, sulcus, preparation). Afterward, the application of fluid silicone continues until the tooth and its adjacents are entirely covered.

For the impression in one step, the fluid silicone is applied in the same way, and on top of that, the putty silicone is applied in the impression tray. In indirect restorations, the supragingival location of the edges simplifies the impression technique, regardless of the way the impression is made.

The digital impression is made with an intraoral optical scanner (Fig. 9.10) following the scanning sequence indicated by the manufacturer. The preparation image can be evaluated in all planes (Fig. 9.11). Most software assesses the limits of the preparation (Fig. 9.12), the obtained morphology (Fig. 9.13), the distance to antagonists, and other information necessary to correct the preparation or create the onlay design.

Difficulties that may arise	Possible solutions
Air voids may appear in the classic impression with silicones	Repeat the impression
For digital impressions, fogging the digital camera	Preheating the optical camera before starting the scan, using the air jet during the scan, and wiping

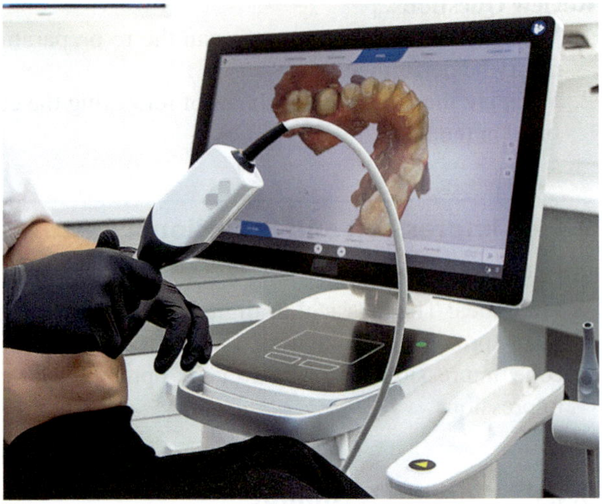

Fig. 9.10 Intraoral digital scanner

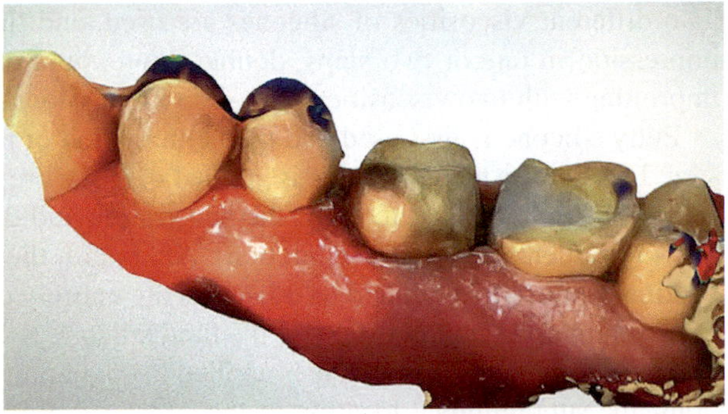

Fig. 9.11 Scanning preparations for a crown and onlay made with Cerec

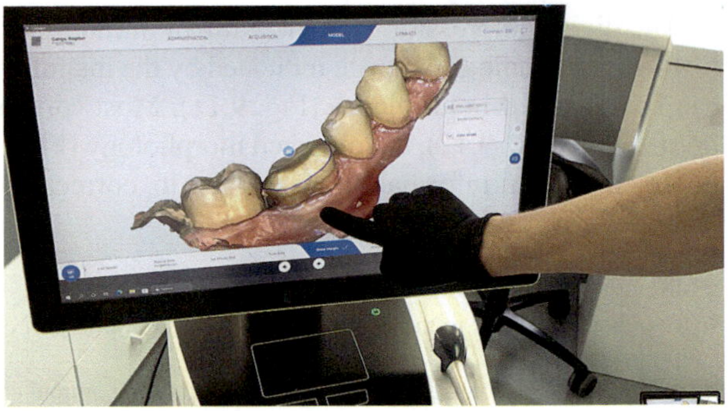

Fig. 9.12 Manual or automatic selection of preparation limits

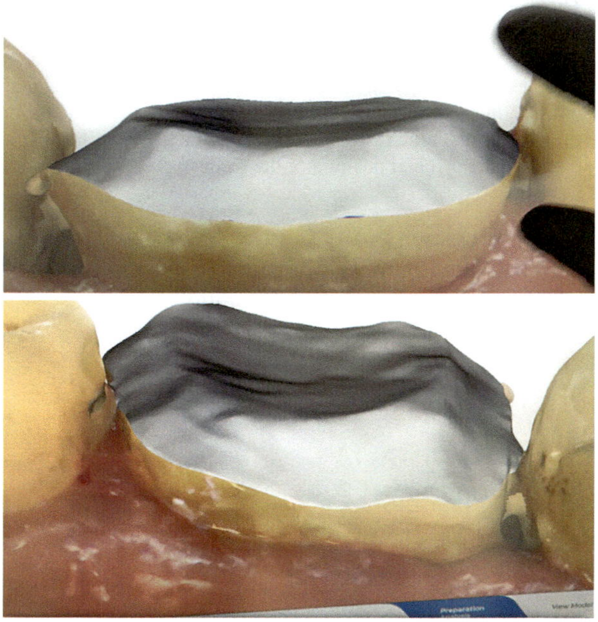

Fig. 9.13 Evaluation of the preparation

9.4.2 Provisional Restoration Between Sessions

Main idea: When two or more sessions are required, the prepared tooth must receive a provisional restoration to stabilize its position and seal the prepared tooth. Stabilizing the position is necessary because the prepared tooth lost contact with the adjacents and antagonists following the preparation.

If the cementation will be done in a different session than the preparation, then a provisional restoration is required (Fig. 9.14). Light-curing materials based on composite resins, such as liquid rubber dams, are most commonly used for this purpose, but there are also provisional composites specially designed for this purpose (Fig. 9.15). Eugenol-based materials are not recommended. The provisional restoration must fill the interdental space to prevent migration of the tooth, adjacent teeth version, and food impaction. The provisional material must be in occlusal contact with the opposing tooth to prevent its extrusion.

Difficulties that may arise	Possible solutions
The drying of the preparation and the application of the liquid rubber dam can lead to difficulties in its removal due to increased adhesion	Avoid excessive preparation drying when immediate dentin sealing has been done with composite resins. These provide excellent adhesion to the liquid dam temporary obturation, which is also a composite resin

Difficulties that may arise	Possible solutions
The dislodging of the provisional restoration between sessions and its absence for several days can lead, in the case of certain patients, to changes in the prepared tooth's position, adjacent, or antagonists. This can cause difficulties in fitting the prosthetic restoration that was made based on the original position of the teeth	Adapting the prosthetic part, if possible or repeating the impression for a new onlay. This time more attention will be paid to the provisional restoration, and the patient will be better instructed to return urgently in the office in case of dislocation of the provisional restoration

Review Questions

1. What is the purpose of a temporary restoration between sessions in the case of preparations for indirect restorations?

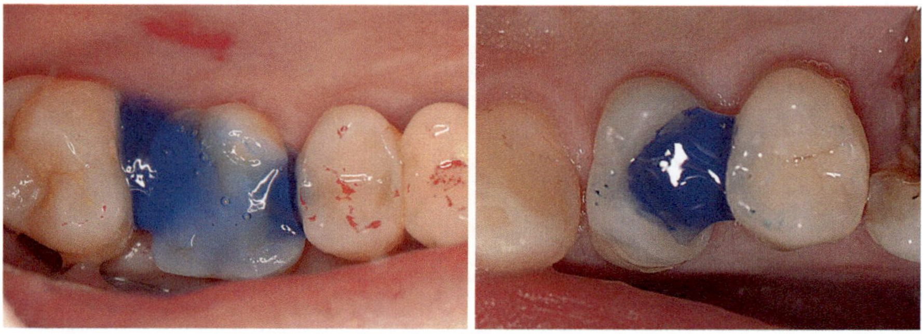

Fig. 9.14 Sealing the preparation and fixing the position of the prepared tooth with provisional restoration (liquid rubber dam)

Fig. 9.15 Light-curing material for temporary restoration of cavities prepared for indirect restorations

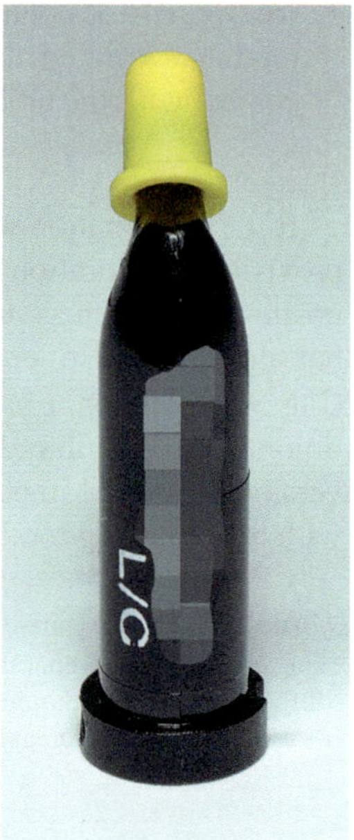

9.5 Cementing

Main idea: The cementation of indirect restorations is carried out under perfect humidity control by isolation with the rubber dam, using light-curing or dual-cure cementing materials.

Cementation of indirect restorations is paramount for long-term success with marginal sealing and retention. This is directly related to the material's properties from which the indirect restoration is made. Thus, depending on the material, the internal surface of the restoration requires treatment with hydrofluoric acid, sandblasting, and applying silane.

Bonding to enamel is superior to bonding to dentin, and ceramics provide superior bonding to composite resin materials. The best quality of tooth cementation can currently be obtained for indirect restorations made of lithium disilicate glass ceramics (e.g., e.max CAD/e.max Press Ivoclar Vivadent; Schaan, Liechtenstein), which is also the most studied type of ceramics in literature.

9.5.1 Cements

Bond strength varies from cement to cement, but total-etch types generally offer the best retention; self-etching systems are intermediate, and self-adhesive types of cement can achieve adhesion approximately equal to self-etching ones [21].

Although there is no consensus on the thickness of the cement layer, a gap of 50–100 microns between the preparation and the restoration allows composite types of cement to achieve good adhesion between the tooth and the indirect restoration.

The most frequently used materials for cementing indirect restorations are [22, 23]:

- Dual-cure cements based on composite resins
- Flowable resin composite materials
- Preheated packable composite resin materials

The polymerization of these materials must consider the possibility of light penetrating the prosthetic restoration. If good light-curing delivery can be obtained (30–60 s on each surface), a pre-warmed conventional composite restoration material can be used for cementation. It has a lower shrinkage coefficient than dual-cure cement, more filler, and a lower shrinkage coefficient. Its preheating increases the conversion rate during polymerization [24]. The use of composite restorative materials for cementing indirect restorations is supported by several long-term studies [25, 26]. Moreover, these materials are easier to handle, and the excess can be removed more easily.

The isolation that provides the best seal and removal of soft parts is rubber dam isolation. For direct and indirect restorations, we recommend isolating a group of teeth to restore the contact points properly. Ligatures are indicated for both stabilization and positioning of the rubber dam sheet. After removal of the provisional restoration and rubber dam isolation, cleaning the cavity by sandblasting is recommended for the complete removal of the provisional material, cleaning of impurities, and creating microretentions. The onlay try-in can then be performed (Fig. 9.16): check the margins, interproximal contacts.

The dentist evaluates the marginal adaptation (Fig. 9.17) and the relationships with the mesially and distally located teeth, the existence of the correct contact points. Occlusal adjustments (static and dynamic occlusion) will be performed after cementation and removal of the rubber dam. It is not recommended to try the inlay in occlusion prior to cementation as it is a risk of fracturing. Onlays can be fixed with wax on rigid instruments (e.g., obturator), or adhesive microbrushes can be used (Fig. 9.18).

Cementation of ceramic onlays goes through the following steps:

- Apply 10% hydrofluoric acid for 20 s for lithium disilicate glass ceramics (e.g., e.max) (Fig. 9.19).
- Abundant washing and drying.
- Apply 35–37% orthophosphoric acid for 10 s to remove salts produced by hydrofluoric acid (not all studies indicate this step) (Fig. 9.20).
- Rinsing with water and drying.
- Silane (Fig. 9.21).
- Adhesive (Fig. 9.22).
- Cement (Figs. 9.23 and 9.24).

Cementation of composite onlays involves the following steps:

- Sandblasting (50 micron aluminum oxide)
- Application of hydrofluoric acid, but not all studies recommend this
- Silane

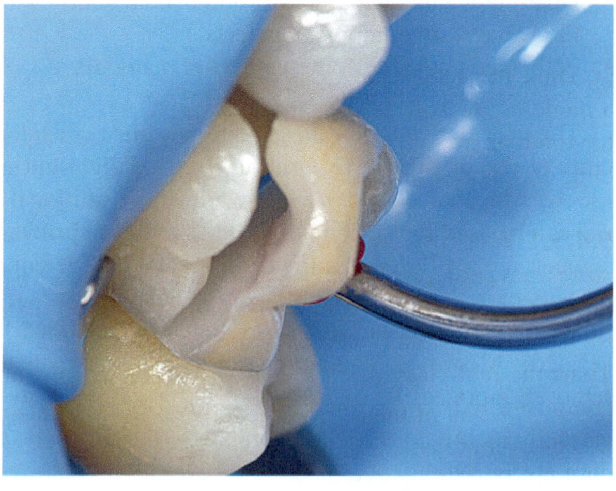

Fig. 9.16 Ceramic overlay fixed on an obturator tip

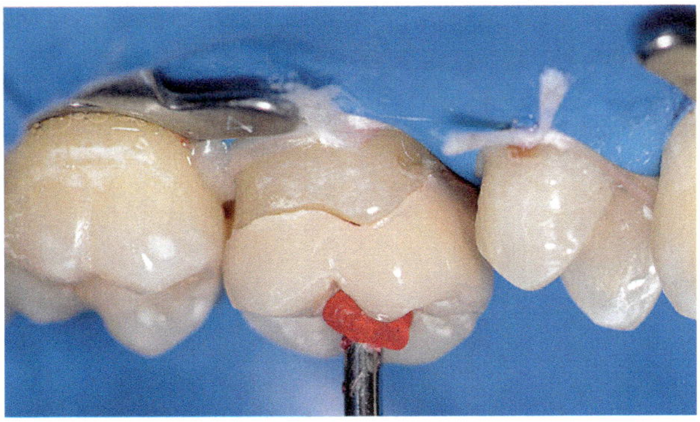

Fig. 9.17 Onlay fit checking, fixed with wax on an obturator tip

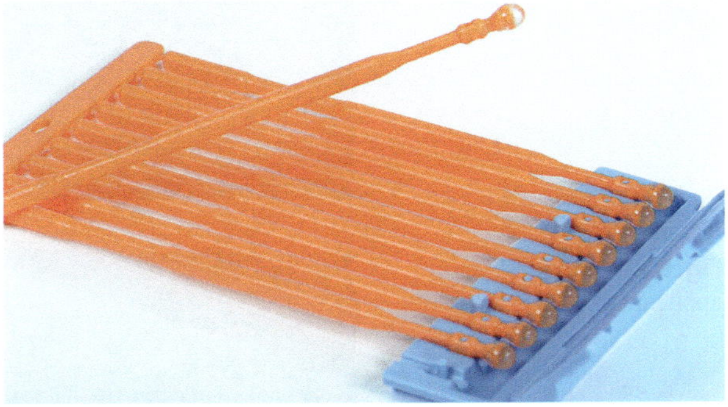

Fig. 9.18 Adhesive stick applicators for indirect restorations and veneers

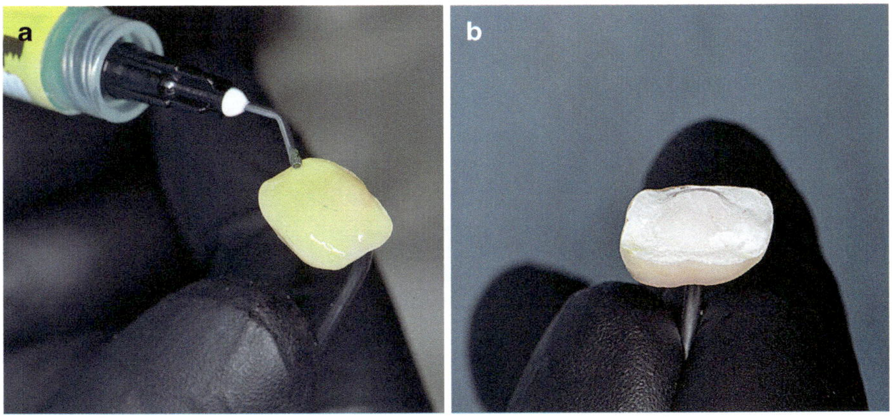

Fig. 9.19 Application of hydrofluoric acid (**a**) and aspect after water rinsing and surface drying (**b**)

- Adhesive
- Cement

The preparation of the tooth for cementation is done after its sandblasting and Teflon isolation of the adjacent teeth (Fig. 9.25) following the same protocol as for direct restorations:

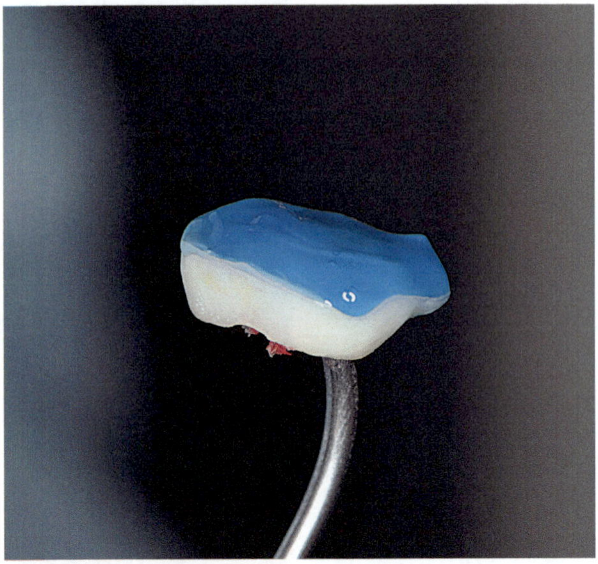

Fig. 9.20 Application of orthophosphoric acid

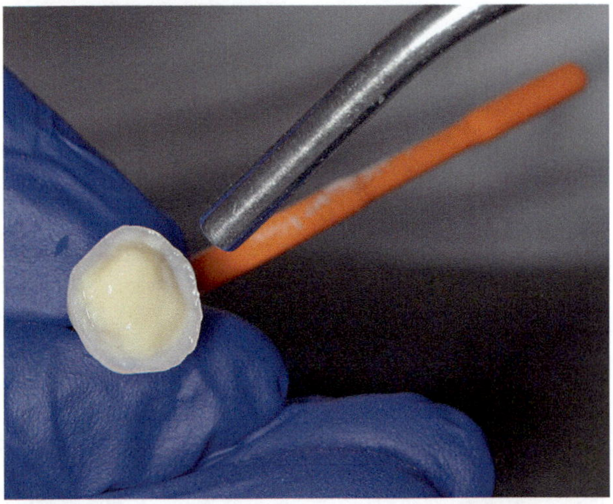

Fig. 9.21 Silane application

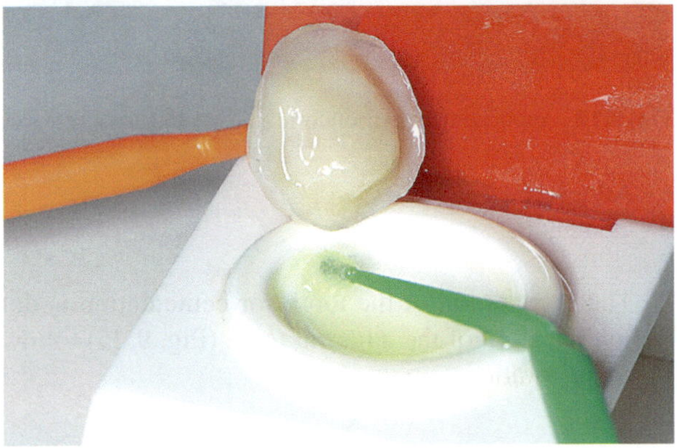

Fig. 9.22 Applying dual-cure adhesive

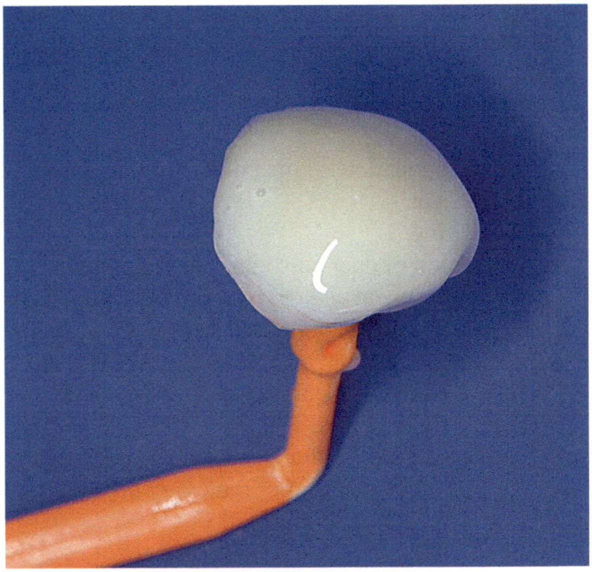

Fig. 9.23 Applying dual-cure cement

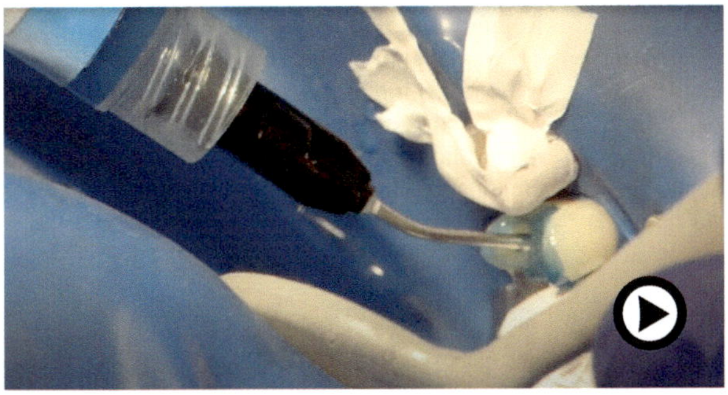

Fig. 9.24 Cementation of ceramic onlays (▶ https://doi.org/10.1007/000-bqx)

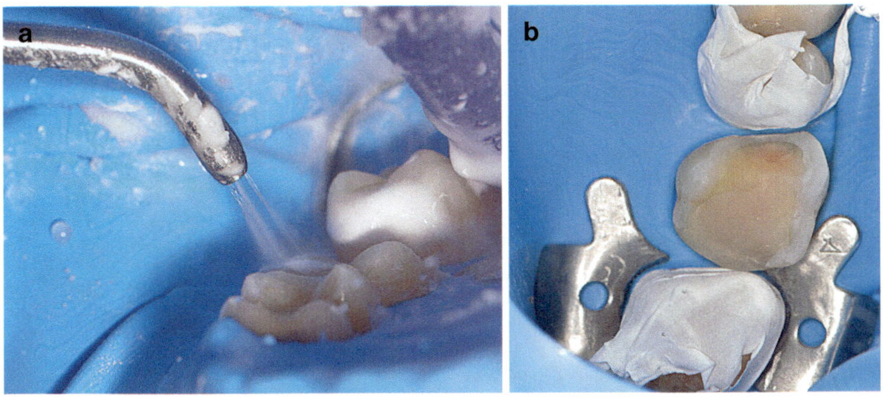

Fig. 9.25 Preparation of the tooth by sandblasting. (**a**) Isolation of adjacent teeth with Teflon tape (**b**)

1. Rubber dam isolation and cavity cleaning with a rotary brush and paste or sand-blasting (Fig. 9.25).
2. Enamel etching for 30 s (Fig. 9.26).
3. Rinsing with water.
4. Drying (Fig. 9.27).
5. Primer application for the infiltration of collagen fibers and the formation of the hybrid layer.
6. Easy drying.
7. Application of dual-cure adhesive (Fig. 9.28).
8. Applying cement and onlay to the tooth (Fig. 9.29).
9. Put pressure on the onlay and remove excess cement from buccal, oral surfaces with microbrushes and interdental with dental floss and microbrushes. Polymerization is ideally carried out with the oxygen barrier (e.g., glycerin gel) (Figs. 9.30 and 9.31).
10. Finishing the edges if applicable and checking the interface limits (Fig. 9.32).
11. Occlusal adjustments after removing the rubber dam (Fig. 9.33).

Difficulties that may arise	Possible solutions
Lack of marginal adaptation	Reintervention of the dental technician
Lack of contact point	Reintervention of the dental technician
Remaining unpolymerized cement in the interdental space	The removal of excess cement is done either before polymerization or after a short polymerization (e.g., maximum of 5 s with a medium power lamp 1100 W/cm^3)
Residual polymerized cement in interdental space	A modified metal abrasive strip can be used by making crenellations with a sharpened bur, similar to a saw with which the interdental cementum film is sectioned

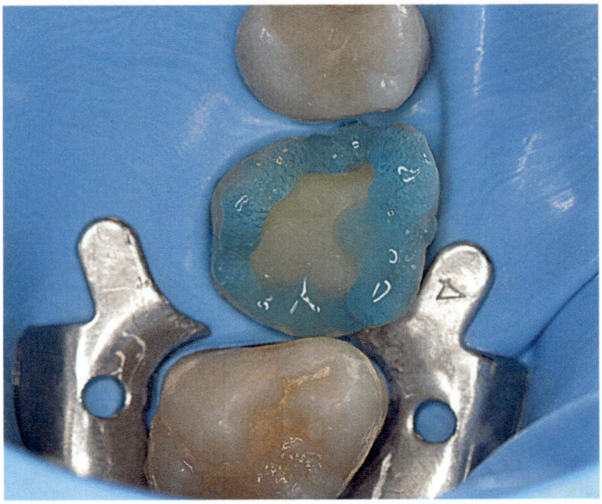

Fig. 9.26 Applying the etching

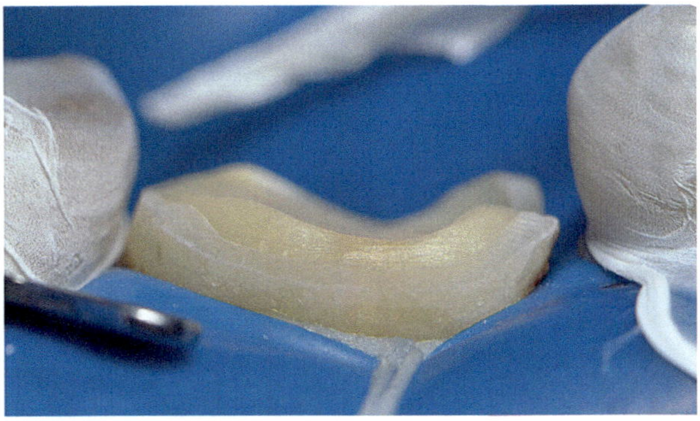

Fig. 9.27 Enamel aspect after drying

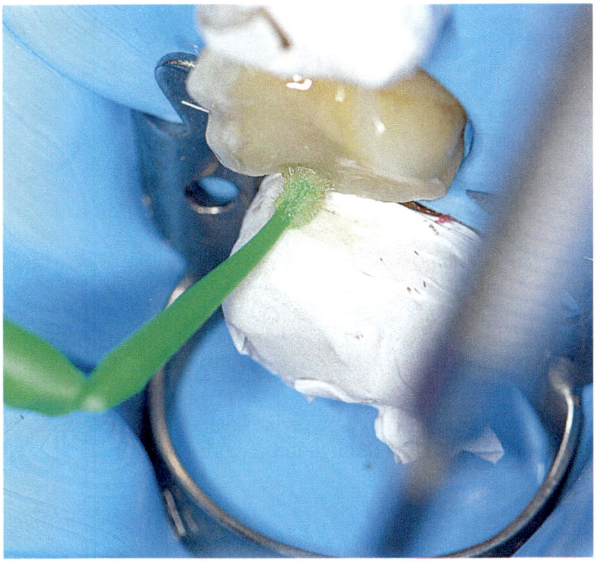

Fig. 9.28 Applying the adhesive to the tooth

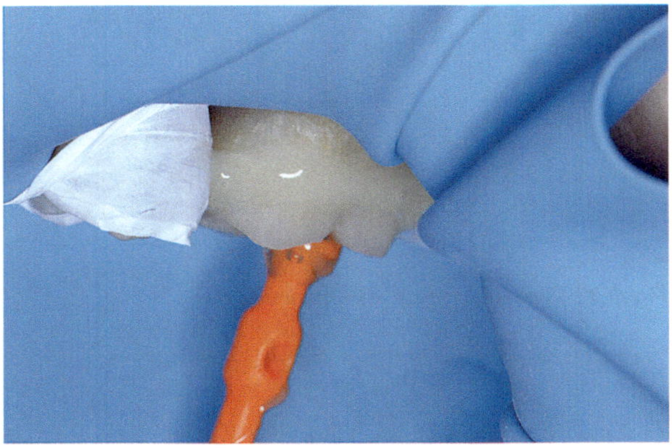

Fig. 9.29 Onlay cementation and reflowing the excess material

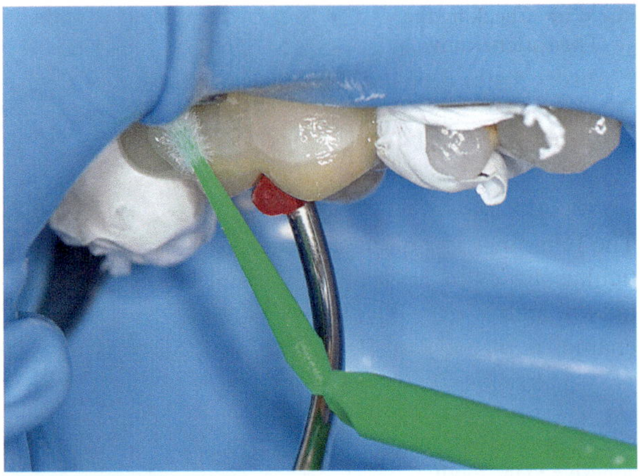

Fig. 9.30 Removing excess cement with a microbrush

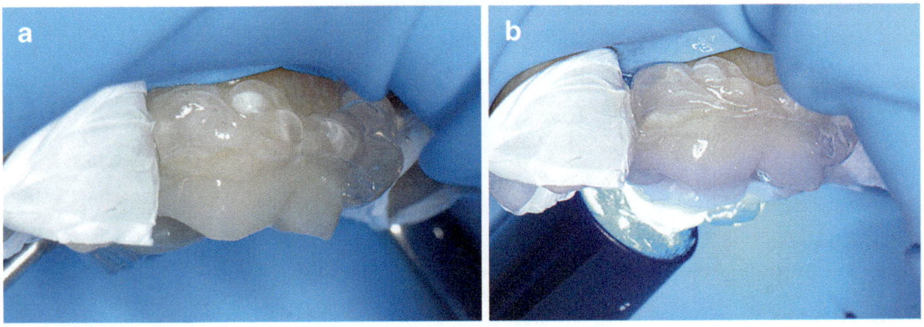

Fig. 9.31 Application of a glycerine layer over the interface area prior to cement polymerization (**a**) and polymerization through the glycerine (**b**)

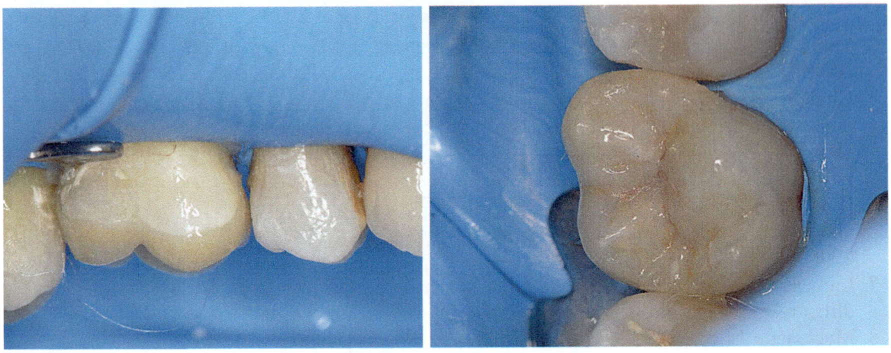

Fig. 9.32 The final aspect after cementation

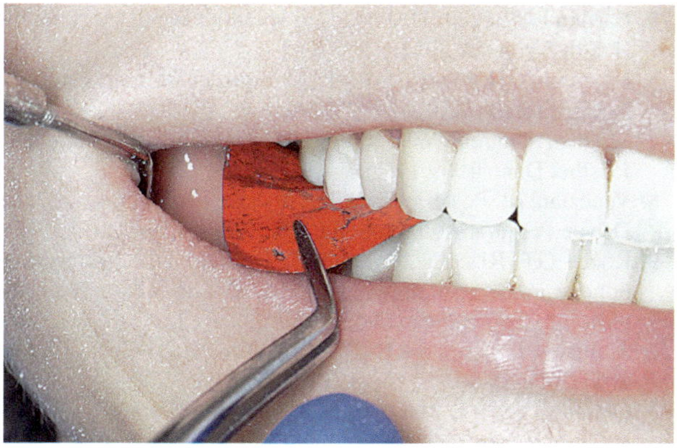

Fig. 9.33 Checking the occlusion after removing the rubber dam

Conclusion

Indirect partial restorations can be considered the treatment of choice for restoring cavities that involve cusps. They are predictable, have good biomechanical properties, and are conservative with the remaining dental tissues. From the point of view of the materials available for performing these restorations, it is impossible to designate material as the gold standard. The choice must be made on a case-by-case basis.

However, based on the results published to date, ceramic (reinforced lithium disilicate ceramic) can be considered the most reliable long-term alternative compared to composite resins, which have inferior properties over time [27].

Review Questions

1. What materials can be used to cement indirect ceramic restorations, and what are the advantages of each type?
2. What are the clinical steps for cementing ceramic and composite resin onlays?
3. What are the steps to prepare the tooth for cementation of an indirect restoration?

References

1. Fron Chabouis H, Smail Faugeron V, Attal JP. Clinical efficacy of composite versus ceramic inlays and onlays: a systematic review. Dent Mater. 2013;29(12):1209–18.
2. Vagropoulou GI, Klifopoulou GL, Vlahou SG, Hirayama H, Michalakis K. Complications and survival rates of inlays and onlays vs complete coverage restorations: a systematic review and analysis of studies. J Oral Rehabil. 2018;45(11):903–20.
3. Santos GC Jr, Santos MJ Jr, Rizkalla AS, Madani DA, El-Mowafy O. Overview of CEREC CAD/CAM chairside system. Gen Dent. 2013;61(1):36–41.
4. Morimoto S, Rebello de Sampaio FB, Braga MM, Sesma N, Özcan M. Survival rate of resin and ceramic inlays, onlays, and overlays: a systematic review and meta-analysis. J Dent Res. 2016;95(9):985–94.

5. Bartlett D, Ricketts D. Advanced operative dentistry. A practical approach. Edinburgh: Elsevier Health Sciences; 2011.
6. Heymann OH, Swift EJ, Ritter AV. Sturdevant's art & science of operative dentistry. 6th ed. St Louis: Elsevier; 2013.
7. Magne P, Douglas WH. Rationalization of esthetic restorative dentistry based on biomimetics. J Esthet Dent. 1999;11(1):5–15.
8. Veneziani M. Posterior indirect adhesive restorations: updated indications and the Morphology Driven Preparation Technique. Int J Esthet Dent. 2017;12(2):204–30.
9. Rocca GT, Rizcalla N, Krejci I, Dietschi D. Evidence-based concepts and procedures for bonded inlays and onlays. Part II. Guidelines for cavity preparation and restoration fabrication. Int J Esthet Dent. 2015;10(3):392–413.
10. Smithson J, Newsome P, Reaney D, Owen S. Direct or indirect restorations? Int Dent Afr Ed. 2011;1(1):70–80.
11. Qanungo A, Aras MA, Chitre V, Mysore A, Amin B, Daswani SR. Immediate dentin sealing for indirect bonded restorations. J Prosthodont Res. 2016;60(4):240–9.
12. Bertschinger C, Paul SJ, Lüthy H, Schärer P. Dual application of dentin bonding agents: effect on bond strength. Am J Dent. 1996;9(3):115–9.
13. Paul SJ, Schaerer P. Effect of provisional cements on the bond strength of various adhesive bonding systems on dentine. J Oral Rehabil. 1997;24:8–14.
14. Hardan L, Devoto W, Bourgi R, et al. Immediate dentin sealing for adhesive cementation of indirect restorations: a systematic review and meta-analysis. Gels. 2022;8(3):175.
15. Josic U, Sebold M, Lins RBE, et al. Does immediate dentin sealing influence postoperative sensitivity in teeth restored with indirect restorations? A systematic review and meta-analysis. J Esthet Restor Dent. 2022;34(1):55–64.
16. Magne P. Immediate dentin sealing: a fundamental procedure for indirect bonded restorations. Esthet Restor Dent. 2005;17:144–54.
17. Elsayed A. Defect-orientated onlay with cavity design optimization and cervical margin relocation: a case report. Int J Comput Dent. 2021;24(1):77–88. PMID: 34006065.
18. Sasse M, Krummel A, Klosa K, Kern M. Influence of restoration thickness and dental bonding surface on the fracture resistance of full-coverage occlusal veneers made from lithium disilicate ceramic. Dent Mater. 2015;31(8):907–15.
19. Politano G, Van Meerbeek B, Peumans M. Nonretentive bonded ceramic partial crowns: concept and simplified protocol for long-lasting dental restorations. J Adhes Dent. 2018;20(6):495–510.
20. Peumans M, Van Meerbeek BV, Lambrechts P, Vanherle G. Porcelain veneers: a review of the literature. J Dent. 2000;28(3):163–77.
21. Burgess JO, Ghuman T, Cakir D. Self-adhesive resin cements. J Esthet Restor Dent. 2010;22(6):412–9.
22. Molin MK, Karlsson SL, Kristiaensen MS. Influence of film thickness on joint bend strength of a ceramic/resin composite joint. Dent Mater. 1996;12:245–9.
23. Silva NR, de Souza GM, Coelho PG, et al. Effect of water storage time and composite cement thickness on fatigue of a glass-ceramic trilayer system. J Biomed Mater Res B Appl Biomater. 2008;84(1):117–23.
24. Park SH, Lee CS. The difference in degree of conversion between light cured and additional heat-cured composites. Oper Dent. 1996;21:213–7.
25. Roggendorf MJ, Kunzi K, Eber J, Roggendorf HC, Frankenberger R, Reich SM. Seven-year clinical performance of CEREC 2 all-ceramic CAD/CAM restorations places within deeply destroyed teeth. Clin Oral Invest. 2012;16:1413–24.
26. Guess PC, Selz CF, Steinhart YN, Stampf S, Strub JR. Prospective clinical split-mouth study of pressed and CAD/CAM all-ceramic partial-coverage restorations: 7-year results. Int J Prosthodont. 2013;26:21–5.
27. Bustamante-Hernández N, Montiel-Company JM, Bellot-Arcís C, et al. Clinical behavior of ceramic, hybrid and composite onlays. A systematic review and meta-analysis. Int J Environ Res Public Health. 2020;17(20):7582.

Failure Management

10

Direct restorations can be damaged over time, indicating complete or partial replacement, and their repair through minimally invasive procedures. This chapter will focus on the decision to partially or fully replace damaged direct restorations and failures of indirect restorations.

10.1 Decision on Partial or Total Replacement

The longevity of direct restorative treatments is a successful evaluation criterion for both patients and dentists. The studies carried out show us that this depends on many factors, among which we can mention [1, 2]:

- Patient-related factors (risk of cavities, age, gender, dental hygiene)
- The number of tooth surfaces included in the restoration and their location
- The arch (maxillary or mandible) and the location of the tooth (anterior or posterior)
- The material used (composite resin, GIc)
- The working technique used (presence or absence of liners or bases)
- Dentist-related factors (attention, working with magnification, etc.)

Of these, the first two have the most significant impact: the individual cavity risk and the number of dental surfaces involved. These factors are associated with two main fail causes of the restorations:

- Marginal or recurrent secondary caries
- Fracture of the composite restoration or the remaining tooth walls

Glass ionomer cement sandwich restorations were the preferred way of achieving adhesion between dentin and composite resin when dentin adhesives still performed poorly. According to some studies, these have an average failure rate at 5 and 10 years of 1.8% and 2.4%, respectively, for posterior composite restorations [1].

Published data confirm that more extensive restorations have a higher risk of failure because each additional surface included in a restoration increases this risk

© The Author(s), under exclusive license to Springer Nature Switzerland AG 2024

M. Bud, *Direct Restorations*, https://doi.org/10.1007/978-3-031-55899-3_10

by 30–40% [1]. Fractures can frequently cause the failure of amalgam and composite resin restorations at the edges of the restoration affecting marginal integrity [3].

In the modern trend of minimally invasive dentistry, repairing composite resin fillings (instead of replacing them entirely) is a widespread procedure that does not yet benefit from a well-established working technique. Despite all its advantages, the repair of direct composite resin restoration is not a simple procedure [4].

So, direct composite resin restorations are repairable (unlike amalgam), which is one of their significant advantages. It is well documented that two masses of composite resins adhere to each other. Therefore, if there is no damage in any other area of the existing restoration, one can opt to remove the damaged portion and add additional composite. Flowable composites are not as mechanically strong but are easier to use to ensure they flow in small spaces that do not directly take occlusal forces. Therefore, it is recommended to use flowable composite only if the repaired area is small, as in the case of prophylactic seals. A packable universal composite is used if the preparation is similar in design to conventional class I or II cavities.

The decision to replace direct restorations with limited defects is frequent for restorations not initially performed by the evaluating dentist [5], as demonstrated in the analysis of the National Health Service in the UK and similar studies in North America [6, 7].

The repair or replacement decision is based on the evaluation of several criteria, among which we can mention:

- Carious risk
- Structural damage
- Catastrophic failure associated with major fractures
- Loss of pulp vitality

One or more limited defects in a restoration do not necessarily mean that the restoration is irreversibly compromised and requires total replacement. Most restoration defects, other than those caused by sudden fractures, develop gradually over long periods [8], allowing the clinician to address the cause of the problem and intervene minimally invasively to correct localized or superficial defects [9]. The life of the restoration can be extended in this way.

The reasons why a filling can be replaced entirely are:

- Allergies to materials
- Galvanism
- Recurrent caries
- Adhesion problems
- Dislocated fillings (Fig. 10.1a)
- Secondary marginal caries with or without fracture of enamel walls (Fig. 10.1b)
- Obvious marginal infiltration with discontinuity and extensive marginal pigmentation (Fig. 10.2)
- Fracture in the mass of the composite or tooth walls (Fig. 10.3)

Fractures involving a coronal composite restoration and tooth walls can sometimes be limited juxtagingivally (Fig. 10.4) or extend subgingivally up to the root level, making subsequent tooth restoration impossible (Fig. 10.5). As a rule,

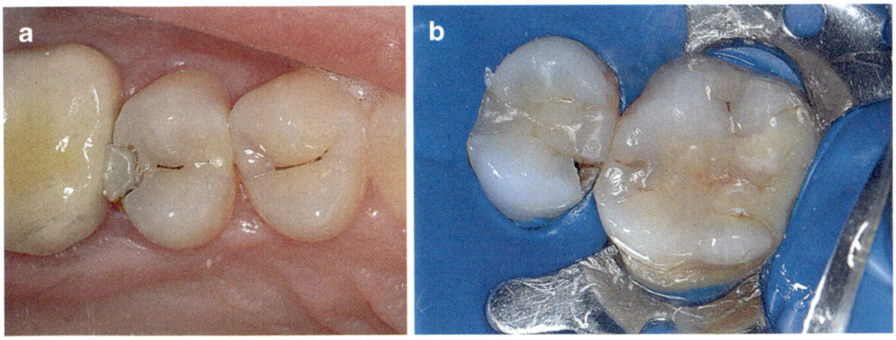

Fig. 10.1 Dislocated composite resin filling (**a**); secondary cavity and fracture of the enamel walls (**b**)

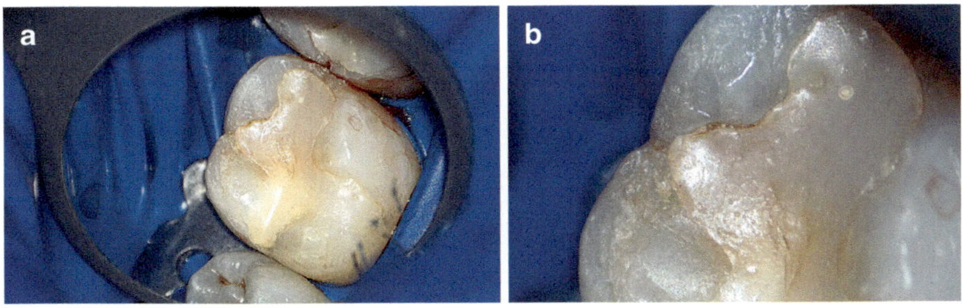

Fig. 10.2 Deficient marginal sealing with gaps at the composite-tooth interface, lack of marginal adaptation. Image without magnification (**a**) and with 1.6× magnification (**b**)

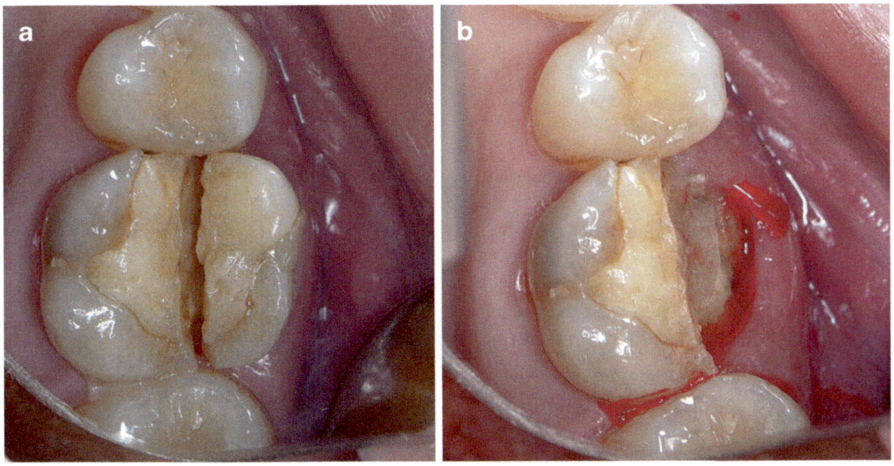

Fig. 10.3 Fracture of the composite restoration extended mesiodistally and in the distal wall (**a**) and the clinical situation after the fractured fragment's removal (**b**)

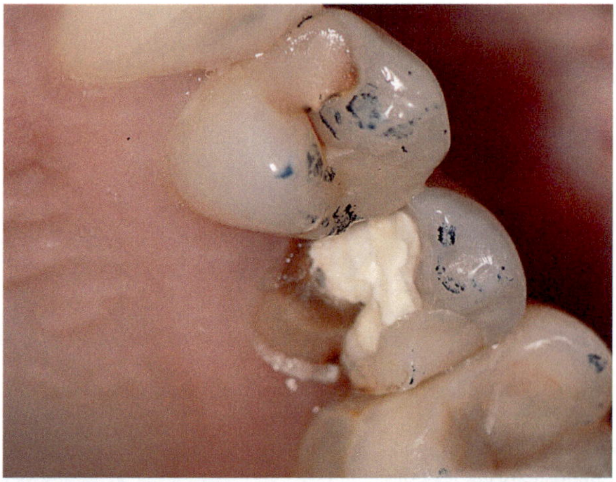

Fig. 10.4 Juxtagingival fracture of the palatal wall of an upper premolar in which a MOD cavity was previously restored with composite resins and cement base

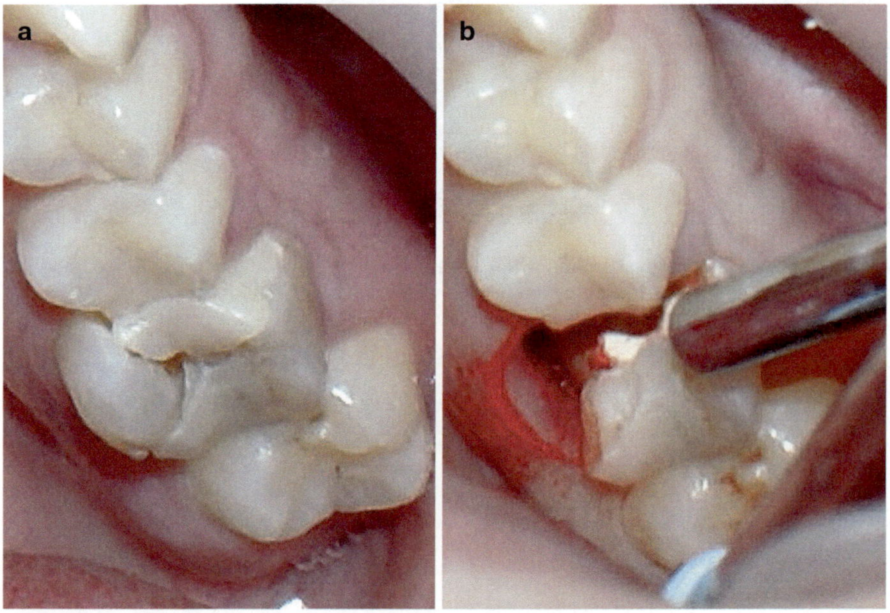

Fig. 10.5 Subgingival fracture of the palatal wall of an upper molar and fracture of the restorative material (**a**) and the clinical aspect after removal of the fractured part (**b**)

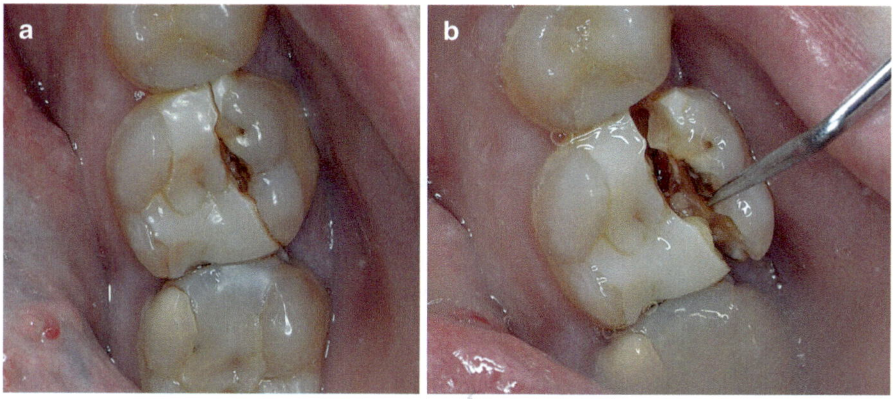

Fig. 10.6 Fracture of the buccal wall of a maxillary first molar previously restored with MOD composite resin, lack of cuspid protection (**a**), and aspect of the mesiodistal fracture line (**b**)

fractures involving vertical tooth walls occur with thin vertical walls without cusp protection (Fig. 10.6), undermined by proximal, oral, and buccal caries, or subjected to intense occlusal forces.

Possible reasons why a filling can be partially replaced or repaired by adding composite:

- Extended extrusions of material that cannot be removed by finishing, especially in the area of the gingival margin
- Lack of contact points between restoration and the adjacent tooth
- Surface voids
- Chipping of composite edges
- Minor enamel fractures adjacent to a corresponding old restoration

The decision for partial or total replacement should be made based on examination tools that maximize or complement the visual examination by naked eye inspection. Among these, we can mention:

- Use of magnification: dental loupes or dental operating microscope.
- Radiographs: bitewing or periapocal.
- Vitality tests: they can change the treatment decision when necrosis is detected.
- Infiltration by staining with caries indicators can identify infected dentin, crack, or fracture lines undetectable to the naked eye.

Conclusion
Partial or total restoration replacement is done when solid reasons and only after careful examinations.

Review Questions
1. What factors do the longevity of direct restorative treatments depend on?
2. What are possible reasons a filling can be replaced?

3. What are possible reasons a filling can be repaired?
4. Examinations underlying the decision to partially or fully replace a direct restoration?

10.2 Failures of Indirect Restorations

Main idea: Indirect restorations can deteriorate over time, requiring repair with composite resins or their complete replacement.

Indirect partial restorations are not without problems, so among the main complications that can occur we mention [10]:

- Dentinal hypersensitivity.
- Marginal and occlusal adaptation problems.
- Loss of marginal integrity with the aspect of microinfiltration and adhesion failure.
- Changes in color and texture due to material wear.
- Antagonistic tooth wear.
- Plaque buildup and gingivitis.
- Secondary decay.
- Total or partial decimation of the restoration (Figs. 10.7 and 10.8).
- Fractures of the material (Fig. 10.9) involving a vertical wall. If the limit of the fracture is juxtagingival or slightly subgingival (1–2 mm), performing a gingivectomy, respectively crown lengthening, can create conditions for appropriate subsequent restoration with a prosthetic crown.
- Coronal fractures can also extend to the root (Fig. 10.10). Such a vertical root fracture indicates tooth extraction.
- Fractures of the tooth walls.

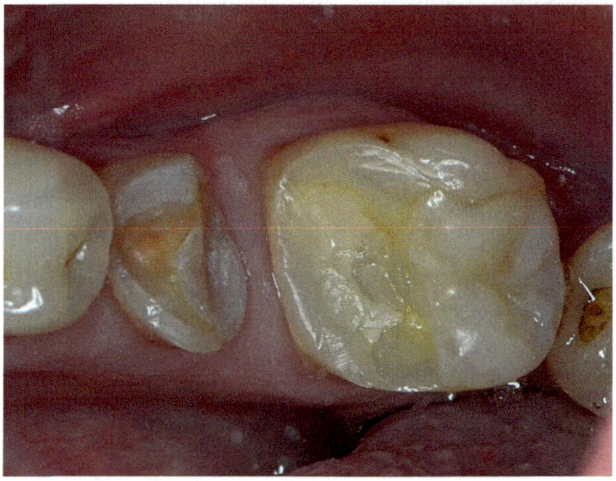

Fig. 10.7 Debonding of an indirect composite restoration on a lower second premolar and partial fracture on a lower first molar

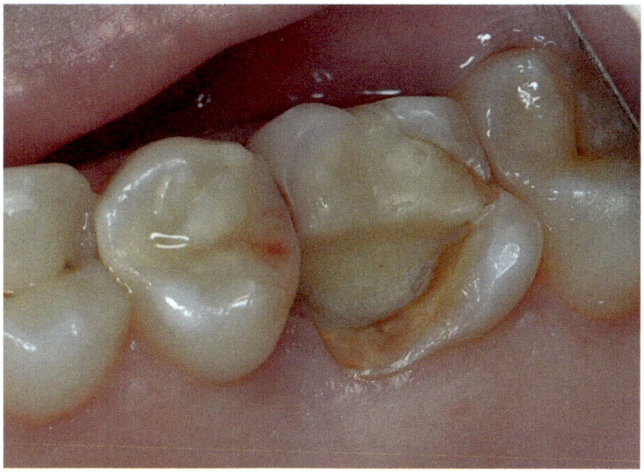

Fig. 10.8 Fracture of an indirect composite restoration on a maxillary first molar with juxtagingival preparation

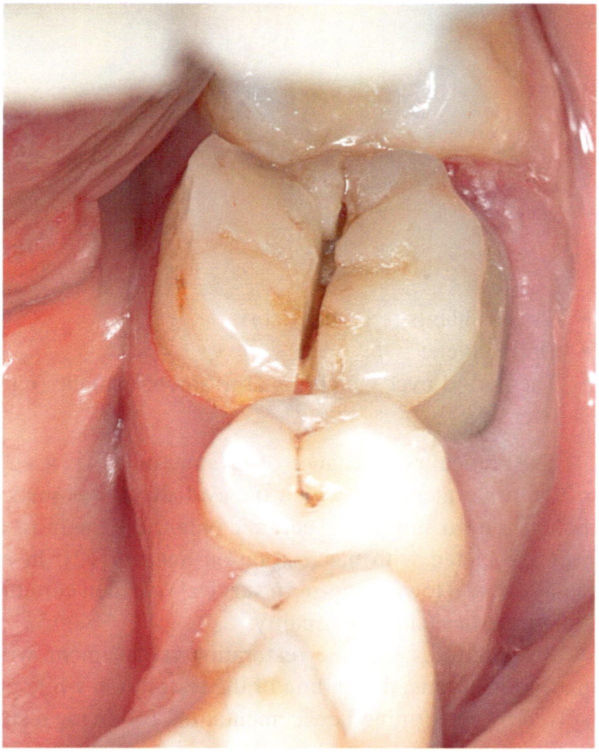

Fig. 10.9 Mesiodistal fracture of an indirect composite restoration and tooth on a mandibular first molar

Onlays are a good, conservative, and predictable option for restoration in the posterior region, with a survival rate of over 90% [11]. The survival rate of indirect restorations is associated with the following:

- The type of material used (e.g., the use of composite, ceramic)
- The condition of the tooth on which the indirect restoration is placed (e.g., endodontically treated teeth have a lower prognosis)

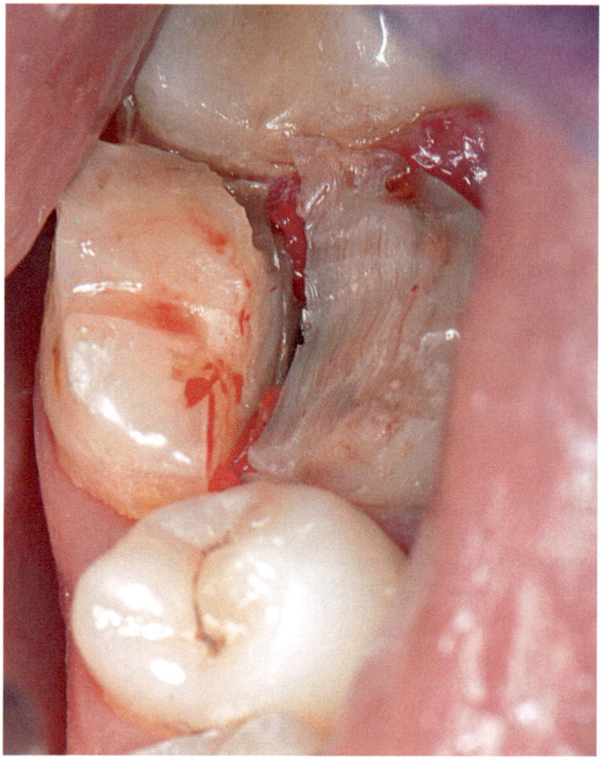

Fig. 10.10 Mesiodistal fracture of an indirect composite restoration on a mandibular first molar extended and at the root level with vertical root fracture

- Vicious habits (e.g., bruxism)
- Oral hygiene
- The period over which the assessment is made (e.g., the survival rate decreases over time)

The clinical performance of ceramic onlays is acceptable (over 90%) regardless of the time interval at which the evaluation was made. The predominant cause of failure is a fracture of the ceramic onlay, and the most commonly observed damage was associated with the restoration margin [12]. In comparison, composite resin onlays have a lower long-term survival rate than ceramic ones due to different material properties and bond quality.

Most failures indicate restoration replacement with a new one, but there are exceptions. Thus, debonding of the restoration while preserving its integrity can be solved by performing new cementation, following a strict adhesive protocol.

Some problems can be fixed by adding composite materials:

- Slight chipping of the onlay
- Chipping of the tooth wall at the restoration limit

Conclusion

As with indirect partial restorations, some complications can compromise the treatment, partially or totally, and their survival rate is dependent on many factors.

Review Questions

1. What are the main complications that can occur with indirect restorations?
2. What is the survival rate of indirect restorations associated with?
3. How do composite versus ceramic onlays perform, and what problems arise with them?
4. How to resolve failures of indirect restorations (replace vs. repair)?

References

1. Opdam NJ, van de Sande FH, Bronkhorst E, et al. Longevity of posterior composite restorations: a systematic review and meta-analysis. J Dent Res. 2014;93(10):943–9.
2. Wierichs RJ, Kramer EJ, Meyer-Lueckel H. Risk factors for failure of direct restorations in general dental practices. J Dent Res. 2020;99(9):1039–46.
3. DaCunha Mello FS, Feilzer AJ, de Gee AJ, Davidson CL. Sealing ability of eight resin bonding systems in a class II restoration after mechanical fatiguing. Dent Mater. 1997;13:372–6.
4. Salamonowicz M, Choromańska M. Repairing modern composite dental fillings. J Stomatol. 2017;70(4):394–404.
5. Bader JD, Shugars DA. Agreement among dentists' recommendations for restorative treatment. J Dent Res. 1993;72(5):891–6.
6. Burke FJ, Lucarotti PS. How long do direct restorations placed within the general dental services in England and Wales survive? Br Dent J. 2009;206(1):E2.
7. Bogacki RE, Hunt RJ, del Aguila M, Smith WR. Survival analysis of posterior restorations using an insurance claims database. Oper Dent. 2002;27(5):488–92.
8. Gordan VV, Riley JL 3rd, Geraldeli S, et al. Dental Practice-Based Research Network Collaborative Group Repair or replacement of defective restorations by dentists in the Dental Practice-Based Research Network. J Am Dent Assoc. 2012;143(6):593–601.
9. Blum IR, Jagger DC, Wilson NHF. Defective dental restorations: to repair or not to repair? Part 1: direct composite restorations. Dent Update. 2011;38(2):78–80, 82–84.
10. Abduo J, Sambrook RJ. Longevity of ceramic onlays: a systematic review. J Esthet Restor Dent. 2018;30(3):193–215.
11. Bustamante-Hernández N, Montiel-Company JM, Bellot-Arcís C, et al. Clinical behavior of ceramic, hybrid and composite onlays. A systematic review and meta-analysis. Int J Environ Res Public Health. 2020;17(20):7582.
12. Vagropoulou GI, Klifopoulou GL, Vlahou SG, Hirayama H, Michalakis K. Complications and survival rates of inlays and onlays vs complete coverage restorations: a systematic review and analysis of studies. J Oral Rehabil. 2018;45(11):903–20.